SERIES 2
PROVISION

Preferred Responses in Ophthalmology

A Self-Assessment Program

Volume II: Discussions

Gregory L. Skuta, MD
Executive Editor

American Academy of Ophthalmology

Lifelong Education for the Ophthalmologist

American Academy of Ophthalmology
655 Beach Street, P.O. Box 7424
San Francisco, CA 94120-7424

Academy Staff
Kathryn A. Hecht, EdD, Vice President, Clinical Education

Programs Department
William M. Hering, PhD, Director, Programs Department
Stephen Moore, PhD, Self-Assessment Program Manager

Publications Department
Hal Straus, Director, Publications Department
Margaret Petela, Managing Editor, Special Projects
Lisa Bogle, Production Manager
Beth T. Berkelhammer, Production Assistant
Rachel Griener, Administrative Assistant

Designed by Mark Ong, Side by Side Studios

This program is supported in part by a grant from Otsuka America Pharmaceutical, Inc.

ProVision: Preferred Responses in Ophthalmology, Series 2, is one component in the Lifelong Education for the Ophthalmologist (LEO) framework, which assists members in planning their continuing medical education. LEO includes an array of clinical education products and programs that members may select to form individualized, self-directed learning plans for updating their clinical knowledge. Active members and fellows who use LEO components may accumulate sufficient CME credits to earn the LEO Award. Contact the Academy's Clinical Education Division for further information on LEO.

This CME activity was planned and produced in accordance with the ACCME Essentials.

Because diagnostic, therapeutic, and practice recommendations (hereinafter "recommendations") may have changed since the publication of this book, because such recommendations cannot be considered absolute or universal in their application, and because the publication process contains the potential for error, the American Academy of Ophthalmology strongly advises that the recommendations in this book be verified, prior to use, with information included in the manufacturers' package inserts or provided by an independent source and be considered in light of a particular patient's clinical condition and history. Caution is especially urged when using new or infrequently used drugs. Including all indications, contraindications, side effects, and alternative agents for each drug or treatment is beyond the scope of this book.

The Academy disclaims responsibility and liability for any and all adverse medical or legal effects, including personal, bodily, property, or business injury, and for damages or loss of any kind whatsoever, resulting directly or indirectly, whether from negligence or otherwise, from the use of the recommendations or other information in this book, from any undetected printing errors or recommendation errors, or from textual misunderstandings by the reader. The ultimate arbiter of any diagnostic or therapeutic decision remains the individual physician's judgment.

Reference to certain drugs, instruments, and other products in this publication is made for illustrative purposes only and is not intended to constitute an endorsement of such drugs, instruments, and other products.

ISBN 1-56055-032-5

CONTENTS

ACKNOWLEDGMENTS

The American Academy of Ophthalmology gratefully acknowledges the contributions of numerous individuals in the development of this program, especially the members of the Self-Assessment Committee.

Self-Assessment Committee

Gregory L. Skuta, MD, *Chair*
Oklahoma City, Oklahoma

Keith D. Carter, MD
Iowa City, Iowa

Susan G. Elner, MD
Ann Arbor, Michigan

Larry P. Frohman, MD
Newark, New Jersey

Edward K. Isbey, Jr, MD
Asheville, North Carolina

Ronald V. Keech, MD
Iowa City, Iowa

Stephen S. Lane, MD
St. Paul, Minnesota

Mark J. Mannis, MD
Sacramento, California

Edward J. Rockwood, MD
Cleveland, Ohio

Contributors

Section 1
Edward J. Rockwood, MD; Beverly C. Forcier, MD; Kathleen A. Lamping, MD
Reviewers: L. Jay Katz, MD; Rebecca K. Morgan, MD

Section 2
Mark J. Mannis, MD
Reviewers: Mark L. McDermott, MD; Michael P. Vrabec, MD

Section 3
Stephen S. Lane, MD; James A. Davison, MD; Harry B. Grabow, MD; Thomas D. Lindquist, MD, PhD; Scott M. MacRae, MD; Samuel Masket, MD; James J. Salz, MD; Theodore P. Werblin, MD, PhD
Reviewers: Douglas D. Koch, MD; Alan Sugar, MD

Section 4
Larry P. Frohman, MD; Anthony C. Arnold, MD; Mark J. Kupersmith, MD; Jonathan D. Trobe, MD
Reviewers: Roy W. Beck, MD; Nancy J. Newman, MD; Jonathan D. Trobe, MD; Floyd A. Warren, MD

Section 5

Keith D. Carter, MD; Ronan M. Conlon, MD, FRCSC; Gene R. Howard, MD; Jeffrey A. Nerad, MD; John J. Woog, MD
Reviewers: George B. Bartley, MD; Robert G. Small, MD

Section 6

Ronald V. Keech, MD; Laurie E. Christiansen, MD; Arlene V. Drack, MD; Christina P. Johnson, MD; David A. Johnson, MD, PhD; G. Frank Judisch, MD; Scott R. Lambert, MD; P. David Reese, MD; Terry L. Schwartz, MD; Sarah J. Stair, MD; Edwin M. Stone, MD, PhD
Reviewers: Steven M. Archer, MD; Mark H. Scott, MD

Section 7

Susan G. Elner, MD; Barbara A. Blodi, MD; Mark W. Johnson, MD; Michael J. Shapiro, MD; Paul A. Sieving, MD, PhD; Andrew K. Vine, MD
Reviewers: Maryanna Destro, MD; Dennis P. Han, MD

Section 8

J. Wayne Beaton, MD; Robert M. Christiansen, MD; Donald C. Fletcher, MD; David L. Guyton, MD; Jack T. Holladay, MD; Jeffrey T. Liegner, MD; Jean Ann Vickery, FCLSA
Reviewers: Cynthia A. Bradford, MD; Stephen R. Russell, MD

PREFACE

The American Academy of Ophthalmology is pleased to offer Series 2 of *ProVision: Preferred Responses in Ophthalmology.* Participation in *ProVision* Series 1, which was released late in 1992, has greatly exceeded original projections, requiring a second printing after the program's second year. In a 1993 survey of *ProVision* Series 1 users, more than 95 percent of respondents either agreed or strongly agreed that *ProVision* had effectively challenged, assessed, and instructed them, and 98 percent indicated that they would recommend *ProVision* to a colleague.

Given the success of *ProVision* Series 1, we are particularly indebted to Dr Thomas A. Weingeist, who, as the first chair of the Self-Assessment Committee and executive editor of *ProVision* Series 1, developed the objectives and organization of this program. Members of the Self-Assessment Committee and the numerous other contributors and formal reviewers for *ProVision* Series 2 listed in the Acknowledgments have volunteered an enormous amount of time and meticulous effort to ensure the quality of this educational product. In addition, the Academy's Practicing Ophthalmologists Advisory Committee on Education and its chair, Dr Hal D. Balyeat, have provided valuable feedback during the preparation of *ProVision* Series 2. As always, the dedication of the Academy staff to successful completion of this project has been critical. Special thanks are due to Stephen Moore, Self-Assessment Program Manager; Margaret Petela, Managing Editor; and Lisa Bogle, Production Manager.

In preparing *ProVision: Preferred Responses in Ophthalmology* Series 2, the committee carefully considered suggestions for improvements that came from users of Series 1, leading clinicians, and professional educators. In keeping with these suggestions, the committee increased the number of sections from seven to eight, each with 50 questions, and included many more color photographs and clinical images. In developing questions and discussions, the committee emphasized areas likely to be encountered by a contemporary comprehensive ophthalmologist, such as phacoemulsification, refractive surgery, infectious disease, ocular oncology, uveitis, and systemic disease.

Although Series 2 offers significant improvements, Series 1 is in no way outdated or superseded; it continues to be the excellent assessment instrument that it always has been. The two products comprise different questions and emphasize different clinical topics. Therefore, practitioners who have not already done so are encouraged to broaden the scope of their self-assessment by also completing *ProVision* Series 1.

All ophthalmologists certified by the American Board of Ophthalmology in 1992 and thereafter will require renewal of their certification every ten years. Time-limited certification, together with other challenges in our profession, makes developing a self-directed lifelong learning program a logical and vital step for all ophthalmologists. We hope that you will find participation in *ProVision* Series 2 a meaningful experience that, together with other elements of the LEO framework, will satisfy your needs for personal assessment and learning and, most importantly, result in the highest possible quality of care for your patients.

Gregory L. Skuta, MD
Oklahoma City, Oklahoma

INTRODUCTION

ProVision and Lifelong Education for the Ophthalmologist (LEO)

In this era of tremendous change in the field of medicine, it is essential for every ophthalmologist to develop a self-directed lifelong learning program. With this in mind, Academy President Dr Ronald Smith officially launched "Lifelong Education for the Ophthalmologist" (LEO) at the 1994 Annual Meeting. The LEO framework encompasses an array of continuing medical education products and programs organized to help ophthalmologists formulate and implement individualized learning plans that address their personal educational goals:

- All ophthalmologists may develop LEO plans to help them become more comprehensive in their practices.
- Subspecialists may develop LEO plans to update their knowledge outside their own subspecialties.
- Members preparing to meet the requirements of certification renewal or managed care groups may develop LEO plans to organize and focus their educational efforts.

Within the LEO framework, the field of ophthalmology is divided into ten areas:

1. Glaucoma
2. Cataract and Anterior Segment Surgery
3. Cornea, External Disease, and Anterior Segment Trauma
4. Ocular Oncology
5. Neuro-Ophthalmology
6. Orbit and Ophthalmic Plastic Surgery
7. Pediatric Ophthalmology and Strabismus
8. Retina, Vitreous, and Posterior Segment Trauma
9. Uveitis and General Medicine
10. Refraction, Contact Lens, and Visual Rehabilitation

Ten Clinical Topic Updates, one for each of these areas, are the latest offerings from LEO. Each is designed to give an overview of its topic, focusing on advances made in the last 5 to 10 years. The Clinical Topic Updates serve as entry points into the LEO framework by assisting ophthalmologists in determining the topics and resources to incorporate in their LEO plans. Call or write the Academy or consult the Academy catalog for availability of the Clinical Topic Updates.

As a tool for assessing ophthalmic knowledge and identifying learning needs, *ProVision* complements the Clinical Topic Updates and serves as another entry point into the LEO framework. Although *ProVision* cannot offer a complete assessment of a practitioner's knowledge and skill, it can indicate areas in which additional study may be warranted. The subspecialty sections in *ProVision* differ somewhat from the ten LEO topics. The developers of Series 2 retained the seven sections from Series 1 and added an eighth, "Optics, Refraction, Contact Lens, and Visual Rehabilitation." Although two of the LEO topics, "Ocular Oncology" and "Uveitis and General Medicine," do not appear as separate sections in Series 2, questions on these topics are included, where appropriate, throughout.

The Academy will continue to develop new LEO products and programs to keep pace with the changing needs of Academy members. LEO Update Courses will be offered during the Annual Meeting and at other times. A LEO project under development is *ProVision Interactive,* a multimedia self-assessment program on CD-ROM. Motion video, audio, computer graphics, and enhanced still photographs will combine to create an interactive environment that realistically simulates patient–physician encounters. Please contact the Academy for information about the availability of these programs.

HOW TO USE
PROVISION SERIES 2

Components and Contents

ProVision consists of two text volumes and one workbook. Volume I, "Questions," provides 50 multiple-choice test items in each of eight sections. The questions in *ProVision* require recall and application of medical knowledge, as well as clinical decision making and judgment. Many of the questions are presented as case studies, providing patient history, symptoms and signs, and test results, including relevant photographs and illustrations. Strong emphasis is placed on awareness of new clinical approaches to the diagnosis and treatment of eye diseases and disorders.

Volume II, "Discussions," duplicates every question and clinical image from Volume I, provides a discussion of each question, and indicates the preferred response. In the discussions, recognized experts in the field explain the clinical and scientific reasons for choosing the preferred response, and give numerous citations to the literature. Lists of all references and pertinent Academy resources are provided at the end of each section in Volume II.

Going beyond standard assessment, *ProVision* emphasizes learning by providing instructional feedback. The term "preferred response" is used instead of "correct answer" to acknowledge the ongoing debate on some clinical points. Because we have included controversial topics, you may not always agree with the preferred response or discussion. The discussions and the preferred responses are based on the information presented in the questions and should not be construed as excluding other acceptable practices.

The Workbook contains

- A Worksheet for recording your responses
- The Program Evaluation and CME Credit Report
- The Self-Evaluation Learning Plan
- A Machine-Scorable Answer Sheet
- The Worksheet Answer Key for self-scoring

The Self-Evaluation Learning Plan and the Machine-Scorable Answer Sheet are provided as alternative ways to obtain Continuing Medical Education credit for *ProVision* and are explained below.

Recommended Approach

The Academy recommends that you work through *ProVision* one section at a time. You need not complete the sections in the order presented, but you should answer all questions for one section in Volume I before reviewing the discussions and preferred responses for that section in Volume II. For maximum benefit, you should read the discussion for every question—whether you chose the preferred response or not—because any discussion may contain some information that is new to you or that relates to another question or discussion. You should record and tally your responses, using the Worksheet and Worksheet Answer Key in the Workbook, and note the specific clinical points made in the discussions that you did not know or with which you disagree. This is the best way for you to identify strengths as well as areas needing further study. (Also please see the section below entitled "Establishing Your Educational Needs.") The Academy recommends that you complete all eight sections, giving special attention to those areas that are *not* a part of your everyday practice. Allow between 3 and 4 hours to complete an entire section (both volumes) in one sitting.

It is also possible to complete all the questions in Volume I before going on to Volume II. If you choose this approach, you may need to set aside approximately 12 hours for Volume I and 16 hours to review the discussions and preferred responses in Volume II. You may instead choose to work through Volume II alone, responding to a question, reading the corresponding discussion, and checking the preferred response before moving to the next question. With this approach, however, you are likely to overestimate your proficiency. Therefore, you should choose this alternative only if you are interested in *ProVision* solely as an educational program. To conduct the most effective self-assessment and to learn the most from the discussions, the Academy encourages you to complete the program as recommended.

Establishing Your Educational Needs

- The questions and discussions in *ProVision* represent only a sample from a larger field of knowledge. Take this into consideration when using *ProVision* to identify areas for further study.
- Do not limit your study solely to those clinical points made in the discussions. Rather, focus on the broader clinical areas of which those points are a part.
- Exercise caution in gauging your knowledge even on questions for which your answer did agree with the preferred response. Verify that your reasoning was clinically valid by studying the discussions for those questions too, not just for the ones you missed.
- The sections are not all equal in difficulty. For this reason, it is not possible to provide an objective performance standard or "passing grade" for any of the sections. Begin establishing your educational needs with any section or sections on which you scored substantially lower than on the other sections—say 25 percent lower.
- Make use of the two lists provided at the end of each section in Volume II. The first is a list of the references cited in support of the specific clinical points made in the discussions themselves. The second is a list of Academy educational resources.
- One self-assessment program cannot identify all areas in which you need more study. *ProVision* Series 1 and the Clinical Topic Updates are useful in identifying other areas needing further study.

Obtaining CME Credit

The American Academy of Ophthalmology is accredited to sponsor Continuing Medical Education (CME) for physicians by the Accreditation Council for Continuing Medical Education. The Academy designates up to 28 Category 1 CME credit hours for participation in *ProVision* Series 2, allowing one credit hour for every hour you spend.

Active members or fellows who participate in LEO may earn the LEO Continuing Education Recognition Award. To qualify, participants must complete 150 hours of Academy-sponsored Category 1 CME credits within a 3-year period, including participation in at least one Academy Annual Meeting or completion of a *ProVision* program. Through an agreement of reciprocity, all LEO Award recipients will be eligible for the American Medical Association's Standard Physician Recognition Award (PRA) certificate.

To apply for your *ProVision* CME credit, you must complete and send to the Academy two forms found in the *ProVision* Workbook:

• The Program Evaluation and CME Credit Report *(both sides)*

Plus one of the following two forms:

• OPTION 1: The Machine-Scorable Answer Sheet *(not the self-scoring Worksheet)*
• OPTION 2: The Self-Evaluation Learning Plan

If you choose to complete the Machine-Scorable Answer Sheet, you will receive a letter from the Academy that gives your scores, the average scores of your peers who also chose Option 1, and some general information about how to interpret your scores. These letters are sent out quarterly. Strict procedures are maintained to ensure the absolute confidentiality of the letters themselves and all information used to generate them. Because the answer sheet is scored by machine, *you must send in the original; photocopies cannot be processed.* Also, please fill in the bubbles completely with blue ink, black ink, or a No. 2 pencil. *Do not send the self-scoring Worksheet for machine scoring.*

If you choose to complete the Self-Evaluation Learning Plan (Option 2), you will formulate specific learning objectives and identify resources and activities that will allow you to accomplish those objectives. There will be no further followup from the Academy.

Although you would receive no additional CME credit for doing so, you may wish to complete both Option 1 and Option 2. You are encouraged also to consider earning additional CME through other Academy publications, programs, and courses, including the courses and seminars available at the Academy's Annual Meeting.

Regardless of the CME credit option you choose, the Academy requires that you also complete the Program Evaluation and CME Credit Report. The Program Evaluation is part of the CME requirement because it is vitally important for the Academy to know your level of satisfaction with *ProVision. Even if you are not applying for CME credit, please fill out the Program Evaluation portion of the form and return it to the Academy.* All evaluation information is processed anonymously. Your candid opinions and comments will help the Academy improve future *ProVision* programs.

GLAUCOMA

Five weeks after a trabeculectomy, a patient presents with a low, scarred bleb and intraocular pressure of 44 mm Hg (see the figure). After instituting therapy with a topical beta blocker, oral carbonic anhydrase inhibitor, and ocular digital massage, the intraocular pressure is 34 mm Hg.

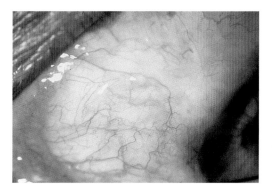

Conjunctival and subconjunctival scarring in the superotemporal quadrant of an eye after unsuccessful glaucoma filtering surgery.

The *most* appropriate next step would be to

a. give subconjunctival 5-fluorouracil injections
b. perform Nd:YAG laser surgery to the internal aspect of the sclerostomy
c. needle the bleb
d. repeat trabeculectomy at a new operative site, using antifibrotic therapy

Discussion

The most common reason for bleb failure is scarring at the episcleral surface of the operative area. Obstruction of the internal aspect of the sclerostomy site can occur with iris, vitreous, and rarely lens. Needling may be beneficial for a high, thick, elevated encapsulated bleb. If the bleb is scarred flat, needling will be of no value. Subconjunctival 5-fluorouracil injections should be administered within the first 2 postoperative weeks and preferably before substantial scarring occurs.[1] In this patient, a repeat trabeculectomy at a new operative site using antifibrotic therapy is the best option.

Preferred Response

d. repeat trabeculectomy at a new operative site, using antifibrotic therapy

A patient complains of itching, redness, and scaling of the eyelids and periorbital skin (see the figure, part A). Conjunctival findings are shown in part B of the figure. He is on topical timolol, dipivefrin, and pilocarpine as well as oral acetazolamide for glaucoma.

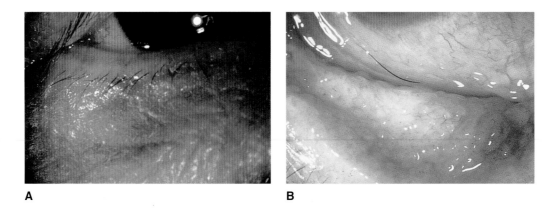

A   **B**

(A) Lower lid erythema, hyperkeratosis, and scaling of a patient with dipivefrin-associated contact dermatitis. **(B)** Fine follicular conjunctival response of a patient with the same condition.

Which of the following actions will *most* likely resolve this problem?

a. discontinue timolol
b. discontinue dipivefrin
c. discontinue pilocarpine
d. prescribe topical dexamethasone ointment

Discussion

Hypersensitivity can develop to any glaucoma medication or preservative. Of those listed, dipivefrin is the most likely agent to cause follicular conjunctivitis and contact dermatitis.[2] Topical corticosteroid ointment may relieve symptoms; however, it is preferable to discontinue the likely offending agent.

Preferred Response

b. discontinue dipivefrin

All of the following can cause a superior visual field defect in automated threshold perimetry *except*

a. glaucoma
b. ptosis
c. lens rim artifact
d. high false-positive rate

Discussion

Glaucoma, ptosis, and lens rim artifact can cause superior visual field defects.[3] A high false-positive rate, which indicates that the patient responded when no stimulus was presented, may be due to a nervous patient and usually causes increased thresholds rather than a visual field defect in automated threshold perimetry.

Preferred Response

d. high false-positive rate

G4

Assuming equal transmission and absorption of laser energy, which time and power setting below would provide energy equal to that delivered by an argon laser with settings of 0.1 sec duration and 500 mW power?

a. 0.05 sec; 2 W
b. 0.02 sec; 1 W
c. 0.02 sec; 2.5 W
d. 1 sec; 5 W

Discussion

The energy delivered by the argon laser in a "perfect" setting is determined by the power in watts or milliwatts, multiplied by the duration in seconds.[4,5] The equation for this relationship is *power × time = energy*. If the power is increased and the time is proportionately decreased, the same amount of energy will be delivered. Answer "c" is the only response demonstrating that relationship in that both these parameters and those provided in the question deliver 50 millijoules of energy.

Preferred Response

c. 0.02 sec; 2.5 W

G5

A 55-year-old man with no previous ocular laser or surgical therapy has advanced glaucomatous visual field loss (see the figure) and cupping. His current intraocular pressure is 37 mm Hg on a beta blocker and pilocarpine. An oral carbonic anhydrase inhibitor was previously tried but was discontinued because the patient complained of malaise and fatigue.

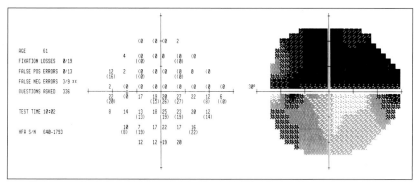

Advanced glaucomatous visual field loss with split fixation and extensive superior visual field loss in a patient with primary open-angle glaucoma.

The next therapeutic step would be to

a. begin a second trial of oral carbonic anhydrase inhibitor and reinforce the need for compliance to prevent visual loss
b. switch from pilocarpine to carbachol to see if intraocular pressure control improved
c. perform laser trabeculoplasty
d. perform trabeculectomy

Discussion

In a patient with advanced glaucomatous visual loss (split fixation) and an intraocular pressure of 37 mm Hg on two medications, laser trabeculoplasty or switching medications cannot be expected to establish a safe pressure.[6,7] Restoring the oral carbonic anhydrase inhibitor is inappropriate not only because it is unlikely to control the pressure adequately but also because it was not previously tolerated. Surgical intervention (trabeculectomy) is the preferred choice in this patient.[8,9]

Preferred Response

d. perform trabeculectomy

A patient with primary open-angle glaucoma underwent trabeculectomy. On the first postoperative day, the visual acuity corrects to 20/80, the bleb is almost flat, the anterior chamber is shallow (see the figure), and the intraocular pressure is 1 mm Hg.

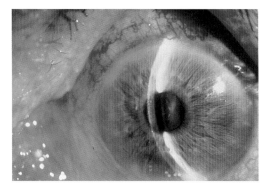

Flat peripheral and shallow central anterior chamber of a patient with bleb leak after recent trabeculectomy.

The *most* likely problem is

a. early failure of bleb with scarring at episcleral surface
b. ciliary body shutdown
c. bleb leak
d. aqueous misdirection (malignant or ciliary-block glaucoma)

Discussion

In a patient with primary open-angle glaucoma in the immediate postoperative period after trabeculectomy, the most common reason for a shallow anterior chamber with a low intraocular pressure and low bleb is a wound leak.[10–12] Early bleb failure and aqueous misdirection could be suspected if the intraocular pressure were elevated after surgery.[13] Ciliary body shutdown can occur but would be less likely than an unrecognized bleb leak in this clinical situation.

Preferred Response

c. bleb leak

G7

Medical management of glaucoma associated with inflammatory ocular disease (uveitis) and active intraocular inflammation could include all of the following *except*

a. pilocarpine
b. beta blocker
c. topical corticosteroid
d. cholinergic antagonist (cycloplegic agent)

Discussion

In a patient with active intraocular inflammation, topical corticosteroid and cycloplegic therapy is appropriate. A topical beta blocker will help reduce intraocular pressure by decreasing aqueous production. Pilocarpine should not be used because it will increase pain and inflammation and may lead to posterior synechiae formation and a poorly dilating pupil, which could progress to pupillary-block glaucoma.[14]

Preferred Response

a. pilocarpine

G8

Which of the following would be the weakest indication for a combined cataract extraction and trabeculectomy in a patient with glaucoma and a visually significant cataract?

a. well-controlled glaucoma (intraocular pressure 13 mm Hg) on a topical beta blocker, miotic agent, and oral carbonic anhydrase inhibitor
b. glaucoma controlled with one medication in an eye with advanced glaucomatous visual field loss
c. an eye with previous trabeculectomy and with intraocular pressure of 18 mm Hg on a beta blocker and miotic agent
d. an eye with a previous history of acute angle-closure glaucoma, treated with laser iridotomy, and now with an intraocular pressure of 17 mm Hg on no medication and with no peripheral anterior synechiae

Discussion

A combined cataract extraction with trabeculectomy can be performed in an eye with well-controlled glaucoma on multiple antiglaucoma medications. A combined procedure is also advantageous for the patient with advanced glaucomatous visual loss, who might suffer further visual loss, including loss of fixation, in the immediate postcataract surgical period if there is substantial intraocular pressure elevation.[15,16] Even in the eye with a previous trabeculectomy, a combined procedure can be helpful if the filter's function is not particularly good or not expected to survive cataract surgery. The patient with normal intraocular pressure on no medication and without substantial peripheral anterior synechiae after an episode of acute angle-closure glaucoma would be the least likely of this group to require a combined procedure.

Preferred Response

d. an eye with a previous history of acute angle-closure glaucoma, treated with laser iridotomy, and now with an intraocular pressure of 17 mm Hg on no medication and with no peripheral anterior synechiae

G9

The weakest indication for antifibrotic therapy in conjunction with glaucoma filtering surgery would be

a. primary trabeculectomy and exfoliation syndrome (pseudoexfoliation) glaucoma
b. neovascular glaucoma
c. glaucoma in pseudophakia
d. previously failed glaucoma filtering surgery

Discussion

The Fluorouracil Filtering Surgery Study (FFSS) demonstrated the value of postoperative subconjunctival 5-fluorouracil in patients undergoing trabeculectomy after previously failed glaucoma filtering surgery and in aphakic or pseudophakic eyes.[17] A number of nonrandomized reports have suggested that 5-fluorouracil also may be beneficial in eyes with neovascular glaucoma.[18] However, filtering surgery with antifibrotic therapy has little chance of success in an eye with neovascular glaucoma unless panretinal laser photocoagulation has been performed and there has been at least some regression of the iris neovascularization. Intraoperative mitomycin-C is an alternative to 5-fluorouracil.[19] Eyes with exfoliation syndrome glaucoma are typically not at a higher risk for failure after primary glaucoma filtering surgery.

Preferred Response

a. primary trabeculectomy and exfoliation syndrome (pseudoexfoliation) glaucoma

G10

All of the following are commonly seen in primary infantile glaucoma *except*

a. increased corneal diameter
b. myopia
c. prominent, anteriorly displaced Schwalbe's line
d. breaks in Descemet's membrane

Discussion

Elevated intraocular pressure in primary infantile glaucoma causes a generalized enlargement of the globe. This can be manifested as an increased corneal diameter, progressive myopia, and breaks in Descemet's membrane. The anterior chamber angle is usually malformed, with a high iris insertion and the appearance of a membrane-like structure over the trabecular meshwork.[20] A prominent, anteriorly displaced Schwalbe's line, known as posterior embryotoxon, can be seen in Axenfeld-Rieger syndrome but is not typically associated with primary infantile glaucoma.

Preferred Response

c. prominent, anteriorly displaced Schwalbe's line

G11

The *most* common reason for long-term visual loss in primary infantile glaucoma is

a. amblyopia
b. corneal edema
c. corneal scarring
d. glaucomatous optic nerve damage

Discussion

Amblyopia is the most common cause of long-term visual loss in eyes with primary infantile glaucoma. Corneal edema often resolves after a surgical procedure to reduce intraocular pressure. Breaks in Descemet's membrane and mild corneal scarring can occur but usually do not cause substantial visual loss. Serious visual loss from glaucomatous optic nerve damage can occur, but it is less common than amblyopia.[20]

Preferred Response

a. amblyopia

G12

All of the following are risk factors for failure after glaucoma filtering surgery *except*

a. pigmentary dispersion
b. iris neovascularization
c. aphakia
d. uveitis

Discussion

Aphakia,[21] uveitis,[22] and iris neovascularization[1] are risk factors for failure of standard glaucoma filtering surgery. Pigmentary dispersion alone is not a risk factor for failure. However, patients with pigmentary dispersion and pigmentary glaucoma tend to be younger,[23] which may represent a risk factor for failure.

Preferred Response

a. pigmentary dispersion

G13

A patient presents 2 years after glaucoma filtering surgery with purulent discharge and endophthalmitis. Which of the following is the *most* likely causative organism?

a. *Staphylococcus epidermidis*
b. *Streptococcus pneumoniae*
c. *Pseudomonas aeruginosa*
d. *Propionibacterium acnes*

Discussion

A late bleb-associated endophthalmitis tends to be caused by *Streptococcus pneumoniae* (pneumococcus) or *Haemophilus influenzae*.[24,25] *Staphylococcus aureus* and *Staphylococcus epidermidis* are more commonly associated with early-onset endophthalmitis after cataract surgery. *Propionibacterium acnes* has been associated with a later-onset endophthalmitis after cataract surgery. *Pseudomonas aeruginosa* causes a fulminant endophthalmitis but is not frequently reported as a causative agent of late bleb-associated endophthalmitis.

Preferred Response   b. *Streptococcus pneumoniae*

A generalized depression of all thresholds is shown on the central field automated perimetric test below.

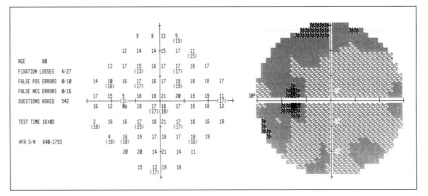

Humphrey full-threshold 30-2 visual field test of a patient with cataract. Note the relatively flat appearance of the visual field, in which central thresholds are only slightly higher than peripheral thresholds.

This finding could be a result of any of the following *except*

a. cataract
b. lens rim artifact
c. miotic agent
d. inaccurate optical correction for near

Discussion   Cataract, miotic therapy, and substantially inappropriate optical correction during perimetry can each cause a contraction of isopters on manual Goldmann perimetry or a generalized depression of thresholds on a central field automated perimetric test.[26,27] A lens rim artifact causes a substantial diminution, often to "0," of a string or ring of peripheral points. Other thresholds are not affected.

Preferred Response   b. lens rim artifact

Of the visual field defects shown, which would be *least* suggestive of glaucoma?

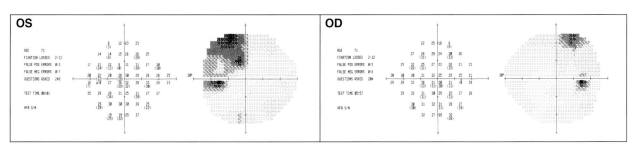

Figure A

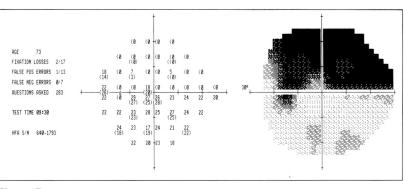

Figure B

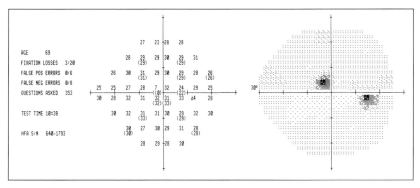

Figure C

(A) Asymmetric early superior bitemporal defect in a patient with pituitary adenoma and early chiasmal compression. **(B)** Altitudinal defect with split fixation in the left eye of a patient with moderately advanced glaucomatous optic nerve damage. **(C)** Dense paracentral scotoma superonasal to fixation in the right eye. **(D)** Diffuse nasal visual field loss in the right eye of a patient with moderate glaucomatous optic nerve damage.

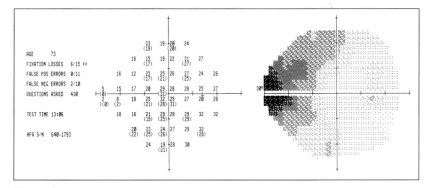

Figure D

a. Figure A
b. Figure B
c. Figure C
d. Figure D

Discussion   Glaucoma causes nerve-fiber-bundle–type visual defects. These may be seen as scotomas within the arcuate region, nasal step, generalized nasal depression (Figure D), paracentral scotomas (Figure C), and, in more advanced visual loss, an altitudinal defect[28] (Figure B). A generalized binasal depression is also a common finding in glaucoma. A bitemporal depression would suggest a chiasmal lesion. Scotomas respecting the vertical midline (Figure A) are suggestive of lesions either involving the chiasm or posterior to the chiasm.

Preferred Response   a. Figure A

The figures below show typical glaucomatous optic nerve changes.

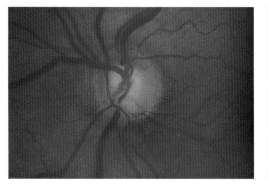

Figure A

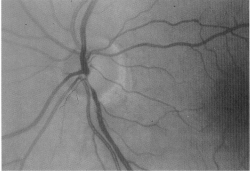

Figure B

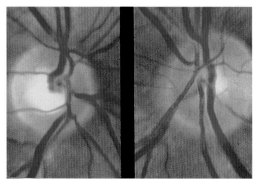

Figure C

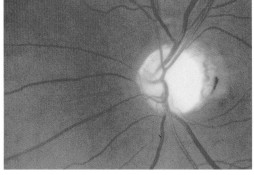

Figure D

(A) Notch in the inferotemporal neuroretinal rim of a patient with glaucoma. **(B)** Diffuse expansion of the optic cup both superiorly and inferiorly, creating an ovoid optic cup in a patient with glaucoma. Note the relatively healthy nasal and temporal optic nerve rim. Also note the bending upward of the superotemporal optic disc vasculature and downward of the inferotemporal vein. **(C)** Left, diffuse optic cup enlargement of the right eye of a patient with unilateral glaucoma. Right, the left optic nerve is normal with almost no optic cup. **(D)** Diffuse pallor of the neuroretinal rim in a patient with history of severe left craniofacial trauma and traumatic optic atrophy.

Typical glaucomatous optic nerve changes can include all of the following *except*

a. notch in neuroretinal rim of the optic nerve (Figure A)
b. vertically oval optic cup (Figure B)
c. unilateral, asymmetric diffuse enlargement of optic disc cup (Figure C)
d. pallor of neuroretinal rim (pallor out of proportion to the degree of cupping) of optic nerve (Figure D)

Discussion

Glaucomatous optic nerve damage can be manifested as a notch in the neuroretinal rim, a vertically oval optic cup, substantial asymmetry of the cup-to-disc ratio, or diffuse enlargement of the optic disc cup.[29] Pallor of the neuroretinal rim suggests a nonglaucomatous cause of optic nerve damage. Pallor may suggest previous optic neuritis, other optic neuropathy, vascular occlusive disease, or neuroretinitis. Very severe intraocular pressure elevation can cause ischemic optic nerve damage and an apparent nonglaucomatous optic atrophy.

Preferred Response

d. pallor of neuroretinal rim (pallor out of proportion to the degree of cupping) of optic nerve (Figure D)

The problem requiring the *most* urgent management after glaucoma filtering surgery is

a. choroidal effusion
b. choroidal hemorrhage
c. shallow anterior chamber with iris-to-cornea touch
d. shallow anterior chamber with lens-to-cornea touch

Discussion

A shallow anterior chamber with lens-to-cornea touch requires immediate intervention. Rapid corneal decompensation and cataract progression can occur if this persists. A shallow anterior chamber with iris-to-cornea touch but without lens-to-cornea touch is a common transient finding after glaucoma filtering surgery and is usually of no consequence.[10] Choroidal effusion is a common finding after glaucoma filtering surgery and usually resolves when intraocular pressure climbs above a hypotonous level.[30] Drainage of choroidal effusion is seldom necessary unless it accompanies lens-to-cornea touch. A choroidal hemorrhage may require drainage; however, in most cases it can be observed or, if necessary, drained at a later time.[31]

Preferred Response

d. shallow anterior chamber with lens-to-cornea touch

Laser trabeculoplasty is indicated for the management of uncontrolled glaucoma in all of the following situations *except*

a. active inflammatory (uveitic) glaucoma
b. exfoliation syndrome glaucoma
c. 35-year-old patient with pigmentary glaucoma
d. chronic primary angle-closure glaucoma with a patent laser iridotomy and one-third of angle closed by peripheral anterior synechiae

Discussion   Exfoliation syndrome glaucoma and primary open-angle glaucoma are appropriate indications for laser trabeculoplasty. A relatively young individual may respond less satisfactorily than an older individual; however, laser trabeculoplasty can still be contemplated in the 35-year-old patient with pigmentary glaucoma. Laser trabeculoplasty cannot be performed in an eye with substantial secondary angle closure, although it is a reasonable option if most of the angle is open. Laser trabeculoplasty should not be performed in an eye with active intraocular inflammation. An exacerbation of inflammation, peripheral anterior synechiae formation, and serious postlaser intraocular pressure elevation may result.

Preferred Response   a. active inflammatory (uveitic) glaucoma

G19

All of the following are associated with chronic angle-closure glaucoma with relative pupillary block *except*

a. hyperopia
b. the presence of exfoliative material in the eye
c. cataract progression
d. peripheral radial iris transillumination defects

Discussion   Chronic primary angle-closure glaucoma is associated with hyperopia and cataract progression, as well as with increasing age. Although exfoliation syndrome glaucoma is usually a secondary open-angle glaucoma, there is also a clinical association of chronic angle-closure glaucoma with exfoliation syndrome.[32,33] Eyes with exfoliation syndrome may have peripupillary iris transillumination defects. Peripheral radial iris transillumination defects are found in eyes with pigmentary dispersion and pigmentary glaucoma in which the anterior chamber angle is typically very deep with slight concavity of the peripheral iris. There is no clinical association of pigmentary glaucoma with chronic angle-closure glaucoma.

Preferred Response   d. peripheral radial iris transillumination defects

G20

All of the following will halt the progression of synechial angle closure in chronic primary angle-closure glaucoma *except*

a. cataract extraction
b. laser iridotomy
c. miotic (cholinergic) therapy
d. posterior lens dislocation

Discussion   Laser iridotomy is the treatment of choice for chronic primary angle-closure glaucoma.[32] A cataract extraction or posterior lens dislocation can relieve relative pupillary block and eliminate a need for iridotomy. Miotic (cholinergic) therapy may increase relative pupillary block by allowing forward movement of the lens against a constricted pupil. Miotic therapy can therefore exacerbate chronic angle-closure glaucoma and precipitate acute angle-closure glaucoma. If miotic therapy is used in the patient with narrow angles or chronic angle-closure glaucoma, it is necessary to perform gonioscopy after institution of miotic therapy to determine if a worsening of angle closure has occurred.

Preferred Response   c. miotic (cholinergic) therapy

A 66-year-old man had uncontrolled intraocular pressure on glaucoma medical therapy with a previous laser peripheral iridotomy for chronic angle closure. Five days after a trabeculectomy, he has a very shallow peripheral and central anterior chamber, patent iridotomy, intraocular pressure of 40 mm Hg, and no evidence of choroidal detachment on ocular B-scan ultrasonography. All of the following may help in the management of this patient *except*

a. miotic (cholinergic) therapy
b. topical beta blocker therapy
c. oral carbonic anhydrase inhibitor therapy
d. vitrectomy

Discussion   Topical beta blocker therapy and oral carbonic anhydrase therapy can reduce intraocular pressure in eyes with aqueous misdirection (malignant glaucoma). Topical cycloplegic (anticholinergic) therapy can reduce the block in aqueous misdirection syndrome by tightening the zonules and causing a posterior displacement of the lens.[13] Miotic (cholinergic) therapy tends to exacerbate the block and increase inflammation. Vitrectomy may be necessary if medical management is not successful.

Preferred Response   a. miotic (cholinergic) therapy

Exfoliation syndrome (pseudoexfoliation) glaucoma is associated with all of the following *except*

a. increased pigmentation of trabecular meshwork
b. zonular dehiscence
c. radial peripheral iris transillumination defects
d. chronic angle closure

Discussion   Eyes with exfoliation syndrome have increased pigmentation of the trabecular meshwork, often in a patchy or nonhomogeneous pattern. Zonular dehiscence can be manifested as spontaneous lens dislocation (see the figures, parts A and B, page 14) or a greater incidence of zonular dialysis and vitreous loss during cataract surgery in eyes with exfoliation syndrome.[34] There is an increased incidence of chronic angle closure in eyes with exfoliation syndrome (see the figure, part C). Radial peripheral iris transillumination defects are found in pigmentary glaucoma and pigmentary dispersion syndrome. Peripupillary iris transillumination defects are more commonly seen in exfoliation syndrome.

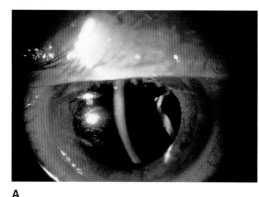

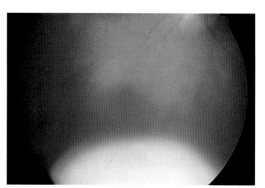

A

B

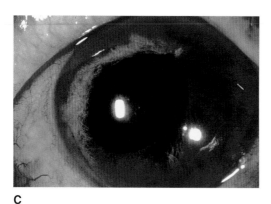

Elderly patient with exfoliation syndrome and spontaneous subluxation of the lens. **(A)** The intact vitreous face. **(B)** The cataractous lens in the posterior segment. **(C)** Superior and temporal iris atrophy after an attack of subacute angle-closure glaucoma in an eye with exfoliation syndrome.

C

Preferred Response   c. radial peripheral iris transillumination defects

G23

The *most* likely abnormality detected on automated perimetry in an ocular hypertensive patient with progressive nuclear sclerotic cataract would be

a. generalized depression, greater centrally
b. increased blind-spot size
c. depressed ring of peripheral points in a central 30° program
d. increased pattern standard deviation

Discussion   A progressive nuclear sclerotic cataract is most likely to cause a generalized depression of a central visual field, greater centrally than peripherally (see the figure, part A).[35] An increased blind-spot size (see the figure, part B) is not expected. The visual field depicted in part B is of a patient with large angioid streaks. Cataracts usually cause an even depression of thresholds rather than focal defects or scotomas. The pattern standard deviation, which highlights localized visual field defects rather than diffuse visual field depression, would probably remain the same in a patient with a progressive nuclear sclerotic cataract. A depressed ring of peripheral points in a central 30° program (see the figure, part C) could be caused by a lens rim artifact, ptosis, and possibly some retinal disorders, such as retinitis pigmentosa or a chorioretinal scar.

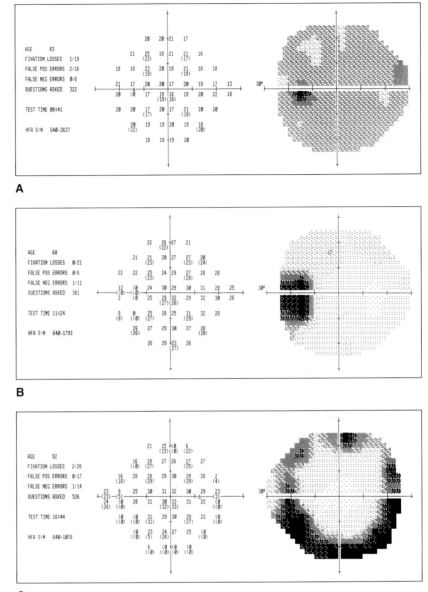

A

B

C

(A) A Humphrey 24-2 visual field test of the left eye in a patient with a moderate nuclear sclerotic cataract. Note the relative flatness of the visual field with absence of focal defects. (B) Enlarged blind spot in the left eye of a patient with large peripapillary chorioretinal atrophy and angioid streaks. (C) Patient with ocular hypertension and a ring of depressed peripheral field points on a Humphrey 24-2 visual field test of the right eye. This represents a lens rim artifact.

Preferred Response   a. generalized depression, greater centrally

G24

All of the following are reasons for an increased mean deviation on automated threshold perimetry *except*

a. cataract progression
b. glaucoma progression
c. high false-positive rate
d. topical miotic (cholinergic) therapy

Discussion

Cataract progression, the addition of topical miotic therapy, and glaucoma progression can each cause an increased mean deviation. A progression of glaucomatous defects may cause an increased mean deviation with or without an increased pattern standard deviation. A high false-positive rate, which indicates that the patient responded when no stimulus was presented, would generally not affect or would decrease the mean deviation. However, if a high false-positive rate is accompanied by supranormal thresholds, the mean deviation may be very small or positive.

Preferred Response

c. high false-positive rate

G25

The *most* important finding suggestive of glaucoma in a patient with elevated intraocular pressure would be

a. cup-to-disc ratio asymmetry of 0.1
b. bilateral cup-to-disc ratio of 0.7
c. very deep optic cup
d. cup-to-disc ratio of 0.4 with notch formation in optic nerve rim

Discussion

Although a cup-to-disc ratio asymmetry of 0.1 to 0.2 may be normal, a difference greater than 0.2 is suggestive of glaucoma. A bilateral cup-to-disc ratio of 0.7 does not necessarily indicate glaucoma. This can be seen in individuals with very large optic nerves and accompanying large optic cups. The depth of the optic cup has very little correlation with glaucoma and glaucomatous optic nerve damage. A cup-to-disc ratio of 0.4 may not arouse much suspicion for glaucoma; however, if accompanied by elevated intraocular pressure and notch formation in the optic nerve rim, it would be strongly suggestive of glaucomatous optic nerve damage.[36]

Preferred Response

d. cup-to-disc ratio of 0.4 with notch formation in optic nerve rim

G26

A 65-year-old man with severe proliferative diabetic retinopathy underwent a very heavy laser photocoagulation treatment session by your retinal associate 1 day previously. Today, the patient presents with mild pain, blurred vision, and an intraocular pressure of 45 mm Hg. Your retinal associate has already treated the patient with a topical beta blocker and oral carbonic anhydrase inhibitor and has referred him to you for further management of elevated intraocular pressure. The patient has no previous history of glaucoma and no evidence of iris neovascularization. On your examination, the anterior chamber appears very shallow and the fellow eye has a deep anterior chamber.

What would be the *most* appropriate initial management step?

a. Perform a laser iridotomy.
b. Perform a laser iridoplasty.
c. Give a topical cycloplegic agent.
d. Perform a trabeculectomy.

Discussion

Very heavy panretinal laser photocoagulation can cause swelling and anterior rotation of the ciliary body, which does not respond to a laser iridotomy. The best initial step would be to administer topical cycloplegic therapy. This, combined with a topical corticosteroid, may cause a posterior rotation and opening of the angle without additional therapy. If the angle closure fails to respond to medical therapy, then a laser iridoplasty would be the next step. Typically, this is performed with the argon laser using a low power, long duration, and large spot size. Examples of parameters are 0.2 to 0.5 sec duration, 200 to 300 mW of power, and 200 to 500 μ spot size. Topical cycloplegia and then laser iridoplasty would be indicated before trabeculectomy.

Preferred Response

c. Give a topical cycloplegic agent.

All of the following statements are true of the topical selective beta blocker betaxolol (Betoptic) *except*

a. It is less effective in lowering intraocular pressure than levobunolol (Betagan) or timolol (Timoptic).
b. It is safer for patients with mild, intermittent asthma attacks.
c. It has more additive effect of lowering intraocular pressure when combined with dipivefrin (Propine) than do the nonselective beta blockers.
d. It can be safely used in patients with congestive heart failure.

Discussion

The nonselective beta blockers levobunolol (Betagan) and timolol (Timoptic) are more effective than betaxolol (Betoptic) in lowering intraocular pressure. The relative beta-1 selectivity of betaxolol allows for safer use in patients with mild, intermittent asthma. A greater additive effect of dipivefrin (Propine) with betaxolol has been demonstrated over dipivefrin with nonselective beta blockers.[37] Beta blockers should not be used in patients with congestive heart failure. Both beta-1 selective and nonselective agents can exacerbate heart failure.

Preferred Response

d. It can be safely used in patients with congestive heart failure.

G28

Laser iridotomy is indicated in all of the following *except*

a. neovascular glaucoma
b. chronic primary angle-closure glaucoma
c. pseudophakic pupillary-block glaucoma
d. inability to adequately view trabecular meshwork in an eye with narrow angle prior to performing laser trabeculoplasty

Discussion

Laser iridotomy is indicated for phakic, pseudophakic, or aphakic pupillary block and for relative pupillary block (acute angle-closure and chronic angle-closure glaucoma). If an angle has no peripheral anterior synechiae but is narrow enough to prevent performance of a laser trabeculoplasty, an iridotomy is appropriate. In neovascular glaucoma, the iris is pulled into the trabecular meshwork by fibrovascular proliferation rather than pushed into the angle by relative pupillary block. The former mechanism would not favorably respond to a laser iridotomy.

Preferred Response

a. neovascular glaucoma

G29

The *most* effective three-drug regimen for an eye with primary open-angle glaucoma would be

a. betaxolol, dipivefrin, pilocarpine
b. levobunolol, pilocarpine, acetazolamide
c. timolol, dipivefrin, carbachol
d. timolol, dipivefrin, acetazolamide

Discussion

Of the multiple-drug regimens listed, a combination of levobunolol (a beta blocker), pilocarpine (a cholinergic agent), and acetazolamide (an oral carbonic anhydrase inhibitor) would provide the greatest intraocular pressure–lowering effect for an eye with primary open-angle glaucoma. The other three options include the combination of a topical beta blocker (betaxolol or timolol) and dipivefrin. There is not much additive effect of a beta blocker with epinephrine or dipivefrin.[29]

Preferred Response

b. levobunolol, pilocarpine, acetazolamide

G30

Two days after a trabeculectomy, a patient has an intraocular pressure of 3 mm Hg with a large bleb, no leak, and shallow but formed anterior chamber. On the third day, she presents stating that she developed moderate pain and decreased vision after bending over. The visual acuity is finger-counting and the intraocular pressure is 37 mm Hg. The bleb is unchanged in appearance. There is a moderate-sized, dark, temporal choroidal detachment. The lens and vitreous are clear, and there is no evidence of a retinal detachment.

All of the following are appropriate actions at this time *except*

a. perform drainage of choroidal hemorrhage
b. add topical beta blocker to reduce intraocular pressure
c. continue topical corticosteroid therapy
d. add cycloplegic therapy

Discussion

After a delayed, postoperative suprachoroidal hemorrhage of limited to moderate size, it is appropriate to continue topical corticosteroid therapy and continue or add cycloplegic therapy. Analgesic therapy for pain is appropriate, and a topical beta blocker and/or oral carbonic anhydrase inhibitor can be employed to control elevated intraocular pressure. In the case described, drainage of choroidal hemorrhage would be the least appropriate action.

Preferred Response

a. perform drainage of choroidal hemorrhage

A 78-year-old man experienced unilateral sudden loss of vision 1 year previously. Currently, he complains of severe pain in that eye. Examination reveals no light-perception vision, intraocular pressure of 72 mm Hg, iris neovascularization, and evidence of a central retinal vein occlusion.

The *least* helpful therapeutic agent at this time would be

a. topical cycloplegic
b. topical corticosteroid
c. topical beta blocker
d. topical cholinergic (miotic) agent

Discussion

The management of a painful blind eye with end-stage glaucoma can include topical cycloplegia (anticholinergic agent) and a corticosteroid agent for comfort. A topical beta blocker may provide relatively little intraocular pressure lowering but may provide some increased comfort. Eyes with end-stage iris neovascularization and neovascular glaucoma have completely or near completely closed angles. A cholinergic agent such as pilocarpine will not successfully reduce intraocular pressure in these eyes and will often increase pain and inflammation.

Preferred Response

d. topical cholinergic (miotic) agent

Which of the following statements is true of apraclonidine (Iopidine)?

a. It is an alpha-1 adrenergic agonist.
b. It commonly causes systemic hypotension.
c. It may cause transient lid retraction.
d. It is associated with macular edema in aphakic eyes.

Discussion   Apraclonidine (Iopidine) can cause conjunctival blanching and lid retraction. Apraclonidine is an alpha-2 adrenergic agonist and, unlike clonidine, does not cause systemic hypotension. Epinephrine and possibly dipivefrin (Propine) are associated with macular edema in aphakic eyes.

Preferred Response   c. It may cause transient lid retraction.

G33   A 21-year-old woman with juvenile open-angle glaucoma and 7 diopters of myopia complains of severe blurring of vision after using 1 drop of pilocarpine. The *most* likely cause of her symptom is

a. a small pupil
b. increased hyperopia
c. increased myopia
d. retinal detachment

Discussion   Young, highly myopic patients may have substantially increased myopia with miotic therapy. This occurs because of a miotic-induced increased convexity of the lens and forward lens movement. All patients with a normal iris develop a small pupil on miotic therapy. This can cause nyctalopia and is more troublesome in older patients with a cataract or other media opacity. Retinal detachment after miotic therapy can occur but would not be the most likely cause of severe visual blurring in this case.

Preferred Response   c. increased myopia

G34   Two years after a successful filtering procedure (full-thickness sclerectomy), a patient complains of pain, tearing, and blurred vision for 2 days. The visual acuity is 20/50, the intraocular pressure is 4 mm Hg, the bleb is flat, and there is a rare cell in the anterior chamber.

The *most* likely explanation of these symptoms and signs is

a. endophthalmitis
b. retinal detachment
c. bleb leak
d. ciliary body detachment

Discussion   The patient with a previously high, thin, ischemic bleb is more prone to develop a late bleb leak. This is usually manifested as mild discomfort, tearing, and blurred vision and may be more likely to occur after full-thickness filtering procedures or trabeculectomy with antifibrotic therapy.[17] Objective signs include a flat bleb (usually with demonstrable leak), mildly decreased visual acuity, low intraocular pressure, and minimal or no anterior chamber inflammation. If severe anterior chamber reaction or hypopyon is seen, endophthalmitis must be suspected. Ciliary body detachment may be seen and is secondary to hypotony and inflammation in an eye with endophthalmitis, retinal detachment, or bleb leak. A retinal detachment could explain many of these findings but would be a less likely cause of this clinical picture.

Preferred Response   c. bleb leak

All of the following statements about chronic primary angle-closure glaucoma are true *except*

a. It can develop in a patient with primary open-angle glaucoma.
b. It can develop in a myopic eye.
c. It often causes no pain.
d. It can be prevented by pilocarpine therapy.

Discussion   Chronic primary angle-closure glaucoma more commonly develops in hyperopic eyes with shorter axial length and crowded peripheral anterior chamber. However, angle-closure glaucoma can develop in the myopic eye, especially one with an enlarging, progressive nuclear sclerotic cataract. Chronic angle-closure glaucoma can develop in an eye with previous primary open-angle mechanism (combined-mechanism glaucoma). Pain is uncommon in chronic angle-closure glaucoma even late in the course of the disease, when substantial intraocular pressure elevation can occur. Pilocarpine therapy usually does not relieve pupillary block. Pupillary block can be increased with miotic therapy, and further angle closure can occur.

Preferred Response   d. It can be prevented by pilocarpine therapy.

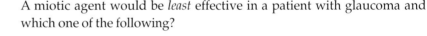

A miotic agent would be *least* effective in a patient with glaucoma and which one of the following?

a. aniridia with open angle
b. angle recession
c. aphakia
d. severe secondary angle closure

Discussion   In the absence of substantial secondary angle closure, aniridia does not reduce the effectiveness of topical miotic (cholinergic) therapy. The effect of miotic agents is mediated through the ciliary muscle and not the pupillary sphincter, which is absent in patients with aniridia. Surgical aphakia does not alter the effectiveness of miotic therapy. Angle trauma and angle recession can decrease the effectiveness of miotic therapy. Eyes with severe synechial angle closure would be the least likely to respond to cholinergic agents and may have a paradoxical rise of intraocular pressure from miotic therapy because of a reduction of nonconventional uveoscleral outflow.

Preferred Response   d. severe secondary angle closure

G37

Glaucoma-like visual field defects can be seen in all of the following conditions *except*

a. cerebrovascular accident
b. buried optic nerve drusen
c. retinal vascular occlusion
d. ischemic optic neuropathy

Discussion

Buried optic nerve drusen, retinal vascular occlusion, and ischemic optic neuropathy all produce optic nerve–type visual field defects that can mimic glaucomatous visual field loss. A cerebrovascular accident would be expected to produce a postchiasmal lesion with a homonymous hemianopic or quadrantic defect.[38]

Preferred Response

a. cerebrovascular accident

G38

A patient with elevated intraocular pressure undergoes automated static threshold perimetry. Most threshold determinations are high (40 dB to 50 dB). What is the *most* likely reason for this?

a. alert but nervous patient
b. drowsy patient
c. media opacity
d. end-stage glaucoma

Discussion

A drowsy patient would be expected to have a high false-negative rate (the patient fails to respond to a previously seen stimulus) and possibly also abnormally low thresholds either diffusely throughout the visual field or in an irregular pattern. Media opacity would also tend to diffusely decrease thresholds. End-stage glaucoma can produce a substantial decrease in some or all thresholded spots. An alert but nervous patient may have high thresholds accompanied by a high false-positive rate (the patient responds when no stimulus is presented).

Preferred Response

a. alert but nervous patient

G39

Lens extraction may resolve glaucoma in all of the following situations *except*

a. microspherophakia
b. phacolytic glaucoma
c. exfoliation syndrome (pseudoexfoliation) glaucoma
d. chronic primary angle-closure glaucoma

Discussion

Lens extraction might resolve glaucoma in microspherophakia, phacolytic glaucoma, and chronic primary angle-closure glaucoma. Exfoliation syndrome glaucoma would not be substantially improved by cataract surgery.

The material is produced by nonpigmented ciliary epithelium and other ocular tissues and can be found in pseudophakic and aphakic eyes on the capsule, vitreous, corneal endothelium, iris, and anterior chamber angle.

Preferred Response   c. exfoliation syndrome (pseudoexfoliation) glaucoma

Which of the following statements is true about corticosteroid-induced intraocular pressure elevation?

a. It usually begins within 1 day after beginning corticosteroid therapy.
b. It is more common in patients with primary open-angle glaucoma than in patients with ocular hypertension.
c. Intraocular pressure usually does not return to baseline levels after discontinuing the corticosteroid.
d. Fluorinated corticosteroids usually cause a greater incidence of intraocular pressure elevation than nonfluorinated corticosteroid preparations.

Discussion   Corticosteroid-induced intraocular pressure elevation usually begins about 2 to 4 weeks after initiation of corticosteroid therapy. Intraocular pressure often returns to baseline levels after discontinuation of the corticosteroid. Fluorinated corticosteroids (eg, fluorometholone) are less likely to cause intraocular pressure elevation than nonfluorinated corticosteroids.[39,40] Corticosteroid responsiveness is more likely in patients with primary open-angle glaucoma than in patients with ocular hypertension or patients without intraocular pressure elevation.

Preferred Response   b. It is more common in patients with primary open-angle glaucoma than in patients with ocular hypertension.

Which of the following is the *most* helpful clue in the diagnosis of chronic primary angle-closure glaucoma?

a. amount of glaucomatous optic nerve damage at presentation
b. gonioscopic findings
c. level of intraocular pressure at presentation
d. ocular symptoms (pain, haloes)

Discussion   Patients with chronic primary angle-closure glaucoma can present with intraocular pressure that is low, normal, or elevated. Ocular symptoms may or may not be present. There may be any degree of glaucomatous optic nerve damage or no damage at all. Gonioscopic findings, preferably with the Zeiss or Posner lens, are the key to the diagnosis of chronic primary angle-closure glaucoma.[33]

Preferred Response   b. gonioscopic findings

A 58-year-old man presents to your office with a history of primary open-angle glaucoma and intraocular pressures of 20 mm Hg OU using a topical beta blocker twice daily and pilocarpine 4%, 3 times daily to both eyes. Gonioscopy reveals open angles and light trabecular pigmentation. You dilate the patient's pupils with two sets of tropicamide 1% and phenylephrine 2.5% drops in each eye. One hour later, you return to perform the dilated examination and the patient complains of blurred vision. There is mild corneal edema, and the intraocular pressure is 44 mm Hg bilaterally.

Which of the following is the *most* likely reason for this acute elevation of intraocular pressure?

a. idiosyncratic reaction to one of the dilating agents
b. hypersensitivity to one of the dilating agents
c. angle closure
d. reversal of intraocular pressure–lowering effect of glaucoma
   medication by one of the dilating agents

Discussion

After dilation of a patient with primary open-angle glaucoma on a topical beta blocker and topical miotic agent, there can be a substantial intraocular pressure elevation, in part because of reversal of the cholinergic effect of the miotic agent.[41] Pigment release may also contribute to intraocular pressure elevation. Hypersensitivity or an idiosyncratic reaction is unlikely. Angle closure can occur after dilation but is a less common cause of elevated intraocular pressure in this clinical situation.

Preferred Response

d. reversal of intraocular pressure–lowering effect of glaucoma
   medication by one of the dilating agents

G43

Topical ocular beta blockers have been reported to cause all of the following side effects *except*

a. heart block
b. exacerbation of myasthenia gravis
c. hypokalemia
d. blockage of the systemic response to hypoglycemia in diabetic patients

Discussion

Topical ocular beta blockers have been reported to cause heart block, exacerbation of myasthenia gravis, and blockage of the systemic response to hypoglycemia in diabetic patients. Hypokalemia is more likely to occur with oral carbonic anhydrase inhibitor therapy, especially with concurrent use of a potassium-depleting diuretic such as furosemide, hydrochlorothiazide, or chlorthalidone.

Preferred Response

c. hypokalemia

G44

Topical ocular beta blockers could have a beneficial effect on all of the following disorders *except*

a. supraventricular tachyarrhythmia
b. systemic hypertension
c. second-degree heart block
d. angina pectoris

Discussion

Oral beta blocker therapy has been used for the control of supraventricular tachycardia and for the treatment of systemic hypertension and angina pectoris. Substantial systemic levels of beta blockers can occur with topical ocular beta blocker therapy. Topical ocular beta blocker therapy can exacerbate second-degree heart block and should be avoided in these patients.

Preferred Response

c. second-degree heart block

G45

All of the following statements are true about dipivefrin (Propine) *except*

a. It is more lipophilic than topical ocular epinephrine formulations.
b. Systemic effects are equally likely with dipivefrin and epinephrine.
c. It is formulated in a lower concentration than the epinephrine formulations.
d. It is more likely to cause contact dermatitis than a topical ocular beta adrenergic antagonist.

Discussion

Dipivefrin (Propine) is more lipophilic than topical ocular epinephrine and therefore penetrates the cornea better. This allows its formulation at a 0.1% strength rather than the typical formulations of epinephrine (0.5%, 1%, and 2%). Dipivefrin is a prodrug that is transformed by corneal esterases into the active agent epinephrine. Contact dermatitis is a common complication of chronic dipivefrin therapy. Dipivefrin has been shown to cause fewer cardiovascular effects than epinephrine.[42]

Preferred Response

b. Systemic effects are equally likely with dipivefrin and epinephrine.

G46

During a trabeculectomy, the block excision is performed 1 mm to 2 mm too far posteriorly. Possible complications of this may include all of the following *except*

a. inadvertent cyclodialysis cleft
b. hemorrhage
c. focal corneal edema
d. vitreous loss

Discussion

A block excision performed too far posteriorly during trabeculectomy may cause an inadvertent cyclodialysis cleft if the scleral spur is penetrated. Intraocular hemorrhage can occur if the major arteriolar circle of the iris is cut. Vitreous loss will occur if the ciliary body is penetrated. Focal corneal edema may occur with a far anteriorly placed block excision and is usually of little consequence. The sclerectomy block excision should be in the "gray" limbal transition zone (see the figure).

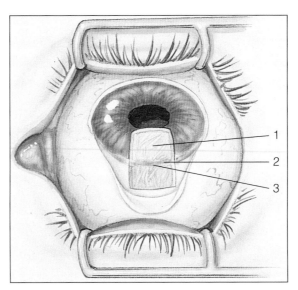

After complete dissection of the trabeculectomy scleral flap (1), the limbal zone is exposed (2). A block excision at or posterior to the anterior margin of sclera (3) will expose or penetrate the ciliary body.

Preferred Response   c. focal corneal edema

G47   A 2-year-old child presents with bilateral findings shown in the figures.

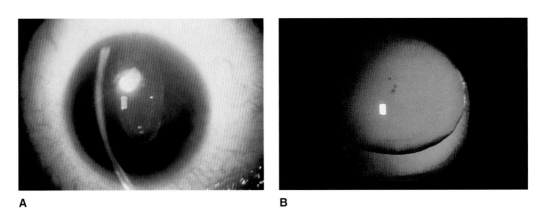

A   **B**

(A) Anterior segment of a patient with aniridia. Note the complete absence of visible iris.
(B) Transillumination of the anterior segment of the same patient, also showing absence of iris, clear lens, and slight superior lens ectopy.

Possible findings would include all of the following *except*

a. peripheral corneal pannus
b. neuroblastoma (Wilms' tumor)
c. angle-closure glaucoma
d. adhesions of peripheral iris to a prominent, anteriorly displaced Schwalbe's line

Discussion   The patient depicted has aniridia, in which there is often a rudimentary iris stub, macular hypoplasia, and nystagmus. Patients with aniridia commonly develop a peripheral corneal pannus. Most cases have an autosomal dominant transmission, but neuroblastoma (Wilms' tumor) is associated with sporadic (nonfamilial) aniridia. One type is associated with mental retardation. The small iris stub can occlude the trabecular meshwork and cause an angle-closure glaucoma. Adhesions of peripheral iris to a prominent, anteriorly displaced Schwalbe's line are seen in Axenfeld-Rieger syndrome.

Preferred Response   d. adhesions of peripheral iris to a prominent, anteriorly displaced Schwalbe's line

G48

Observe the optic nerve in the photograph below.

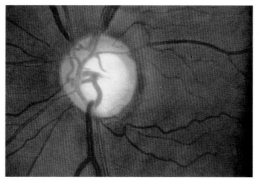

Left optic nerve of a patient with primary open-angle glaucoma, showing diffuse cupping with notch formation inferotemporally and greatest damage from the 5 o'clock to 6 o'clock position.

Which of the four visual field tests would best match this optic nerve?

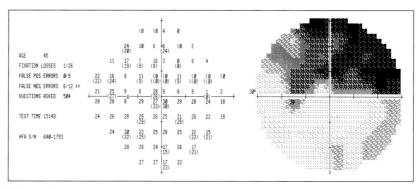

Figure A

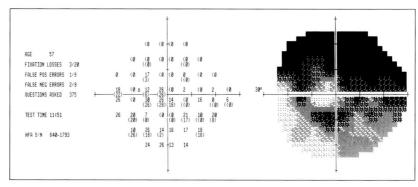

Figure B

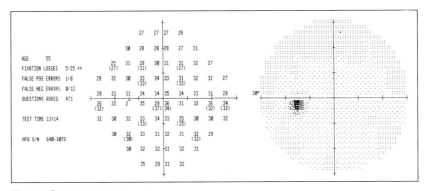

Figure C

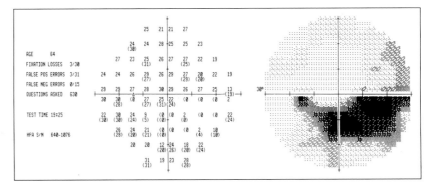

Figure D

(A) Visual field of the eye with the optic nerve depicted in the photograph. Note the large superior visual field defect corresponding to the inferotemporal optic nerve damage. **(B)** Central island of vision with inferior and inferotemporal remnant. This patient would be expected to have a notch formation of the left optic nerve both superiorly and inferiorly, which might be somewhat greater inferiorly. **(C)** Normal visual field test in an eye with ocular hypertension and no glaucomatous optic nerve damage. **(D)** Inferior arcuate defect of a patient with glaucoma who had a notch of the superotemporal neuroretinal rim.

a. Figure A
b. Figure B
c. Figure C
d. Figure D

Discussion

The left optic nerve depicted in the photograph above has an inferotemporal thinning of the optic nerve rim and notch formation from the 5 o'clock to 6 o'clock position. The superior visual field loss in Figure A would match this optic nerve damage. The visual field in Figure B would require an optic nerve with advanced damage of the superior and inferior neural-retinal rim. The visual field in Figure C is normal, and the visual field in Figure D would be found in a patient with a defect in the superior portion of the optic nerve.

Preferred Response   a. Figure A

A 35-year-old woman presents with the clinical findings in the right eye shown in the figures. The intraocular pressure is 38 mm Hg, and gonioscopy shows extensive peripheral anterior synechiae in that eye.

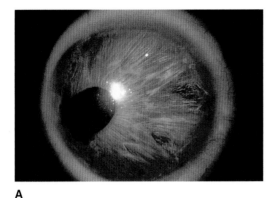

A

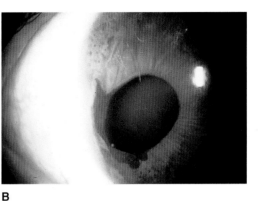

B

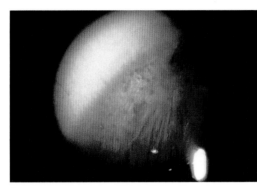

C

(A) Anterior segment appearance of a patient with an iridocorneal endothelial syndrome. Note corectopia and early tearing of the iris nasally and inferonasally. **(B)** Higher-power view of the same eye inferotemporally, showing ectropion uveae and peripheral anterior synechiae. **(C)** Superotemporal area of the same eye, showing iris "nevi"—protrusions of iris stroma created by proliferation of the endothelial-like membrane on the iris surface.

Which one of the following is *most* likely to provide the greatest reduction of intraocular pressure?

a. acetazolamide
b. laser iridotomy
c. laser trabeculoplasty
d. topical corticosteroid

Discussion   This patient has an iridocorneal endothelial (ICE) syndrome. Of the choices, acetazolamide would provide the greatest reduction of intraocular pressure. Laser iridotomy would be neither necessary nor appropriate. Eyes with ICE syndrome have glaucoma secondary to an angle-closure mechanism; however, there is no pupillary block. Laser trabeculoplasty cannot be performed in an eye with extensive primary or secondary angle closure. As active intraocular inflammation is not associated with an ICE syndrome, topical corticosteroid therapy would not help.

Preferred Response   a. acetazolamide

Which of the gonioscopic photographs shown below would represent a normal anatomic finding?

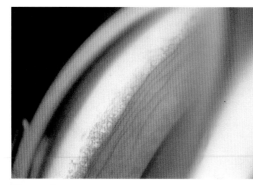

Figure A

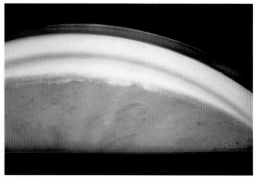

Figure B

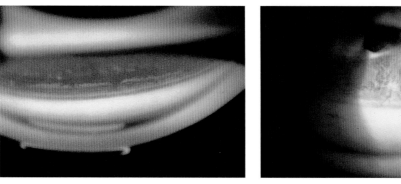

Figure C

Figure D

(A) Gonioscopy of a normal angle with extensive iris processes (uveal trabecular meshwork). **(B)** Scattered low to midtrabecular peripheral anterior synechiae in an eye with previous bouts of anterior uveitis. **(C)** Increased trabecular pigmentation and angle recession in an eye with previous blunt ocular trauma. **(D)** Peripheral iris and angle neovascularization in an eye with proliferative diabetic retinopathy.

    a. Figure A
    b. Figure B
    c. Figure C
    d. Figure D

Discussion   Figure A shows a heavy layer of uveal trabecular meshwork, or iris processes, a normal anatomic finding. Figure B shows scattered peripheral anterior synechiae in an eye with previous episodes of acute anterior uveitis. Figure C shows traumatic angle recession, and Figure D shows rubeotic vessels in the angle on the trabecular meshwork of a patient with proliferative diabetic retinopathy.

Preferred Response   a. Figure A

References

1. Heuer DK, Parrish RK II, Gressel MG, et al: 5-Fluorouracil and glaucoma filtering surgery. III. Intermediate follow-up of a pilot study. *Ophthalmology* 1986; 93:1537–1546.

2. Coleiro JA, Sigundsson H, Lockyer JA: Follicular conjunctivitis on dipivefrin therapy for glaucoma. *Eye* 1988;2:440–442.

3. Anderson DR: *Automated Static Perimetry.* St. Louis: CV Mosby Co; 1992.

4. Shields MB: *Textbook of Glaucoma.* 3rd ed. Baltimore: Williams & Wilkins; 1992.

5. Higginbotham EJ, Shahbazi MF: Laser therapy in glaucoma: an overview and update. *Int Ophthalmol Clin* 1990;30:187–197.

6. Glaucoma Laser Trial Research Group: The Glaucoma Laser Trial. 1. Acute effects of argon laser trabeculoplasty on intraocular pressure. *Arch Ophthalmol* 1989; 107:1135–1142.

7. Glaucoma Laser Trial Research Group: The Glaucoma Laser Trial. 2. Results of argon laser trabeculoplasty versus topical medicines. *Ophthalmology* 1990;97: 1403–1413.

8. Cairns JE: Indications for surgery in glaucoma. *Glaucoma* 1981;3:307.

9. Grant WM, Burke JF Jr: Why do some people go blind from glaucoma? *Ophthalmology* 1982;89:991–998.

10. Stewart WC, Shields MB: Management of anterior chamber depth after trabeculectomy. *Am J Ophthalmol* 1988;106:41–44.

11. Cain W Jr, Sinskey RM: Detection of anterior chamber leakage with Seidel's test. *Arch Ophthalmol* 1981;99:2013.

12. Sugar HS: Complications, repair, and reoperation of antiglaucoma filtering blebs. *Am J Ophthalmol* 1967;63:825–833.

13. Levene R: A new concept of malignant glaucoma. *Arch Ophthalmol* 1972;87: 497–506.

14. Ritch R, Shields MB, Krupin T, eds: *The Glaucomas.* St Louis: CV Mosby Co; 1989.

15. Mills RP: Combined cataract extraction and trabeculectomy. In: Mills RP, Weinreb RN, eds: *Glaucoma Surgical Techniques.* Ophthalmology Monograph 4. San Francisco: American Academy of Ophthalmology; 1991.

16. Shields MB: Combined cataract extraction and guarded sclerectomy: reevaluation in the extracapsular era. *Ophthalmology* 1986;93:366–370.

17. Fluorouracil Filtering Surgery Study Group: Fluorouracil filtering surgery study one-year follow-up. *Am J Ophthalmol* 1989;108:625–635.

18. Rockwood EJ, Parrish RK II, Heuer DK, et al: Glaucoma filtering surgery with 5-fluorouracil. *Ophthalmology* 1987;94:1071–1078.

19. Skuta GL, Beeson CC, Higginbotham EJ, et al: Intraoperative mitomycin versus postoperative 5-fluorouracil in high-risk glaucoma filtering surgery. *Ophthalmology* 1992;99:438–444.

20. Hoskins HD Jr, Kass MA: *Becker-Shaffer's Diagnosis and Therapy of the Glaucomas.* 6th ed. St Louis: CV Mosby Co; 1989.

21. Heuer DK, Gressel MG, Parrish RK II, et al: Trabeculectomy in aphakic eyes. *Ophthalmology* 1984;91:1045–1051.

22. Patitsas CJ, Rockwood EJ, Meisler DM, et al: Glaucoma filtering surgery with postoperative 5-fluorouracil in patients with intraocular inflammatory disease. *Ophthalmology* 1992;99:594–599.

23. Wilensky JT: Diagnosis and treatment of pigmentary glaucoma. *Focal Points.* Vol V, Module 9. San Francisco: American Academy of Ophthalmology; 1987.

24. Katz LJ, Cantor LB, Spaeth GL: Complications of surgery in glaucoma: early and late bacterial endophthalmitis following glaucoma filtering surgery. *Ophthalmology* 1985;92:959–963.

25. Mandelbaum S, Forster RK, Gelender H, et al: Late onset endophthalmitis associated with filtering blebs. *Ophthalmology* 1985;92:964–972.

26. Rebolleda G, Muñoz FJ, Victorio JMF, et al: Effects of pupillary dilation on automated perimetry in glaucoma patients receiving Pilocarpine. *Ophthalmol* 1992; 99:418–423

27. Goldstick BJ, Weinreb RN: The effect of refractive error on automated global analysis program G-1. *Am J Ophthalmol* 1987;104:229–232.

28. *Glaucoma.* Basic and Clinical Science Course, Section 10. San Francisco: American Academy of Ophthalmology; 1993–1994.

29. Rockwood EJ: Medical treatment of open angle glaucoma. *Focal Points.* Vol XI, Module 10. San Francisco: American Academy of Ophthalmology; 1993.

30. Savage JA: Glaucoma filtration surgery. In: Higginbotham EJ, Lee DA, eds: *Management of Difficult Glaucoma: A Clinician's Guide.* Boston: Blackwell Scientific Publications; 1994.

31. Givens K, Shields MB: Suprachoroidal hemorrhage after glaucoma filtering surgery. *Am J Ophthalmol* 1987;103:689–694.

32. *Primary Angle-Closure Glaucoma.* Preferred Practice Pattern. San Francisco: American Academy of Ophthalmology; 1992.

33. Wand M: Diagnosis and management of angle-closure glaucoma. *Focal Points.* Vol VI, Module 10. San Francisco: American Academy of Ophthalmology; 1988.

34. Skuta GL, Parrish RK II, Hodapp E, et al: Zonular dialysis during extracapsular cataract extraction in pseudoexfoliation syndrome. *Arch Ophthalmol* 1987; 105:632–634.

35. Lam BL, Alward WLM, Kolder HE: Effect of cataract on automated perimetry. *Ophthalmology* 1991;98:1066–1070.

36. *Glaucoma Suspect.* Preferred Practice Pattern. San Francisco: American Academy of Ophthalmology; 1989.

37. Weinreb RN, Ritch R, Kushner FH: Effect of adding betaxolol to dipivefrin therapy. *Am J Ophthalmol* 1986;101:196–198.

38. Walsh TJ, ed: *Visual Fields: Examination and Interpretation.* Ophthalmology Monograph 3. San Francisco: American Academy of Ophthalmology; 1990.

39. Stewart RH, Kimbrough RL: Intraocular pressure response to topically administered fluorometholone. *Arch Ophthalmol* 1979; 97:2139–2140.

40. Kass MA, Cheetham J, Duzman E, et al: The ocular hypertensive effect of 0.25% fluorometholone in corticosteroid responders. *Am J Ophthalmol* 1986;102:159–163.

41. Shaw BR, Lewis RA: Intraocular pressure elevation and pupillary dilation in open angle glaucoma. *Arch Ophthalmol* 1986;104:1185–1188.

42. Kerr CR, Hass I, Drance SM, et al: Cardiovascular effects of epinephrine and dipivalyl epinephrine applied topically to the eye in patients with glaucoma. *Br J Ophthalmol* 1982;66:109–114.

Additional Resources From the AAO

Academy Statements   *The Clinical Effectiveness of Automated Perimetry.* Ophthalmic Procedures Assessment. 1989. (Item No. 112001)

Excess Risk of Glaucomatous Blindness Among Black Americans. Public Health Note. 1993.

Laser Peripheral Iridotomy for Pupillary-Block Glaucoma. Ophthalmic Procedures Assessment. 1994. (Item No. 112006)

Laser Trabecular Surgery for Open-Angle Glaucoma. Ophthalmic Procedures Assessment. 1989. (Item No. 112007)

Basic and Clinical Science Course   *Glaucoma.* Section 10. Updated annually.

Focal Points   Camras CB: *Diagnosis and Management of Complications of Glaucoma Filtering Surgery.* Vol XII, Module 3. 1994. (Item No. 029012)

Deutsch TA, Goldberg MF: *Traumatic Hyphema: Medical and Surgical Management.* Vol II, Module 5. 1984. (Item No. 029002)

Drake MV: *A Primer on Automated Perimetry.* Vol XI, Module 8. 1993. (Item No. 029011)

Drance SM, Keltner JL, Johnson CA: *Automated Perimetry.* Vol I, Module 11. 1983. (Item No. 029001)

Faye EE: *Management of the Partially Sighted Patient.* Vol V, Module 6. 1987. (Out of print)

Fellman RL, Spaeth GL, Starita RJ: *Gonioscopy: Key to Successful Management of Glaucoma.* Vol II, Module 7. 1984. (Item No. 029002)

Gross RL: *Cyclodestructive Procedures for Glaucoma.* Vol X, Module 4. 1992. (Item No. 029010)

Heuer DK, Lloyd MA: *Management of Glaucoma with Poor Surgical Prognoses.* Vol XIII, Module 1. 1995. (Item No. FP95)

Hodapp EA, Anderson DR: *Treatment of Early Glaucoma.* Vol IV, Module 4. 1986. (Item No. 029004)

Hoskins HD Jr, Migliazzo CV: *Filtering Surgery for Glaucoma.* Vol IV, Module 9. 1986. (Item No. 029004)

Jampel HD: *Normal (Low) Tension Glaucoma.* Vol IX, Module 12. 1991. (Item No. 029009)

Kass MA: *Medical Treatment of Open-Angle Glaucoma.* Vol I, Module 2. 1983. (Item No. 029001)

Kolker AE: *Laser Therapy for Glaucoma.* Vol I, Module 13. 1983. (Item No. 029001)

Lieberman MF: *Glaucoma and Automated Perimetry.* Vol XI, Module 9. 1993. (Item No. 029011)

Lynch MG, Brown RH: *Systemic Side Effects of Glaucoma Therapy.* Vol VIII, Module 4. 1990. (Out of print)

Miller KN, Carlson AN, Foulks GN, et al: *Associated Glaucoma and Corneal Disorders.* Vol VII, Module 4. 1989. (Item No. 029007)

Panek WC: *Role of Laser Treatment in Glaucoma.* Vol XI, Module 1. 1993. (Item No. 029011)

Quigley HA: *Nerve Fiber Layer Assessment in Managing Glaucoma.* Vol VI, Module 5. 1988. (Item No. 029006)

Ritch R: *Exfoliation Syndrome.* Vol XII, Module 9. 1994. (Item No. 029012)

Rockwood EJ: *Medical Treatment of Open-Angle Glaucoma.* Vol XI, Module 10. 1993. (Item No. 029011)

Schwartz B: *Optic Disc Evaluation in Glaucoma.* Vol VIII, Module 12. 1990. (Out of print)

Shields MB: *Trends in the Therapy of Secondary Glaucomas.* Vol III, Module 4. 1985. (Out of print)

Van Buskirk EM, Weleber RG: *Intraocular Lenses in Glaucoma.* Vol IV, Module 7. 1986. (Item No. 029004)

Walton DS: *Childhood Glaucoma.* Vol VIII, Module 10. 1990. (Out of print)

Wand M: *Diagnosis and Management of Angle-Closure Glaucoma.* Vol VI, Module 10. 1988. (Item No. 029006)

Wand M: *Diagnosis and Treatment of Neovascular Glaucoma.* Vol III, Module 8. 1985. (Out of print)

Wilensky JT: *Diagnosis and Treatment of Pigmentary Glaucoma.* Vol V, Module 9. 1987. (Out of print)

LEO Clinical Topic Update   Brandt JD: *Glaucoma.* 1995. (Item No. 0212210)

Monographs   Mills RP, Weinreb RN, eds: *Glaucoma Surgical Techniques.* Ophthalmology Monograph 4. 1991. (Item No. 0210201)

Walsh TJ, ed: *Visual Fields: Examination and Interpretation.* Ophthalmology Monograph 3. 1990. (Item No. 0210090)

Preferred Practice Patterns   *Glaucoma Suspect.* 1989. (Item No. 110005)

Primary Angle-Closure Glaucoma. 1992. (Item No. 110017)

Primary Open-Angle Glaucoma. 1992. (Item No. 110019)

Slide-Script   Coleman AL: *Glaucoma: Diagnosis and Management.* Eye Care Skills for the Primary Care Physician Series. 1994. (Item No. 0240314)

Videotapes   Chen CJ: *Management of Suprachoroidal Hemorrhage With Perfluorophenanthrene.* Annual Meeting Series. 1994. (Item No. 0252033)

Minckler DS: *Angle-Closure Glaucoma.* Clinical Skills Series. 1989. (Item No. 0250833)

Sherwood MB: *Management of High-Risk Glaucoma.* Clinical Skills Series. 1994. (Item No. 0250963)

Van Buskirk EM: *Glaucoma Filtration Surgery: Trabeculectomy and Variations.* Clinical Skills Series. 1988. (Item No. 0250763)

Wilson RP: *Management of Combined Cataract and Glaucoma.* Classic Series. 1989. (Item No. 0250843)

EXTERNAL DISEASE AND CORNEA

E1

A 6-year-old boy has developed a pink mass on the inside of the lower lid that has enlarged rapidly (see the figure). The mass is associated with marked mucus production.

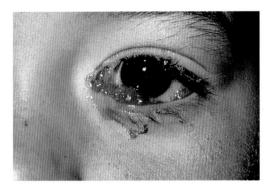

Benign conjunctival papilloma in a child.

The *most* likely diagnosis is

a. squamous cell carcinoma
b. rhabdomyosarcoma
c. conjunctival papilloma
d. lymphogranuloma venereum

Discussion

This child has the characteristic findings of a benign conjunctival papilloma. Squamous cell carcinoma is rare in this age group, is usually unifocal, and is usually located at the limbus rather than the fornix or palpebral conjunctival surface. Orbital rhabdomyosarcoma in children rarely may extend into the conjunctiva and first appear clinically in that location; although unlikely, rhabdomyosarcoma should always be a consideration, and this possibility mandates the submission of any specimen for pathologic examination. There is no history to suggest lymphogranuloma venereum. True pedunculated mucous membrane papillomas in children are usually multiple and bilateral. They have a distinct predilection for the conjunctival fornix and the palpebral conjunctiva and are often less inflamed than cancerous conjunctival tumors.[1]

Preferred Response

c. conjunctival papilloma

E2

The *most* likely cause of the lesion in the patient in Question E1 is

a. actinic trauma
b. viral infection
c. herpes simplex
d. *Chlamydia psittaci*

Discussion

Childhood conjunctival papillomas are of probable viral origin. This most likely accounts for their characteristic clinical appearance, including multifocal lesions, and their bilaterality and frequent recurrence. There is no relationship between childhood conjunctival papillomas and herpes simplex infection or infection by chlamydial organisms. Actinic trauma (ultraviolet exposure) is associated with dysplastic conjunctival lesions in adults.

Preferred Response

b. viral infection

E3

All of the following features are characteristic of the condition diagnosed in the patient in Question E1 *except*

a. tendency to recur and spread to other sites on the ocular surface after excision
b. predilection for the conjunctival fornix
c. frequent malignant degeneration
d. occurrence at multiple sites in a single eye

Discussion

Childhood conjunctival papillomas are not predisposed to malignant degeneration. Histopathologically, they do not show the dysplasia of neoplastic lesions but demonstrate acanthotic epithelium that contains goblet cells and has a fibrovascular central core. Although the course of these lesions is usually self-limited (2 to 3 years), treatment may be necessary. Surgical excision is often accompanied by rapid and exuberant regrowth in multiple locations. If the lesion does not resolve spontaneously, cryoablation may be effective utilizing applications at −60° to −70° over the entire surface of the growth, which will subsequently involute.

Preferred Response

c. frequent malignant degeneration

E4

A 57-year-old farmer is referred to the ophthalmologist by a family practitioner for management of chronic conjunctivitis that has been unresponsive to topical antibiotics or antibiotic/corticosteroid combinations for more than 10 weeks. The patient has a painless red eye that produces a mucoserous discharge. His ocular lesion is shown in the figure.

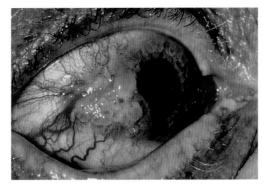

Squamous cell carcinoma of the conjunctiva straddling the limbus and associated with marked inflammation.

The *most* likely diagnosis is

a. squamous cell carcinoma of the conjunctiva
b. ocular pemphigoid
c. drug toxicity
d. acanthosis nigricans

Discussion

Although the appearance of squamous cell carcinomas of the conjunctiva is highly variable, they usually appear in middle age, with a fairly even distribution between ages 40 and 70. They are 5 times more common in men than in women, and there is a strong suggestion that they are related to actinic trauma. Exposure to ultraviolet light is considered the main predisposing factor to the development of squamous cell carcinoma of the conjunctiva. These tumors are usually located within the palpebral fissure on the bulbar conjunctiva, usually at the nasal or temporal limbus.[2] They may occur rarely on the palpebral conjunctiva or in the cul-de-sac. They are often associated with inflammation and may masquerade as a chronic infection. Since these lesions are sometimes treated for long periods as an infectious conjunctivitis before a conjunctival malignancy is suspected or recognized, drug toxicity may be a consideration in the differential diagnosis. Drug toxicity is, however, more likely to appear as a diffuse conjunctival hyperemia. Pemphigoid characteristically occurs in a more elderly population and is characterized by foreshortening of the fornices. Acanthosis nigricans is a rare paraneoplastic disorder with characteristic papilliform lesions of the lid margin.

Preferred Response

a. squamous cell carcinoma of the conjunctiva

Lesions of the type shown in the figure in Question E4 tend to have all of the following characteristics *except*

a. They are most commonly unifocal.
b. They tend to be slow growing.
c. They are generally exophytic.
d. They invade the intraocular space 50% of the time.

Discussion

Malignant epithelial lesions of the conjunctiva are commonly solitary and focal, with histologic dysplasia appearing in a relatively confined space with an abrupt transition from tumor to normal tissue. They are generally very slow growing and spread locally only. For this reason, they usually may safely be observed for growth or change before the decision for excision is reached. The growth of these tumors is almost always superficial and exophytic. Initially the process is intraepithelial. Even when it converts from carcinoma in situ to penetrate the basement membrane, the tough corneal-scleral connective tissue acts as an effective barrier. Invasion of the intraocular space is extremely rare.

Preferred Response

d. They invade the intraocular space 50% of the time.

The figure shows a corneal lesion with a fimbriated border pattern.

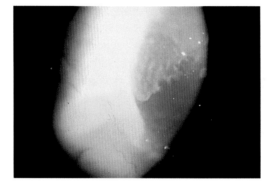

Corneal epithelial dysplasia associated with squamous cell carcinoma of the conjunctiva.

This lesion is *most* likely to be

a. squamous dysplasia
b. corneal nevus
c. fibrous outgrowth
d. leukoplakia

Discussion

The appearance of squamous cell dysplasia and neoplasia of the conjunctiva is highly variable. As noted previously, squamous cell carcinoma is most commonly focal and solitary. There is generally significant vascular engorgement. Leukoplakia is an opaque or gelatinous whitening produced by keratinized, acanthotic epithelium on the surface of a mucous membrane and is a frequent expression of squamous cell carcinoma of the conjunctiva (see the figure below, part A). Another presentation of squamous cell carcinoma is a papillomatous form, which usually appears at the limbus and is often associated with significant inflammation (see the figure below, part B). When dysplasia or neoplasia extends onto the cornea, the lesion may appear as a gray opacification of the corneal epithelium with characteristic fimbriated edges (see the figure above).[3]

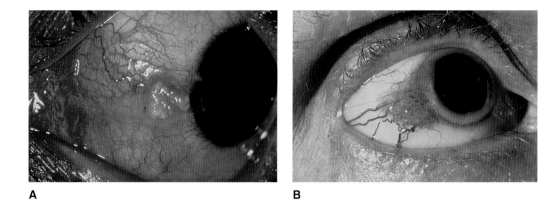

A   **B**

Squamous cell carcinoma. **(A)** Leukoplakia. **(B)** Papillomatous form.

Preferred Response   a. squamous dysplasia

The *most* appropriate surgical management of squamous cell carcinoma of the conjunctiva is

a. wide marginal conjunctivectomy with deep anterior sclerectomy
b. beta-irradiation
c. superficial excision with adjuvant cryoablation
d. cryoablation alone

Discussion   As noted previously, these lesions are superficial and exophytic. Local excision of the lesion can and should be carried out without deep scleral resection or keratectomy, since such a maneuver may actually weaken the barrier to invasion of the intraocular space. A wide no-touch surgical excision with supplementary cryoablation is the method most commonly advocated. Superficial extension of the tumor onto the cornea is removed by denuding the affected tissue with absolute alcohol on a cotton-tipped applicator. It is important to orient the excised specimen for the pathologist after excision to facilitate histopathologic assessment. Irradiation does not have a role in the management.

Preferred Response   c. superficial excision with adjuvant cryoablation

E8   A 25-year-old Hispanic woman has noticed a change in a brown spot on her right eye. Although she states that the spot has been present since she was 14 years old, she and her family have noticed a distinct enlargement and deepening of the pigment over the last 4 months (see the figure on page 40). She is concerned that the lesion may represent a developing cancer. Aside from the lesion, her external examination is unremarkable.

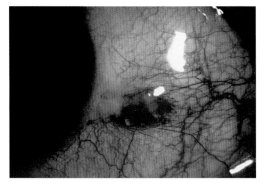

Benign nevus of the conjunctiva.

The *most* likely diagnosis of the lesion is

a. nevus of Ota
b. malignant melanoma of the conjunctiva
c. benign conjunctival nevus
d. squamous cell carcinoma

Discussion   No mention is made of periocular skin pigmentation; therefore, nevus of Ota (oculodermal melanocytosis) is not considered in this case. A squamous cell carcinoma would not likely be pigmented and is usually associated with some degree of inflammation. Malignant melanoma, although not excluded from the differential diagnosis, would likely appear more aggressively and with deeper pigmentation. Congenital, benign nevi, as seen in this patient, are apparent in only 50% of cases after the first decade of life. They may change their size and pigmentation during childhood and at times of hormonal transition. By age 30, only 75% of such nevi have become apparent. Only two-thirds of nevi are pigmented; within a given nevus, the pigment may vary from black to brown to a salmon color, to portions with no pigmentation whatsoever. The lesion may also have a characteristic cystic appearance. Nevi near the limbus are usually flat, but they may be elevated further out on the globe. Nevi represent benign tumors of nevus cell origin and are commonly sharply demarcated. An increase in pigment does not necessarily mean growth of the lesion.[1,4]

Preferred Response   c. benign conjunctival nevus

Initial management of the lesion in Question E8 might include all of the following *except*

a. baseline photographic documentation
b. excisional biopsy
c. review of old facial photographs
d. cryoablation

Discussion   Since congenital, benign nevi often do not become clinically obvious until the third or fourth decade of life, they may not be noticed by the patient until they reach a critical degree of pigmentation. For this reason, it is often helpful to obtain old pictures of the patient to see if the lesion is long-standing but unnoticed. Documentation of the appearance of a nevus by clinical photographs is extremely important, and accurate measurements of its size should be recorded. Because the lesion is benign, it is reasonable to follow it longitudinally with baseline and serial photographs for comparison. If the pigmentation is objectionable cosmetically or emotionally to the patient, the nevus may be excised as a simple ellipse of conjunctiva. Adjuvant cryoablation is unnecessary. Excision is also appropriate if the lesion shows significant growth and there is concern that malignant degeneration is a possibility.

Preferred Response   d. cryoablation

A 38-year-old blond woman who works as a forest ranger reports first noting the appearance of a brown lesion on the right eye 4 months ago. Since then the lesion has grown in size and darkened in pigmentation (see the figures). She denies any inflammation or ocular discomfort.

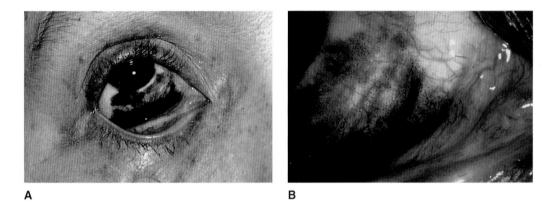

A   **B**

(A) Malignant melanoma of the conjunctiva arising from primary acquired melanosis. **(B)** Detail of the lesion.

The *most* likely diagnosis of this lesion is

a. congenital melanosis of the conjunctiva
b. primary acquired melanosis
c. benign nevus
d. ochronosis

Discussion   The rapid appearance of this lesion, its size and granularity, and its pigmentation in a lightly pigmented individual are strongly suggestive of primary acquired melanosis (PAM). Congenital melanosis of the conjunctiva would be unusual in a blond individual and would certainly have been noticed early in life. This lesion is far too large and rapidly changing for a benign nevus. The appearance of this lesion should arouse strong suspicion for potential malignant transformation. It is important to remember that PAM may wax and wane, enlarging and regressing over time. All suspicious lesions of PAM should be biopsied to determine the presence or absence of atypia or neoplasm.[5-7] Ochronosis, or alkaptonuria, is a rare autosomal-recessive metabolic disorder characterized by the presence of pigmentation of the cartilage and other connective tissues. Ocular manifestations include pigment in the sclera, conjunctiva, and limbal cornea and would not be consistent with a rapidly changing lesion, as in this case.

Preferred Response   b. primary acquired melanosis

The patient described in Question E10 has been advised by her grandmother, who is being treated for glaucoma, that these lesions run in the family, as evidenced by the pigmented lesions she has had in her own eye (shown below) for several years.

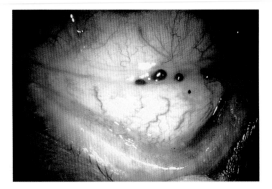

Adrenochrome deposits of the conjunctiva secondary to epinephrine use.

These lesions in the grandmother *most* likely represent

a. conjunctival nevi
b. malignant melanoma
c. adrenochrome deposits
d. congenital melanosis

Discussion   The small brown-black lesions seen in the patient's grandmother, who is on glaucoma therapy, represent adrenochrome deposits in the conjunctiva. The appearance of the lesions, their chronicity, and the use of an antiglaucoma drop (presumably containing epinephrine) strongly suggest this diagnosis. Such deposits represent the oxidation products of epinephrine and are seen most commonly on the palpebral and forniceal conjunctiva. Although usually asymptomatic, adrenochrome deposits may irritate the cornea mechanically. They may also blacken corneal scars, the eyelid margin, the caruncle, and hydrophilic contact lenses. Their appearance is distinctly different from both benign nevi and pigmented lesions of the conjunctiva with malignant potential.[1]

Preferred Response   c. adrenochrome deposits

E12

The patient in Question E10 returned 1 month later with a palpable mass in the upper lid. Eversion of the upper lid revealed the deeply pigmented mass pictured below.

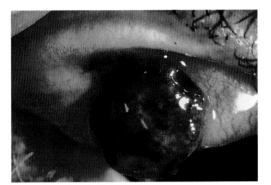

Malignant melanoma of the superior tarsal conjunctiva.

The *most* likely diagnosis is

a. adrenochrome deposit
b. pyogenic granuloma
c. acanthosis nigricans
d. malignant melanoma

Discussion

Acanthosis nigricans is an exceptionally rare paraneoplastic lesion in the eye, usually manifested as a papillomatous response on the conjunctiva and lid margin and sometimes accompanied by a distant neoplastic lesion. Primary malignant melanoma of the conjunctiva is uncommon and represents less than 1% of malignant ocular tumors. It is seen most commonly in adults between ages 30 and 70 and occurs with equal frequency in men and women. It most commonly occurs near the limbus in the interpalpebral space but may be seen in the fornix and less frequently (as in this case) on the palpebral conjunctiva.[5] Dilated conjunctival vessels associated with the pigmented mass may be seen. A malignant melanoma may originate from a pre-existing nevus, de novo, or most commonly from primary acquired melanosis (PAM). Roughly 17% of patients with PAM develop malignant melanoma of the conjunctiva. A thickened lesion that appears within the flat granular lesion of PAM should be considered malignant transformation. Pyogenic granuloma would likely be associated with more inflammation. Because the patient is not using a topical epinephrine-containing agent, adrenochrome deposits are ruled out.

Preferred Response

d. malignant melanoma

The appropriate management of malignant melanoma of the conjunctiva is

a. observation only, since there is a negligible mortality rate from these tumors
b. excision with adjunct cryoablation of raised pigmented lesions
c. PUVA (psoralens plus ultraviolet A) therapy
d. beta-irradiation

Discussion

Observation alone is not warranted in lesions of this nature. PUVA (psoralens plus ultraviolet A light) therapy has no place in the management of malignant melanoma, nor is beta-irradiation an appropriate modality. The optimal management of malignant melanoma has been controversial. The most common approach is combined excisional biopsy and adjunct cryoablation.[8–11] Cryotherapy is selectively effective against melanocytic proliferation and appears to render recurrence less likely than if excision alone is used. The procedure should be performed using a no-touch technique under the operating microscope, with care taken to include 3 to 4 mm of adjacent normal conjunctiva. Double freeze-thaw applications are then applied to the surrounding conjunctiva. In exceptional cases of widespread malignant melanoma of the conjunctiva, orbital exenteration may be indicated.

Preferred Response

b. excision with adjunct cryoablation of raised pigmented lesions

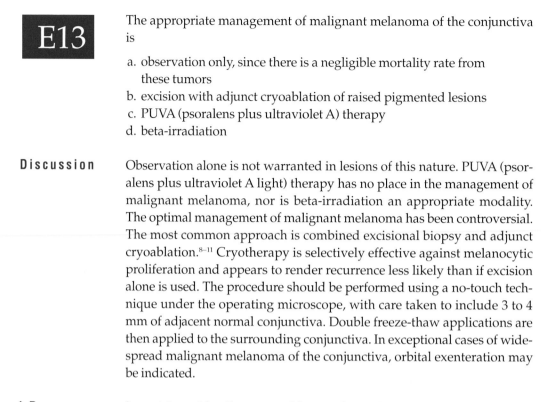

A college basketball player who wears extended-wear soft contact lenses presents at the ophthalmologist's office after 2 days of pain, redness, and photophobia. He noticed an enlarging spot on his cornea (see the figure) 24 hours prior to coming to the doctor's office.

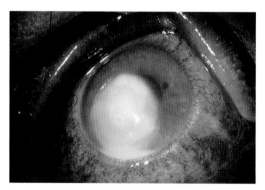

Pseudomonas corneal ulcer secondary to use of extended-wear soft contact lenses.

The *most* appropriate initial step in managing this problem is

a. immediate treatment with a single broad-spectrum topical antibiotic
b. subconjunctival injection of antibiotics
c. diagnostic scrapings of the corneal lesion for Gram stain and culture
d. treatment with an antibiotic/corticosteroid combination

Discussion

The initial management step for any lesion suspected of being a bacterial corneal ulcer is to order the appropriate microbiologic workup.[12]

Although certain groups of microbes generate a typical clinical presentation, clinical presentation alone cannot be used as the basis for the choice of therapy. Initial choice of treatment is based on Gram-stain findings, with modification of therapy contingent on the results of culture and sensitivity data. The choice of medication should be as specific as possible. The unavailability or absence of Gram-stain findings may indicate the use of broad-spectrum therapy, such as an aminoglycoside (eg, gentamicin) in combination with a cephalosporin (eg, cefazolin), to cover pathogens from both the Gram-positive and Gram-negative groups. It is now recognized that frequent topical instillation of fortified antibiotics is as effective as or more effective than serial subconjunctival injections. Treatment with a corticosteroid in the initial phases of a suspected bacterial keratitis is not warranted.

Preferred Response   c. diagnostic scrapings of the corneal lesion for Gram stain and culture

The patient in Question E14 is initially managed on the basis of the results of the Gram stain performed in the ophthalmologist's office (see the figure).

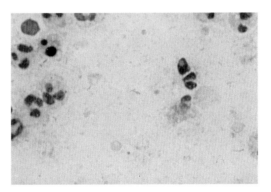

Gram stain demonstrating polymorphonuclear leukocytes and small pleomorphic Gram-negative rods consistent with *Pseudomonas* species.

The findings are *most* consistent with

a. *Pseudomonas aeruginosa*
b. *Neisseria gonorrhoeae*
c. *Streptococcus pneumoniae*
d. *Staphylococcus aureus*

Discussion   The stain shows slender Gram-negative rods consistent with *Pseudomonas aeruginosa*. This finding is consistent with the clinical picture with which the patient presented, ie, a raised mucoid infiltrate, rapid progression of the lesion, and a history of soft contact lens wear. *Neisseria gonorrhoeae* is also an aggressive Gram-negative organism; however, it is seen on Gram stain as a Gram-negative intracellular diplococcus. Both *Streptococcus pneumoniae* and *Staphylococcus aureus* are Gram-positive cocci, the former occurring as bean-shaped, encapsulated diplococci or in chains and the latter as rounded cocci often seen in clusters.

Preferred Response   a. *Pseudomonas aeruginosa*

A thorough discussion of the history of the contact lens habits of the patient in Question E14 revealed that he wore the lenses 24 hours a day and removed them for cleaning every 2 weeks. At the time of removal, he used chemical disinfection and then, to ensure sterility, stored the lenses in distilled water overnight prior to reinsertion. He noted that he did not routinely clean his storage apparatus.

All of these historical points are significant for the development of contact-lens–related infection *except*

a. 24-hour wear
b. use of distilled water for sterility
c. failure to maintain clean storage apparatus
d. chemical disinfection

Discussion

Epidemiologic data have recently demonstrated that overnight wear of soft contact lenses increases the risk of developing bacterial keratitis eightfold.[13,14] Patients are often confused about the difference between sterile water and distilled water that can be purchased at the grocery store. The ophthalmologist should provide the patient with explicit instructions to use commercially prepared sterile saline for the storage of lenses in combination with proper employment of sterilization systems, as well as proper maintenance of storage containers. Properly employed, chemical sterilization is effective for the vast majority of pathogens associated with corneal infection in contact lens use.

Preferred Response   d. chemical disinfection

A 62-year-old woman has been followed for corneal decompensation from Fuchs' dystrophy. She has demonstrated gradual progression from asymptomatic cornea guttata to stromal edema and frank bullous keratopathy over 4 years. She now complains of severe pain, photophobia, and tearing that has lasted for 5 days. Her cornea appears as shown in the figure.

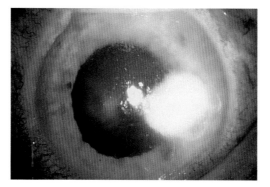

Staphylococcal ulcer.

The *most* likely diagnosis would be

a. *Pseudomonas* keratitis
b. herpes simplex keratitis
c. staphylococcal marginal keratitis
d. Terrien's marginal degeneration

Discussion

The findings in this patient are consistent with staphylococcal marginal keratitis. Inferior marginal lesions of this type are found most commonly with concomitant blepharitis, particularly with the hallmarks of staphylococcal lid disease, such as marginal ulcerations, collarettes, irregular or broken lashes, and a history of recurrence or chronicity. Most common in the middle-aged population, such inferior marginal lesions are occasionally seen in younger patients with neutrophil dysfunction. *Pseudomonas* rarely causes a marginal keratitis and causes an infection that is much more aggressive than in this patient. Herpes simplex may present as marginal lesions that are both ulcerated and infiltrated but that are usually found in the absence of typical concomitant lid disease. The staphylococcal lesions in this case must be differentiated from the lesions of herpes simplex, since the management principles are quite different. Terrien's marginal degeneration is a marginal inflammatory disease, but it is commonly asymptomatic, is not ulcerated, and is characterized by thinning, vascular incursion, and lipid deposition. The natural course of staphylococcal marginal keratitis is breakdown of the overlying epithelium with healing in 2 to 4 weeks. Recurrences are common.[15]

Preferred Response

c. staphylococcal marginal keratitis

The management of the disorder diagnosed in the patient in Question E20 includes all of the following *except*

a. topical corticosteroids
b. lid hygiene
c. topical antibiotic
d. prophylactic antiviral drops

Discussion

Since the cause of the patient's ulcers is a hypersensitivity reaction to staphylococcal antigenic toxins, the approach to management must be twofold: eradication of bacterial colonization of the lids and treatment of the corneal inflammatory response. Cultures should be made of the corneal lesions and of the lid margin. A positive lid-margin culture and a negative corneal culture would suggest that these are indeed hypersensitivity lesions. Treatment with intensive lid hygiene and an antistaphylococcal antibiotic drop (eg, trimethoprim sulfate) or an ointment such as bacitracin will manage the underlying colonization of the lids. The intense inflammatory response in the cornea is effectively aborted by use of a mild topical corticosteroid (eg, fluorometholone). Such treatment must, however, be employed in patients whose followup can be assured and only once the diagnosis has been clearly established, since the peripheral lesions of herpes simplex can resemble these lesions. Antiviral prophylaxis is not indicated.

Preferred Response   d. prophylactic antiviral drops

A debilitated 63-year-old man who lives on the streets had developed a red, painful eye 5 days prior to seeing an ophthalmologist. His cornea at the time of examination is shown in the figure, part A. The results of Gram staining of corneal scrapings are shown in part B of the figure.

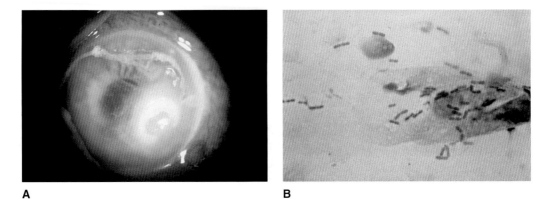

A   B

(A) Paracentral ulcer secondary to *Moraxella* species. **(B)** Large Gram-negative diplobacilli consistent with *Moraxella lacunata.*

The organism *most* likely involved is

a. *Pseudomonas aeruginosa*
b. *Klebsiella pneumoniae*
c. *Moraxella lacunata*
d. *Neisseria gonorrhoeae*

Discussion   Large Gram-negative diplobacilli are characteristic of *Moraxella lacunata.* Occasionally, these diplobacilli will stain Gram positive as well. This organism is found primarily in individuals debilitated from alcohol abuse, chronic disease, or old age and is, in that sense, an opportunistic organism. The ulcer produced is less rapidly aggressive than those produced by other Gram-negative species, but it will proceed to perforation if left untreated. It is characteristically found in the midperipheral cornea and is variably associated with hypopyon. Susceptibilities vary, but *Moraxella* is generally sensitive to aminoglycosides. *Pseudomonas aeruginosa* produces a raised mucoid infiltrate and appears on Gram staining as slender pleomorphic rods. *Klebsiella* is an uncommon corneal pathogen that is usually the result of enteric contamination of the eye and is characterized by cigar-shaped Gram-negative rods. *Neisseria gonorrhoeae* produces a hyperacute and rapidly progressive keratoconjunctivitis and is characterized by intracellular Gram-negative diplococci.

Preferred Response   *c. Moraxella lacunata*

A 47-year-old electrician was working under a house when some dirt was dislodged from a beam overhead and fell into his eye. He flushed out the eye on the site and went about his work. Two days later, he developed a red, painful eye and mild photophobia. Symptoms became progressively worse over the next week. He was seen by a family practitioner, who gave him an eyedrop containing antibiotic and corticosteroid. He then noticed a white spot in the center of his cornea while shaving and saw the ophthalmologist. The lesion in the photograph did not stain with fluorescein.

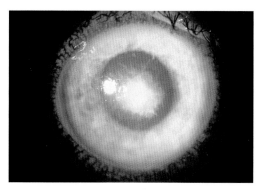

Fungal keratitis
(Aspergillus).

The history and appearance of the lesion are *most* consistent with

a. fungal keratitis
b. *Acanthamoeba* keratitis
c. herpes simplex keratitis
d. Gram-negative ulcer

Discussion   Contaminated trauma to the eye can be associated with a number of pathogens, including fungi, *Acanthamoeba*, atypical mycobacteria, and herpes simplex virus. Fungal infections are the most common and are often seen in the context of injury with organic matter, such as abrasions from plants or tree branches. *Acanthamoeba* is seen most commonly, although certainly not exclusively, in contact lens wearers. Chronic suppurative lesions may also be induced by atypical mycobacteria and are commonly associated with traumatic contact with soil or contaminated water. Finally, approximately 20% of ocular herpes infections follow traumatic injury. Based on clinical morphology alone, it would therefore be difficult to pinpoint the precise cause of this lesion. The history of soil-contaminated trauma, the whitish infiltrate with small satellite lesions, the intact epithelium, and the relatively indolent progress of the lesion that was accelerated by the addition of topical corticosteroids suggest that this is a fungal lesion.

Preferred Response   a. fungal keratitis

E24

The appropriate laboratory workup of the ulcer presented in Question E23 would include all of the following measures *except*

a. scraping for Giemsa stain
b. plating on Sabouraud's agar
c. plating on blood agar to be maintained at room temperature
d. plating on nonnutrient agar with a lawn of *E coli*

Discussion

A Giemsa stain, or variant thereof, is the best readily available stain for the detection of fungal elements in a smear. One may find budding yeast or hyphal elements that stain a deep indigo. Gram staining may also detect these elements as "Gram-positive" figures in the smear. Sabouraud's agar is designed to maximize the growth of fungi while inhibiting other microbes from growing. Fungi may also grow well on blood agar if it is kept at room temperature; the warm temperature (37°C) utilized in most incubators produces an environment too warm for fungal growth. Nonnutrient agar with heat-killed *E coli* is the preparation used for demonstrating the growth of *Acanthamoeba* organisms. Occasionally, corneal biopsy is necessary to diagnose fungal infection.[16]

Preferred Response

d. plating on nonnutrient agar with a lawn of *E coli*

E25

The patient in Question E23 developed fungal cultures positive for *Aspergillus*. Based on the initial laboratory workup and later on the cultures, he was treated with an antimicrobial. All of the following classes of drugs might be considered *except*

a. imidazoles (eg, miconazole and ketoconazole)
b. polyenes (eg, amphotericin B and natamycin)
c. macrolides (eg, tetracycline and erythromycin)
d. pyrimidines (eg, flucytosine)

Discussion

All of the above-mentioned antimicrobial classes are utilized against fungal infection except the macrolides. The macrolides, including tetracycline and erythromycin among others, are utilized effectively against bacterial infections. Imidazoles (miconazole, ketoconazole), polyenes (amphotericin B, natamycin), and pyrimidines (flucytosine) are used against a spectrum of fungal organisms. Fungi exhibit varying degrees of susceptibility to the drug classes, and the choice of drug depends on the classification of the fungus.[17]

Preferred Response

c. macrolides (eg, tetracycline and erythromycin)

E26

Despite aggressive therapy with antifungal agents, the lesion of the patient in Question E23 progressed and began to melt centrally. Medications were stopped and the cornea was scraped and recultured. Once again, hyphal elements were seen and *Aspergillus* grew on agar plates. At this point the *most* reasonable therapeutic option would be

a. therapeutic penetrating keratoplasty
b. lamellar keratoplasty
c. treatment with propamidine isethionate
d. chemical cautery

Discussion

Fungal keratitis that does not respond to the spectrum of available anti-fungal preparations and threatens the integrity of the cornea may be an indication for therapeutic keratoplasty. The purpose of this procedure is to excise the nidus of infection and reestablish corneal integrity before the fungus gains access to the anterior chamber. This represents a last resort in the management of such cases. Lamellar keratoplasty is contraindicated in such infections, since it does not eradicate the organisms and the fungi tend to thrive in the lamellar interface. Propamidine is utilized in the face of *Acanthamoeba* infection. Chemical cautery is no longer utilized for the management of infectious corneal ulcers.

Preferred Response

a. therapeutic penetrating keratoplasty

A 32-year-old Caucasian man complains to the ophthalmologist of bilateral intermittent redness, lacrimation, and foreign-body sensation. The most recent episode has been associated with extreme, almost disabling, photophobia. His lesion is shown in the figure.

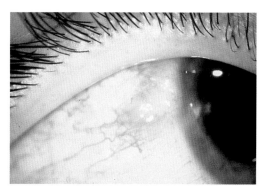

Limbal phlyctenule of probable staphylococcal origin.

This lesion is *most* consistent with

a. superior limbic keratoconjunctivitis
b. phlyctenulosis
c. Thygeson's superficial punctate keratitis
d. staphylococcal marginal keratitis

Discussion

The history and findings are most consistent with phlyctenulosis. Believed to be a local conjunctival and/or corneal immune response to bacterial antigen, this problem is often bilateral and may affect either the cornea or the conjunctiva or both. The limbus is the usual site of the disease. Phlyctenules may be solitary or multiple. Classically, the phlyctenule is a grayish, gelatinous nodule that ulcerates over 10 to 15 days and is associated with a wedge-shaped spate of vessels. Superior limbic keratoconjunctivitis is quite different in appearance and is limited to the superior limbus with hypertrophic conjunctiva and adjacent filamentary keratitis; it is also characterized by intense irritation. Thygeson's disease is a chronic disorder of unknown etiology characterized by recurring and evanescent clusters of corneal epithelial lesions. Staphylococcal marginal keratitis, although linked to phlyctenulosis etiologically, appears quite different clinically.[15]

Preferred Response b. phlyctenulosis

The most common cause of the condition diagnosed in Question E27 is

a. tuberculosis
b. *Staphylococcus aureus*
c. *Moraxella* infection
d. *Streptococcus pneumoniae*

Discussion Phlyctenulosis is most commonly associated with chronic infection with *Staphylococcus aureus* and probably represents a hypersensitivity response to staphylococcal antigen. In the past, it was most commonly linked to tuberculin antigen. However, today, nontuberculous phlyctenulosis is much more common. Although other organisms have been associated with the disease (including other bacteria, parasites, and several viruses), phlyctenulosis associated with staphylococcal infection is the only clinically significant type seen today.

Preferred Response b. *Staphylococcus aureus*

A 73-year-old man presents to the ophthalmologist with a 10-day history of accelerating discomfort and red eye. The patient exhibits signs of intense pain. Examination reveals a sharply demarcated peripheral corneal ulceration with a central overhanging edge (see the figure).

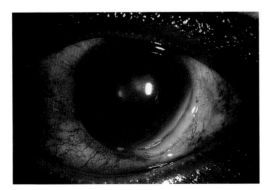

Mooren's ulcer, demonstrating gray, overhanging central edge and circumferential ulceration.

The *most* likely diagnosis is

a. Terrien's marginal degeneration
b. staphylococcal marginal keratitis
c. senile marginal furrow
d. Mooren's ulcer

Discussion

The most likely diagnosis in this case is Mooren's ulcer. This idiopathic condition, which occurs unilaterally and primarily in the elderly, is characterized by painful ulceration and ectasia of the peripheral cornea. The findings begin as a grayish infiltrate in the peripheral cornea, progressing to subsequent breakdown of the overlying epithelium and anterior stroma. There is circumferential and central progression with characteristic undermining of the central wall of thinned tissue, resulting in an overhanging central edge. The adjacent conjunctiva is usually inflamed and engorged, and there may be a mild to moderate anterior uveitis. A second, more severe form occurs as bilateral ulceration in younger patients, particularly blacks. This form of the disease, seen more commonly in Africa, is much more aggressive and poorly responsive to therapy. Terrien's marginal degeneration is nonulcerating, occurs in younger patients, and is not symptomatic with severe pain, as is Mooren's ulcer. Senile marginal furrow is an asymptomatic thinning of the limbus in the elderly.[18,19]

Preferred Response

d. Mooren's ulcer

Therapeutic approaches for the ulcer shown in Question E29 include all of the following *except*

a. topical corticosteroids
b. systemic immunosuppressive agents
c. conjunctival resection
d. topical nonsteroidal anti-inflammatory agents

Discussion

The management of Mooren's ulcer is difficult and often unsatisfactory. Accordingly, many different treatments have been employed. Medical treatments have included topical corticosteroids, collagenase inhibitors, cyclosporine A, and heparin. Systemic medication may include immunosuppressive agents, such as corticosteroids, cyclophosphamide, and methotrexate. Perhaps the most effective surgical treatment is excision or ablation of the adjacent conjunctiva. Other surgical approaches have included lamellar keratoplasty, delimiting keratotomy, cyanoacrylate application, and conjunctival flaps. Nonsteroidal anti-inflammatory agents have no role to date in the management of this disease.[18,20,21]

Preferred Response

d. topical nonsteroidal anti-inflammatory agents

A 66-year-old woman presents with redness, pain, and decreased vision in the left eye that has lasted for 2 weeks. She is noted to have an area of ulceration and extreme thinning at the limbus (see the figure, part A, page 56), and, in addition, she has a moderately dry eye. Her hands appear as shown in part B of the figure.

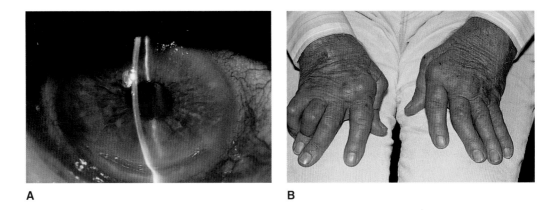

A   **B**

(A) Marginal corneal ulcer seen in association with rheumatoid arthritis. **(B)** Characteristic joint deformities in advanced rheumatoid arthritis.

The *most* likely diagnosis in this case is

a. rheumatoid marginal corneal ulceration
b. Mooren's ulcer
c. Terrien's marginal degeneration
d. sclerokeratitis

Discussion   Rheumatoid arthritis is the collagen vascular disorder that most commonly affects the peripheral cornea. Seen most commonly in elderly women, ocular involvement in the disease includes keratoconjunctivitis sicca, episcleritis, scleritis, and a variety of corneal problems. The peripheral cornea is most commonly involved and may be affected by sclerosing keratitis, furrowing, acute stromal keratitis, and keratolysis. This case represents rheumatoid marginal corneal ulceration. The typical joint and systemic manifestations of rheumatoid arthritis distinguish this patient's ocular condition from Mooren's ulcer (see Question E29) and from Terrien's marginal degeneration, which occurs in a younger population, is nonulcerating, and is not associated with underlying systemic disease. The peripheral corneal manifestations of rheumatoid arthritis often occur in association with adjacent scleritis.

Preferred Response   a. rheumatoid marginal corneal ulceration

All of the following treatments are appropriate for the management of the problem of the patient in Question E31 *except*

a. conjunctival resection
b. topical corticosteroids
c. topical collagenase inhibitors
d. lamellar keratoplasty

Discussion   The management of marginal furrowing and ulceration in rheumatoid disease is a difficult problem. The primary goal is to control aggressively any contiguous scleral inflammation. However, topical corticosteroids should not be used in either furrowing or peripheral keratolysis, since they may potentiate collagenolytic factors. Topical collagenase inhibitors (eg, N-acetylcysteine), bandage contact lenses, and application of cyano-acrylate glue have all been utilized effectively. Also, the eye must be kept adequately hydrated. Surgically, resection of the adjacent conjunctiva has been proven effective. Lamellar or penetrating keratoplasty may be required for restoration of ocular integrity or for visual rehabilitation.

Preferred Response   b. topical corticosteroids

A 43-year-old woman presents with irritation and a gritty sensation in both eyes. These symptoms have been present for several months but have worsened during the dry summer season and tend to worsen as the day goes on. She is otherwise in good health. The figure shows the result of fluorescein staining.

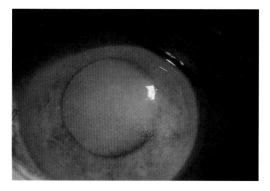

Paracentral and inferior punctate keratopathy demonstrated by fluorescein staining in a patient with aqueous-deficiency dry eye.

All of the following abnormalities in a patient with aqueous-deficiency dry eye might be expected *except*

a. decreased tear meniscus
b. abnormal Schirmer test
c. diminished tear break-up time
d. increased mucus in the precorneal tear film and/or filamentary keratitis

Discussion   The primary corneal changes in aqueous-deficiency dry eye consist of inferior peripheral and paracentral staining, a decreased tear meniscus, and a diminished Schirmer test. The characteristic staining is best demonstrated with rose bengal vital staining, although fluorescein stain will also highlight punctate keratopathy. In classic aqueous deficiency, there is a diminution in the height of the tear meniscus and a decrease in the wetting of the Schirmer strip. The decrease in aqueous production may produce a relative excess of mucus on the corneal surface due to the loss of a dilutional effect. This may result in mucous plaques or filament formation. Tear break-up time is an indicator of the adequacy of the mucinous component of the tear film and generally reflects mucin-deficiency rather than aqueous-deficiency dry eye. Even in fairly significant aqueous deficiency, the tear break-up time may be normal unless there is significant epithelial surface disruption or substantial concomitant meibomian gland disease, which can destabilize the tear film.

Preferred Response   c. diminished tear break-up time

E34

Appropriate therapy of keratitis sicca includes all of the following *except*

a. application of mucolytic agents
b. punctal occlusion
c. topical corticosteroids
d. tear substitutes

Discussion

Standard initial therapy of dry eye begins with the application of artificial tears. Tear substitutes alone, however, may not be adequate to control surface keratopathy. In such cases, occlusion of either two or all four of the puncta may be an effective adjunct to management. Mucolytic agents, such as 10% N-acetylcysteine, applied 2 to 3 times daily may be helpful in reducing symptoms from mucous plaques on the corneal surface. Topical corticosteroids should be used with extreme caution in patients with dry eye and resulting surface keratopathy because of their potential to retard wound healing and to potentiate collagenolytic activity. Corticosteroids have no place in the primary treatment of keratitis sicca.[1]

Preferred Response

c. topical corticosteroids

E35

A 26-year-old woman who wears rigid gas-permeable lenses 14 to 16 hours a day complains of a scratchy sensation after 6 to 8 hours of wearing time. Examination of the corneal surface reveals the staining pattern shown in the figure.

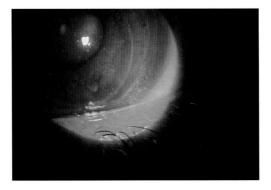

3 and 9 o'clock staining associated with incomplete blinking in a contact lens wearing patient.

All of the following statements about this condition are true *except*

a. It is referred to as 3 and 9 o'clock staining.
b. It may result from peripheral desiccation of the cornea.
c. It is uncommon in wearers of gas-permeable contact lenses.
d. It can be managed by lubrication, alterations in lens design, or conversion to hydrogel lenses.

Discussion

The term 3 and 9 o'clock staining is used to describe peripheral desiccation of the cornea. It occurs in up to 80% of patients who wear gas-permeable lenses. Symptoms that may accompany 3 and 9 o'clock staining include itching, increased lens awareness, and a dry sensation. The phenomenon of 3 and 9 o'clock staining may be caused by tear-film instability from incomplete blinking, aqueous insufficiency, or a poor lens-edge–corneal relationship. The resultant poor wetting of the corneal periphery produces the characteristic interpalpebral punctate corneal staining and associated symptoms. Treatment measures include the addition of artificial tears, reassessment of the lens–cornea relationship and change in the lens design, blinking exercises, or conversion to a hydrogel lens.

Preferred Response   c. It is uncommon in wearers of gas-permeable contact lenses.

A 34-year-old man visits the ophthalmologist 3 weeks after being fit with new rigid gas-permeable contact lenses. He complains of hazy vision, particularly after removing the lenses and using his glasses. Examination of the cornea reveals the findings shown in the figure.

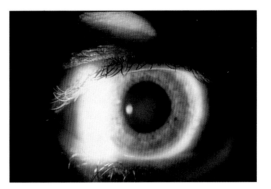

Central epithelial edema (Sattler's veil) due to corneal hypoxia from a tight-fitting contact lens.

The cause of this problem is

a. a lens that is too loosely fit
b. hypersensitivity to proteins on the lens surface
c. epithelial hypoxia
d. stromal edema

Discussion   Referred to as Sattler's veil, this patient's problem represents central corneal epithelial edema that results from hypoxic stress. Sattler's veil may occur with either rigid or hydrogel lenses and is best observed using sclerotic scatter or retroillumination techniques. There is usually a central circular clouding with a distinct demarcation from the clearer peripheral cornea. When epithelial edema of this type occurs with hydrogel lenses, it is usually more evenly spread across the cornea and is therefore somewhat more difficult to see. Patients may complain of hazy vision or spectacle blur that usually dissipates after 30 to 60 minutes. Epithelial edema of this type is usually associated with a tight lens fit. There is no relationship between the development of focal edema and hypersensitivity reactions to lens protein. Contact-lens–induced hypoxia can also produce stromal edema. However, significant light scatter is not produced until greater than 15% stromal swelling occurs.

Preferred Response   c. epithelial hypoxia

A 67-year-old woman complains of foreign-body sensation, tearing, and photophobia in her left eye, in which the vision has been poor for several years. The figure shows the result of biomicroscopic examination.

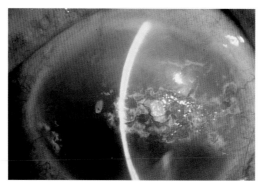

Calcific band keratopathy.

The *most* likely diagnosis is

a. calcific band keratopathy
b. Salzmann's nodular degeneration
c. central cloudy cornea of François
d. spheroid degeneration

Discussion

The history and corneal appearance are consistent with calcific band keratopathy. The five main causes of this degenerative phenomenon are chronic inflammation, hypercalcemia, hereditary band keratopathy, hyperphosphatemia, and chronic mercurial exposure. The clinical picture is quite different in Salzmann's nodular degeneration. Salzmann's degeneration is also the late sequela of a keratitis and may not appear until years after the active disease. However, it presents as midperipheral gray white or bluish gray smooth, rounded nodules, often in a circular configuration. Central cloudy cornea of François is a deep central shagreen that is bilateral and hereditary and has no effect on vision. Spheroid degeneration is characterized by translucent golden brown spherules in the superficial stroma. These deposits represent proteinaceous material and result from the combined effect of genetic predisposition, actinic exposure, age, and environmental trauma.[1]

Preferred Response

a. calcific band keratopathy

Management of the condition diagnosed in the patient in Question E37 includes all of the following *except*

a. bandage contact lens
b. chelation with disodium EDTA
c. application of silver nitrate
d. scraping

Discussion

The first management principle in dealing with calcific band keratopathy is to determine the underlying cause. This may require both historical and laboratory workup, including serum calcium, phosphorus, and uric acid.

If the deposition is either visually disabling or, as is more common, symptomatic with foreign-body sensation, tearing, and photophobia, one may employ a therapeutic lens for relief of irritation. More long-lasting treatment requires removal of the calcific deposit. This can be accomplished by applying disodium EDTA in a 0.05 mol/L to 0.25 mol/L concentration topically to soften the calcium. The deposit can then be more easily scraped from the corneal surface. The epithelium is then allowed to heal over the defect with the use of a patch or a bandage lens; this procedure often provides relief from pain and restoration of useful vision. Chemical cautery with silver nitrate, although applicable in such conditions as superior limbic keratoconjunctivitis and as prophylaxis against infection in the neonate, has no role in the management of calcific band keratopathy.

Preferred Response   c. application of silver nitrate

A 12-year-old boy underwent penetrating keratoplasty for complications of herpes simplex keratitis. He was managed with a routine regimen of prednisolone acetate and a prophylactic regimen of topical antiviral medication for the first several weeks. His postoperative course was uncomplicated until he developed an area of focal injection near a graft suture and an adjacent superficial anterior stromal crystalline deposit in the clear cornea (see the figure).

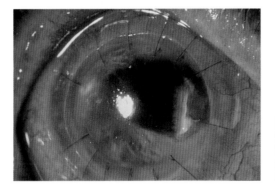

Infectious crystalline keratopathy caused by *S viridans* in a patient with a corneal graft and on chronic topical corticosteroids.

The *most* likely diagnosis is

a. recurrent herpes simplex keratitis
b. bacterial keratitis
c. fungal keratitis
d. steroid crystallization

Discussion   This patient's lesion most likely represents bacterial infection in the setting of localized immune suppression. Identified as infectious crystalline keratopathy, this lesion is commonly caused by *Streptococcus viridans* or one of the variety of generally nonpathogenic staphylococci. Commonly, this infection is accompanied by a minimal surrounding inflammatory response and most often occurs in the setting of a compromised host. For this reason it is seen, although not exclusively, in the setting of the postgraft patient who is often on long-standing topical corticosteroid treatment. Although there is roughly a 20% recurrence rate of herpes simplex in the patient graft, recurrences do not occur in the form of a crystalline keratopathy. Fungal infection should be ruled out in such cases, but it is less likely in this setting. Corticosteroids are not reported to leave crystalline deposits.[22–24]

Preferred Response   b. bacterial keratitis

The *least* appropriate antibiotic for the management of the condition of the patient in Question E39 is

a. vancomycin
b. cefazolin
c. gentamicin
d. penicillin

Discussion   All of the agents mentioned above are effective against *Streptococcus* species with the notable exception of gentamicin. Resistance to gentamicin by *Streptococcus pneumoniae* as well as other *Streptococcus* species has been demonstrated. The most appropriate antibiotic for use in streptococcal infection is a fortified cephalosporin or vancomycin. Penicillin is not commonly used topically, but it can be compounded for use in such a case.

Preferred Response   c. gentamicin

All of the following may produce crystalline deposits in the cornea *except*

a. systemic paraproteinemias
b. cystinosis
c. chlorpromazine
d. streptococcal infection

Discussion   Crystalline deposits in the cornea may be produced by systemic metabolic abnormalities, such as cystinosis. In this condition, multiple refractile crystals are deposited throughout the cornea and conjunctiva. These findings are associated with both the infantile nephropathic form as well as the benign adult form of cystinosis. Systemic paraproteinemias, such as multiple myeloma, may also be characterized by crystalline corneal deposits. Streptococcal infection in the form of crystalline keratopathy may also manifest as crystalline deposition, as mentioned in Question E39. Other causes of crystalline keratopathy include cholesterol deposition; Schnyder's crystalline dystrophy; calcium oxalate (*Dieffenbachia* plant sap exposure); Bietti's marginal crystalline dystrophy; other drugs, such as indomethacin, chloroquine, and thioridazine; gout; and uremia. Chlorpromazine in higher doses for long periods produces a brownish tan powderlike deposit in the deep stroma of the cornea; the deposition is not, however, crystalline.[1]

Preferred Response   c. chlorpromazine

A 19-year-old college student complains of poor vision. He states that he has long been nearsighted but that his glasses have recently required several changes, and even with his most recent correction, he is having difficulty. Examination reveals a best-corrected acuity of 20/40 with spectacle correction. The results of slit-lamp biomicroscopy are shown in the figures.

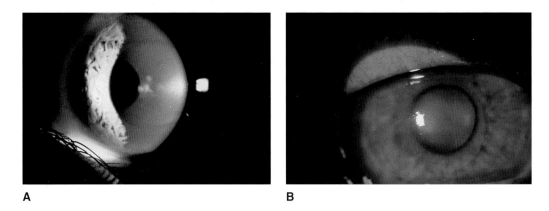

A   **B**

Basal epithelial iron ring (Fleischer ring) in keratoconus, viewed in broad oblique illumination **(A)** and with cobalt-blue illumination **(B)**.

The *most* likely diagnosis is

a. keratoconus
b. pellucid marginal degeneration
c. Terrien's marginal degeneration
d. keratoglobus

Discussion

The patient's history and corneal appearance on biomicroscopy are most consistent with keratoconus. Progressive myopia, multiple spectacle or contact lens changes, and a qualitatively unsatisfactory best-corrected acuity suggest early keratoconus. The presence of a distinct Fleischer ring representing iron deposition at the level of the basal epithelium is diagnostic of this disorder. Pellucid marginal degeneration is a distinct disorder in the spectrum of noninflammatory ectasias of the cornea. However, it differs from keratoconus in that the thinnest area of the cornea is not at the apex of the cone, but rather in a crescentic distribution near the inferior limbus. The effect of this pathologic configuration is that the patient with pellucid marginal degeneration presents with progressive and marked against-the-rule astigmatism. Generally, there is no circular iron deposition or apical reticular scarring as in keratoconus. Keratoglobus is a diffuse thinning of the ocular coats, including cornea and sclera. Patients with keratoglobus often have a markedly steepened cornea, a blue sclera, and a tendency for corneal rupture with trauma. There is also an association with collagen fragility syndromes. Terrien's marginal degeneration is an inflammatory condition that includes peripheral vascularization, intracorneal lipid deposition, and nonulcerative thinning and ectasia of the corneal periphery.[25]

Preferred Response

a. keratoconus

E43

Other findings associated with the condition found in the patient in Question E42 include all of the following *except*

a. pre-Descemet's striae
b. apical reticular scarring and thinning
c. peripheral vascularization
d. inferior corneal steepening

Discussion

Keratoconus is a noninflammatory ectasia. Corneal vascularization is, therefore, not a characteristic of this disease. Other characteristic findings in keratoconus include an abnormal, scissoring retinoscopic reflex; inferior keratometric/topographic steepening from downward displacement of the cone; subepithelial/anterior reticular stromal scarring; Vogt's striae in the deep stroma that disappear with application of digital pressure through the upper lid; irregular astigmatism; and, in more advanced cases, outward conical protrusion of the lower lid in down gaze (Munson's sign).[25]

Preferred Response

c. peripheral vascularization

E44

Of the computer-assisted topographic analyses shown below, which is *most* likely to correspond with the patient in Question E42?

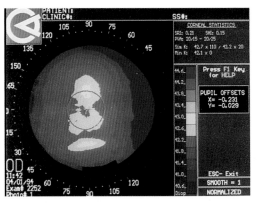

Figure A

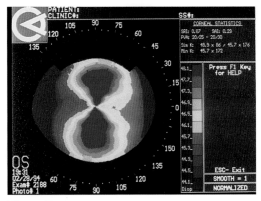

Figure B

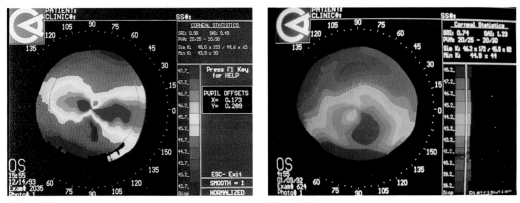

Figure C

Figure D

Patterns seen in computer-assisted topographic analysis. **(A)** Normal cornea. **(B)** With-the-rule astigmatism. **(C)** Against-the-rule astigmatism. **(D)** Keratoconus.

a. Figure A
b. Figure B
c. Figure C
d. Figure D

Discussion

Computer-assisted topographic analysis is often much more sensitive than either keratometry or photokeratoscopy. Commonly, the "warmer" (red) colors signify steeper areas, while the "cooler" (blue) colors represent flatter dioptric powers. Each topogram is accompanied by a color scale that correlates the hue in the topogram with a dioptric power. In keratoconus, there is characteristic inferior steepening consistent with the pattern in topogram D. In addition, one may also note significant surface irregularity, indicated either by the color topograms or by the numerical indices provided in the software. Topogram A indicates a normal spherical cornea. Topogram B demonstrates with-the-rule astigmatism, with the steepest arc along the vertical meridian. Topogram C demonstrates against-the-rule astigmatism, with the steepest arc along the horizontal meridian.

Preferred Response

d. Figure D

A patient with keratoconus is fit with a rigid gas-permeable contact lens. The patient's fluorescein pattern is shown below.

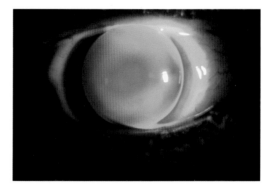

Characteristic fluorescein staining pattern seen in a patient with a contact lens with marked central bearing.

Which of the following characteristics does the fluorescein pattern demonstrate?

a. central bearing
b. peripheral touch
c. a lens that is too steep
d. tight lens syndrome

Discussion

The fluorescein pattern seen in this contact lens fit demonstrates marked central bearing, with exclusion of fluorescein from the central cornea where the corneal epithelium directly touches the back of the contact lens. This indicates that the steepest posterior curvature of the lens is considerably flatter than the corneal curvature. Peripheral touch would be indicated if there were thinning of the pooled fluorescein at the periphery of the lens. The fluorescein pattern in a lens that is too steep not only would show a central accumulation of fluorescein rather than the central thinning that is shown in this photograph, but also might demonstrate an air bubble under the steep lens between its posterior surface and the corneal apex. Tight lens syndrome is a clinical syndrome, not a lens fitting pattern. In tight lens syndrome, either a rigid or soft lens is fit too tight or tightens on the cornea, leading to hypoxia and inflammation.

Preferred Response   a. central bearing

The lens–cornea relationship in the patient in Question E45 is the best achievable fit leading to stability of position and acceptable vision. The *most* appropriate measure at this point in the patient's management is to

a. abandon contact lens fitting and suggest keratoplasty
b. let the patient try the lens
c. consider a central flattening procedure to facilitate lens fit
d. perform radial keratotomy

Discussion   Contact lens fitting in keratoconus requires different criteria for success than routine fitting in the myope. A certain degree of central bearing on the corneal apex may be quite acceptable under these circumstances if well tolerated by the patient both visually and optically. The appropriate step is, therefore, to let the patient try the lens. He must be monitored closely; however, if the lens is well tolerated and the vision is good, there is no evidence that such a fit is deleterious to the cornea. Keratoplasty after contact lens fit in keratoconus is indicated only if the lens fit does not correct the patient adequately to meet his or her visual needs or if, even with acceptable vision, the lens cannot be functionally retained in the eye because of the steep cornea. Central flattening procedures, such as thermokeratoplasty or epikeratoplasty, are rarely indicated, since the vast majority of keratoconus patients can be fit with either single-cut or specially designed lenses. Radial keratotomy is contraindicated in a patient with keratoconus, because the process will progress despite temporary correction of the myopia provided by the refractive surgery. In addition, the thinning of the cornea seen in keratoconus may make keratotomy a hazardous procedure.

Preferred Response   b. let the patient try the lens

The patient in Question E45 is happy with the fit of his contact lenses. However, 6 months later, he calls the office and agitatedly explains that he saw his family practitioner for a red eye that he developed 3 days ago. The family doctor told him that he had a serious corneal infection, prescribed antibiotics, and referred him to you for treatment. The lesion appears as shown in the figure. There is no epithelial defect, and the anterior chamber is deep and has only slight flare and a few cells. However, you note photophobia, tearing, conjunctival hyperemia, and vision decreased to bare finger-counting.

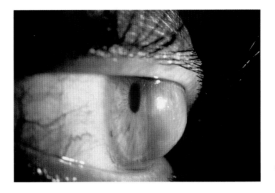

Acute corneal hydrops in keratoconus.

The *most* likely diagnosis is

a. bacterial keratitis
b. *Acanthamoeba* keratitis
c. acute corneal hydrops
d. corneal perforation

Discussion   The patient is suffering from acute corneal hydrops. This represents an acute ingress of aqueous into the corneal stroma associated with a break in Descemet's membrane. The patient usually experiences acute visual loss, ocular irritation, photophobia, and conjunctival hyperemia. There may be an accompanying mild iritis. The hydropic cornea can be dramatic in clinical appearance, with the sudden appearance of a dense, thickened, white spot in the cornea, which at first glance may resemble an infectious keratitis. Bacterial keratitis must, of course, be considered; however, the lack of an overlying ulceration and purulent discharge makes this most unlikely. Likewise, although *Acanthamoeba* infection is most commonly associated with contact lens wear, it is likely to be much slower in onset and to be associated with considerably greater pain than hydrops. Perforation is extremely rare in keratoconus and would be characterized by a leakage site in the cornea and a flat or shallow anterior chamber.[25]

Preferred Response   c. acute corneal hydrops

The *most* appropriate management of the problem in Question E47 is

a. keratoplasty
b. cyclopentolate and topical hypertonic salt solution
c. therapeutic contact lens
d. antibiotics

Discussion   Patients with acute hydrops are best managed symptomatically with cycloplegia and topical hypertonic saline drops and ointment. The former will manage the mild accompanying iritis, and the latter may help to reduce the swelling of the corneal epithelium somewhat. However, the patient must be told that time is necessary for the posterior cornea to re-seal and for the accumulated fluid to be "pumped out" by the endothelium. Because the epithelium is intact, there is no real rationale for a therapeutic contact lens. Antibiotics have no role once it has been determined that an infection is not present. Keratoplasty is not indicated in the setting of acute hydrops. The ophthalmologist should wait until corneal swelling has subsided. At that point, if there is residual scarring and contact lens fitting is no longer feasible, a keratoplasty can be performed.

Preferred Response   b. cyclopentolate and topical hypertonic salt solution

A 65-year-old woman complains of deep, boring pain of 3 days' duration. She denies any visual deficits, but she is unable to sleep because of the accelerating pain. Her eye is shown in the figure.

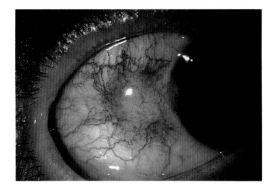

Anterior scleritis.

The clinical picture is *most* consistent with

a. interstitial keratitis
b. nodular scleritis
c. conjunctivitis
d. anterior uveitis

Discussion   The lesion shown in the figure is most consistent with anterior nodular scleritis. Anterior scleritis may be diffuse or nodular. In either case the symptoms are characterized by deep, boring pain. In nodular scleritis, the nodule is elevated, has a deep red or violaceous appearance, may or may not have an overlying episcleritis, and is clearly distinguishable from overlying conjunctival and episcleral hyperemia. Such lesions are multiple in 40% of cases and, if directly contiguous to the cornea, may induce a sclerokeratitis. Interstitial keratitis in its active form is characterized by corneal inflammation, opacity, and vascular engorgement. Conjunctivitis is clearly distinguishable from scleritis both by symptoms and by the vascular layer that is engorged. Anterior uveitis occurs in 30% of patients with scleritis; however, if it occurs without scleritis, one would more likely see circumcorneal flush and anterior chamber inflammation rather than a scleral nodule.

Preferred Response   b. nodular scleritis

All of the following laboratory tests would be appropriate in the workup of the patient in Question E49 *except*

a. serum glucose
b. fluorescent treponemal antibody absorption (FTA-ABS)
c. antinuclear antibody (ANA)
d. rheumatoid factor (RF)

Discussion

In approximately 50% of patients with scleritis, an associated systemic disease can be identified. A variety of systemic diseases have been associated, including syphilis, tuberculosis, herpes zoster, gout, and the group of collagen vascular diseases including rheumatoid arthritis, systemic lupus erythematosus, polyarteritis nodosa, and Wegener's granulomatosis. The FTA-ABS to look for evidence of syphilis infection, active or inactive, is appropriate. A positive ANA, although nonspecific, may lead to more specific testing for diagnosis of underlying disease. Rheumatoid arthritis is commonly associated with scleritis and can be detected serologically using a rheumatoid factor. Serum glucose does not add to the specificity of the diagnosis in such a case. The investigation of possible underlying disease and subsequent treatment may be very important in patients with scleritis, particularly those with necrotizing scleritis.[26]

Preferred Response

a. serum glucose

References

1. *External Disease and Cornea.* Section 8 of Basic and Clinical Science Course. San Francisco: American Academy of Ophthalmology; 1994.
2. Cha SB, Shields JA, Shields CL, et al: Squamous cell carcinoma of the conjunctiva. *Intl Ophthalmol Clin* 1993;33:19–24.
3. Waring GO III, Roth AM, Ekins MB: Clinical and pathologic description of 17 cases of corneal intraepithelial neoplasia. *Am J Ophthalmol* 1984;97:547–559.
4. Jay B: Naevi and melanomata of the conjunctiva. *Br J Ophthalmol* 1964;49:169–204.
5. De Potter P, Shields CL, Shields JA: Malignant melanoma of the conjunctiva. *Intl Ophthalmol Clin* 1993;33:25–30.
6. Folberg R, McLean IW, Zimmerman LE: Conjunctival melanosis and melanoma. *Ophthalmology* 1984;91:673–678.
7. Reese AB: Precancerous and cancerous melanosis. In: Boniuk M: *Ocular and Adnexal Tumors: New and Controversial Aspects.* St. Louis: CV Mosby Co; 1964.
8. Shields JA, Shields CL, Augsburger JJ: Current options of management of conjunctival melanoma. *Orbit* 1986;6:25–30.
9. Jakobiec FA, Brownstein S, Wilkinson RD, et al: Combined surgery and cryotherapy for diffuse malignant melanoma of the conjunctiva. *Arch Ophthalmol* 1980;98:1390–1396.
10. Jakobiec FA, Brownstein S, Albert W, et al: The role of cryotherapy in the management of conjunctival melanoma. *Ophthalmology* 1982;89:502–515.
11. Jakobiec FA, Rini FJ, Fraunfelder FT, et al: Cryotherapy for conjunctival primary acquired melanosis and malignant melanoma: experience with 62 cases. *Ophthalmology* 1988;95:1058–1070.
12. Jones DB: Decision-making in the management of microbial keratitis. *Ophthalmology* 1981;88:814–820.
13. Schein OD, Glynn RJ, Poggio EC, et al: The relative risk of ulcerative keratitis among users of daily-wear and extended-wear soft contact lenses: a case-control study. *N Engl J Med* 1989;321:773–778.

14. Palmer ML, Hyndiuk RA: Contact lens-related infectious keratitis. *Intl Ophthalmol Clin* 1993;33:23–49.

15. Friedlaender MH: *Allergy and Immunology of the Eye.* New York: Raven Press; 1993.

16. Forster RK: Fungal diseases. In: Smolin G, Thoft RA, eds: *The Cornea: Scientific Foundations and Clinical Practice.* Boston: Little, Brown & Co; 1987.

17. Johns KJ, O'Day DM: Pharmacologic management of keratomycoses. *Surv Ophthalmol* 1988;33:178–188.

18. Schanzlin DJ: Mooren's ulceration. In: Smolin G, Thoft RA, eds: *The Cornea: Scientific Foundations and Clinical Practice.* Boston: Little, Brown & Co; 1987.

19. Robin JB, Schanzlin DJ, Verity SM, et al: Peripheral corneal disorders. *Surv Ophthalmol* 1986;31:1–36.

20. Brown SI: Mooren's ulcer: treatment by conjunctival excision. *Br J Ophthalmol* 1975;59:675–682.

21. Brown SI, Mondino BJ: Therapy of Mooren's ulcer. *Am J Ophthalmol* 1984;98:1–6.

22. Gorovoy MS, Stern GA, Hood CI, et al: Intrastromal noninflammatory bacterial colonization of a corneal graft. *Arch Ophthalmol* 1983;101:1749–1752.

23. Meisler DM, Langston RH, Naab TJ, et al: Infectious crystalline keratopathy. *Am J Ophthalmol* 1984;97:337–343.

24. Stern GA: Infectious crystalline keratopathy. *Intl Ophthalmol Clin* 1993;33:1–7.

25. Krachmer JH, Feder RS, Belin MW: Keratoconus and related noninflammatory corneal thinning disorders. *Surv Ophthalmol* 1984;28:293–322.

26. Watson P: Diseases of the sclera and episclera. In: Tasman W, Jaeger EA: *Duane's Clinical Ophthalmology.* Philadelphia: JB Lippincott Co; 1990.

Additional Resources From the AAO

Academy Statements

Acanthamoeba Keratitis in Contact Lens Wearers: Homemade Saline Solution, Swimming, Hot Tubs. Clinical Alert. 1987.

Contact Lens Advisory: Keratitis and Extended-Wear (Overnight) Contact Lens Use. Clinical Alert. 1989.

Homemade Saline Solutions and Acanthamoeba Keratitis. Public Health Note. 1992.

Basic and Clinical Science Course

External Disease and Cornea. Section 8. Updated annually.

Focal Points

Belin MW: *Optical and Surgical Correction of Keratoconus.* Vol VI, Module 11. 1988. (Item No. 029006)

de Luise VP: *Management of Dry Eyes.* Vol III, Module 3. 1985. (Out of print)

Rowsey JJ, Hays JC: *Corneal Astigmatism: Topographic and Surgical Insights.* Vol V, Module 4. 1987. (Out of print)

Preferred Practice Patterns

Blepharitis and the Dry Eye in the Adult. 1991. (Item No. 110011)

Conjunctivitis. 1991. (Item No. 110012)

Slide-Scripts

External Disease and Cornea: A Multimedia Collection. 1994. (Item No. 0260054)

Tang RA: *Ocular Manifestations of Systemic Disease.* Eye Care Skills for the Primary Care Physician Series. 1989. (Item No. 0240339)

Young SE: *Managing the Red Eye.* Eye Care Skills for the Primary Care Physician Series. 1994. (Item No. 0240310)

Videotape

Abbott RL: *Surgical Intervention in Corneal and External Diseases.* Clinical Skills Series. 1989. (Item No. 0250813)

CATARACT AND ANTERIOR SEGMENT SURGERY

A patient is noted to have the cataract shown in the slit-lamp photograph below.

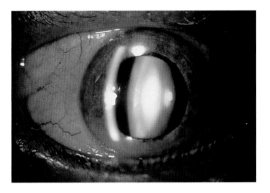

Nuclear sclerotic cataract.

Cataracts of this type may be associated with all of the following *except*

a. early loss of near (reading) vision
b. a myopic shift
c. monocular diplopia
d. difficulty seeing road signs at dusk

Discussion

The normal lens nucleus hardens and becomes more pigmented with age. These changes may be inferred by the biomicroscopist when it is noted in the optical section that the nucleus has lost its lamellar structure and is becoming amber in color. The transition from a normally aging nucleus to a nuclear sclerotic cataract is a subtle one marked not by easily observable morphologic changes but rather by changes in visual function. The first functional change is usually a myopic shift in refraction. This results in the "second sight" that enables some patients to discard their reading glasses. Blurring is at first more for distance vision (particularly in dim illumination) than for near, even when optimal spectacle correction is used. Monocular diplopia is also a frequent complaint.

Preferred Response

a. early loss of near (reading) vision

On pupillary dilation, a patient shows the characteristic lens change shown in the figure.

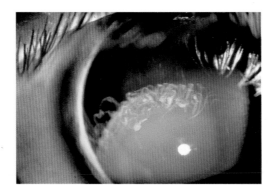

Inferiorly dislocated lens with equatorial zonular remnants.

The *least* likely diagnosis is

a. Marfan syndrome
b. homocystinuria
c. Weill-Marchesani syndrome
d. Sturge-Weber syndrome

Discussion

The differential diagnosis of ectopia lentis includes Marfan syndrome, homocystinuria, Weill-Marchesani syndrome, hyperlysinemia, sulfate oxidase deficiency, congenital syphilis, trauma, Ehlers-Danlos syndrome, and exfoliation syndrome. Sturge-Weber syndrome is not associated with spontaneous lens dislocation.

Preferred Response

d. Sturge-Weber syndrome

An 80-year-old woman underwent uneventful phacoemulsification and polymethylmethacrylate (PMMA) IOL implantation. She was noted to have an axial length of 21.8 mm and exfoliation syndrome with a maximally dilated pupil of 5.5 mm preoperatively. A 4.5 mm capsulorhexis was performed at surgery and a 5.5 mm optic, 12 mm overall length IOL was placed within the capsular bag. Three weeks after surgery, a contraction of the capsulorhexis opening to approximately 3.5 mm is noted, as shown in the figure.

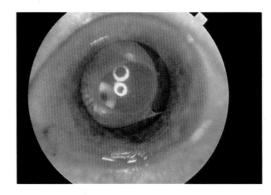

Capsular contraction with decreased anterior capsule diameter.

The *most* appropriate management for this patient is

a. continued observation
b. perform multiple radial anterior Nd:YAG capsulotomies
c. perform Nd:YAG posterior capsulotomy
d. increase topical corticosteroid to reduce contraction

Discussion Capsule contraction syndrome has been described in patients with previous uveitis, exfoliation syndrome, advanced age, and retinitis pigmentosa. Its cause is an imbalance of the forces that affect shrinkage of the capsular bag anatomy. Fibrotic contraction forces are favored over zonular traction, which normally maintains capsular bag diameter. These forces are in opposition indefinitely, but most of the contracture seems to occur in the first 3 to 6 months. The earlier it is recognized, the earlier intervention may be accomplished to preserve zonular integrity and reduce unwanted IOL shift or visual aberrations from the encroaching capsulorhexis edge. The figure below shows the same patient at 2 months after five radial anterior capsulotomies were created with a power setting at 1.2 millijoules. Notice the larger anterior capsular diameter. A course of continued observation may result in further contraction and lead to decreased visual acuity. Posterior capsulotomy and topical corticosteroids will not relieve the contraction phenomenon.[1]

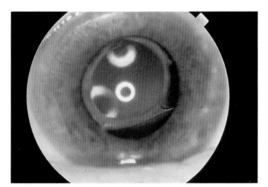

Following Nd:YAG radial anterior capsulotomies, the anterior capsule diameter is significantly increased.

Preferred Response b. perform multiple radial anterior Nd:YAG capsulotomies

Two years after uncomplicated phacoemulsification with deliberate sulcus placement of a three-piece posterior chamber lens with polypropylene haptics, a healthy adult patient notes intermittent obscurations of vision. Examination during an episode of decreased vision demonstrates a microhyphema and elevation of intraocular pressure to 30 mm Hg. Red reflex examination at the slit lamp reveals the finding shown in the figure.

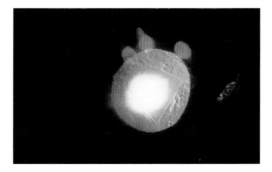

Iris transillumination defect secondary to intraocular lens chafe.

The *most* likely diagnosis is

a. iris neovascularization
b. peripheral uveitis
c. pseudophakic iris chafing syndrome
d. iris nevus syndrome

Discussion   Posterior iris chafing by the loop or the optic portion of sulcus-fixated posterior chamber lens implants may cause a spectrum of disorders, including iris-pigment epithelial "window defects," pigment dispersions with or without intraocular pressure elevation, intermittent microhyphemas with transient visual obscurations, and the uveitis-glaucoma-hyphema (UGH) syndrome. It appears that secondary pigmentary glaucoma is more likely with planar haptic designs than with angulated haptics. Optic and haptic materials may play a role in the development of the disorder. Implantation of both supporting haptics of the implant within the capsular bag is suggested to prevent posterior iris chafing. In iris neovascularization, one would expect to see fine iris vessels, which are not present here. Iris transillumination defects are not normally seen in peripheral uveitis or in the iris nevus syndrome, where the iris is studded with multiple nevi.[2,3]

Preferred Response   c. pseudophakic iris chafing syndrome

A 23-year-old woman requests refractive surgery. She is a −3.00 myope. Keratometry reading in the right eye is 44.00 D/45.00 D × 90°. Keratometry reading in the left eye is 45.00 D/48.00 D × 120° with +2 distortion of the keratoscopic mires OS.

The *most* appropriate advice to give her is to

a. have radial keratotomy (RK) in the right eye and an RK with transverse incision in the left
b. discontinue her contact lenses indefinitely
c. discontinue her contact lenses for 2 to 3 weeks and return for corneal topography
d. increase artificial tears, since they may help the irregular mires

Discussion   This patient may have distortion of corneal mires in the left eye based on either contact-lens–induced corneal warpage or early keratoconus. It would be best to have her discontinue the lenses for 2 to 3 weeks and then reevaluate the keratometry and, if possible, perform corneal topography. Topography that is characteristic of keratoconus may be diagnostic. Refractive surgery is not indicated in patients with keratoconus because the long-term effects of a corneal weakening procedure, such as radial keratotomy, or a subtraction procedure, such as excimer photoablation, are unknown. Artificial tears would not affect corneal irregularity unless there was irregular drying of the surface.

Preferred Response   c. discontinue her contact lenses for 2 to 3 weeks and return for corneal topography

An 18-year-old patient presents with complaints of a decrease in vision for the past several months. Examination shows the eyelids to be thickened, with weeping fissures at the lateral canthi. Slit-lamp examination demonstrates a cataract located anteriorly (see the figure). The patient also complains of multiple skin lesions that are dry, erythematous, and very pruritic.

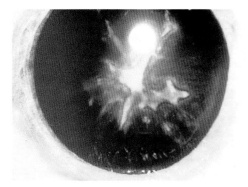

Stellate-shaped anterior subcapsular cataract.

This constellation of findings is *most* characteristic of

a. herpes simplex
b. vernal keratoconjunctivitis
c. atopic disease
d. systemic lupus erythematosus

Discussion

Anterior subcapsular cataracts with the characteristic "stretched bear rug" configuration seen here occur in approximately 10% of patients with atopic disease. The skin lesions of atopic dermatitis are dry, erythematous, vesicular, and pruritic. Scratching leads to excoriations, weeping, scaling, and crusting. The face and eyelids can be affected in more severe cases. Corneal findings include punctate keratitis, marginal ulceration, vascularization, and stromal opacification. Vernal keratoconjunctivitis is not associated with cataract formation except secondarily as a result of chronic topical corticosteroid use. The skin rash is not characteristic of lupus, in which an erythematous rash appears on the nose and cheeks in a "butterfly" distribution. Herpes simplex is characterized by dendritic keratitis and a vesicular skin rash.

Preferred Response

c. atopic disease

A 65-year-old patient has developed progressive nuclear sclerosis in both eyes and is having difficulty with reading and near work. Refraction is OD –1.25 –1.50 × 155 = 20/50, and OS –5.50 –2.00 × 25 = 20/40. Six years ago he had radial keratotomies performed in both eyes. Prior to his radial keratotomy (RK), he was –5.00 sphere in the right eye and –5.50 sphere in the left eye. He had four-incision RK in each eye with a goal of emmetropia in the right eye and mild myopia in the left eye for near vision. Two years after his RKs, his right eye was 20/60 uncorrected, and his left eye was 20/200. Refraction was OD +2.50 −1.50 × 135 = 20/30; OS −2.75 −0.50 × 180 = 20/30. His original keratometry was OD 42.50 D/43.00 D; OS 42.50 D/43.00 D. His present keratometry is OD 38.50 D/37.50 D; OS 42.00 D/41.50 D. His axial length measurements are OD 25.71 mm and OS 25.94 mm.

The *least* acceptable course of action would be to

a. obtain computerized video keratography of both eyes
b. proceed with the cataract surgery utilizing his present keratometry and axial length measurements
c. calculate his true corneal power by subtracting his refractive effect (original spherical equivalent *minus* two-year post-RK spherical equivalent) from his original keratometry
d. calculate his corneal power by placing a plano contact lens of known curvature on his cornea and refracting over it

Discussion   Standard keratometry following radial keratotomy (RK) is notoriously inaccurate in estimating the true corneal power. In most cases, the keratometry is steeper than the known refractive effect following the radial keratotomy. In a normally shaped cornea, the corneal mires are approximately 3 mm apart. Following RK, the refractive effect in diopters is usually greater than the change in keratometry. Thus, if measured keratometry is entered in the intraocular lens (IOL) calculation, the predicted power of the IOL for emmetropia will usually be underestimated.

In the present case, the video keratography (36.10 D in the right eye, Figure A, and 40.46 D in the left eye, Figure B) agrees with the theoretical keratometry based on original refraction and K readings and the post-RK refraction. This was calculated as follows:

For the right eye: The patient was originally a −5.00 sphere. Post-RK, he was a +1.75 spherical equivalent (SE) for 6.75 D of refractive effect. His original keratometry was 42.75 D less 6.75 D of refractive effect to equal a theoretical K of 36.00 D. This correlates well with the video keratograph showing a central K of 36.10 D.

For the left eye: His left eye was originally a −5.50 sphere. Following his radial keratotomy, he was a −3.00 SE for 2.50 D of refractive effect. His original keratometry was 42.75 D minus 2.50 D of refractive effect to equal a theoretical K of 40.25 D. This correlates with the video keratograph showing a central K of 40.46 D. Contrast these Ks with the average standard keratometry Ks of OD 38.00 D, OS 41.75 D.

It is well known that following radial keratotomy, some patients receive a multifocal effect on the cornea, and this patient may be using these areas for his distance vision. Although video keratography will in general provide more accurate readings than the actual keratometry, patients should be cautioned that, because of their previous radial keratotomy, there is some reduction in accuracy of IOL calculations.[4]

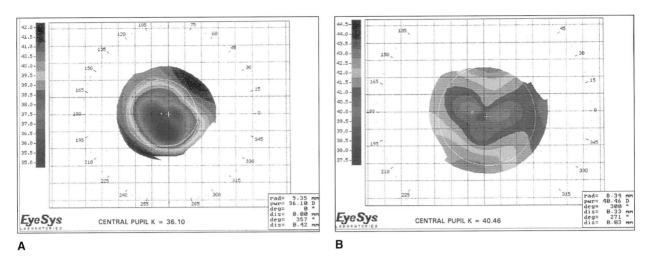

A   **B**

(A) Video keratograph of right eye indicating central corneal curvature of 36.10 D. **(B)** Video keratograph of left eye indicating central corneal curvature of 40.46 D.

Preferred Response   b. proceed with the cataract surgery utilizing his present keratometry and axial length measurements

C8   The lens change shown in the figure is often associated with anterior polar cataracts in what associated disease or syndrome?

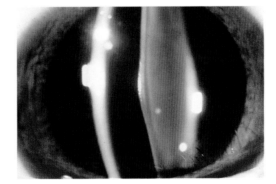

Anterior lenticonus.

a. Lowe syndrome
b. Alport syndrome
c. rubella
d. Down syndrome

Discussion   Alport syndrome is a hereditary renal disease generally transmitted in an autosomal dominant fashion. The disorder is more severe in males. Nerve deafness is a prominent feature of Alport syndrome. The most significant ocular abnormalities in this disorder are anterior lenticonus, as shown in the figure, and anterior polar cataracts. The most common ocular complication of Lowe syndrome is the presence of congenital cataracts and posterior lenticonus. Lenticonus is not a feature of either rubella or Down syndrome.

Preferred Response   b. Alport syndrome

All of the following statements about the rubella syndrome are true *except*

a. The retina often demonstrates a "salt and pepper" appearance.
b. It often includes bilateral nuclear sclerotic cataracts.
c. Virus-induced iridocyclitis may occur if all cortical and nuclear lens material is not removed during the initial cataract surgery.
d. It occurs when the mother is infected during the third trimester.

Discussion

The rubella syndrome occurs when the mother is infected during the first trimester of pregnancy. Associated findings include microphthalmos, shallow anterior chamber, a "salt and pepper" appearance of the fundus, hearing loss, patent ductus arteriosis and other heart and valve abnormalities, and genitourinary defects. Histologically, the characteristic finding in rubella cataract is retention of fetal cell nuclei in the cataractous lens nucleus. The rubella virus may be present in the lens for up to 3 years after birth. All cortical and nuclear material must be removed during cataract surgery to avoid virus-induced iridocyclitis.

Preferred Response

d. It occurs when the mother is infected during the third trimester.

C10

The subtraction video keratograph shown in the figure demonstrates the difference between the preoperative video keratograph (top left, A) and the postoperative video keratograph (bottom left, B). Blue on scale represents little to no dioptric change; red represents significant change.

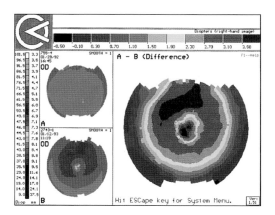

Subtraction video keratograph demonstrating a central island.

This video keratograph demonstrates

a. central flattening induced by excimer laser photoablation
b. the result of a myopic ablation on a patient with keratoconus
c. a "central island" with a central nipple (steepening) of tissue
d. "bow tie" regular astigmatism

Discussion

Central islands following photorefractive keratectomy (PRK) have been seen in approximately 20% to 30% of patients in some series. The characteristic video keratographic picture is a central dark, round spot (demonstrating a minimal dioptric change) surrounded by a central red or yellow area (demonstrating a significant and uniform dioptric change) on a subtraction image. A normal myopic ablation would show a uniform area of flattening in the cool color zone, the blues or purples. A "bow tie" configuration of regular astigmatism would be in the configuration of a bow tie, with the area of the tie being steeper than the surrounding areas. The etiology of central islands in photorefractive keratectomy is currently unknown. The most popular theory is that central tissue is not ablated because of hydration differences between the central and peripheral portions of the cornea. Other theories that have been popularized include irregular beam energies across the cornea and the formation of central vortex plumes of debris blocking the incoming beam. Blowing a gas across the surface of the cornea during the ablation may minimize this. Many patients demonstrating a central island topographically are asymptomatic with excellent uncorrected vision. Good results have been reported for patients who are symptomatic and have undergone repeat PRK to the central nipple area.

Preferred Response   c. a "central island" with a central nipple (steepening) of tissue

An intraoperative technique is shown in the figure.

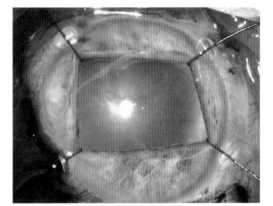

Intraoperative photograph demonstrating the use of iris hooks to increase pupillary diameter.

This technique would be *most* advantageous in patients with

a. a dislocated crystalline lens
b. exfoliation syndrome
c. phacolytic glaucoma
d. positive vitreous pressure

Discussion   The figure demonstrates the use of polypropylene iris retractor hooks, which have proven to be beneficial in increasing the pupillary diameter, thereby facilitating cataract extraction. Studies have shown that pupils in exfoliation syndrome dilate submaximally.[5] This is presumably related to iris infiltration and fibrosis from the exfoliation. The other three conditions listed are not associated with submaximal pupillary dilation. Other methods of increasing the pupillary diameter for facilitation of cataract extraction include radial sphincterotomies and sector iridectomies.

Preferred Response   b. exfoliation syndrome

A 32-year-old woman presents with 20/40 vision in both eyes correctable to 20/25 bilaterally and a lens opacity (see the figure).

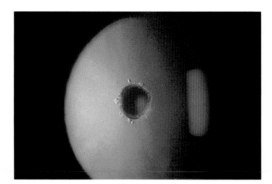

Posterior polar cataract.

If the lens opacity becomes progressive, which one of the following complications is this patient's eye prone to develop?

a. postoperative uveitis
b. postoperative choroidal detachment
c. intraoperative capsular rupture
d. intraoperative zonular dialysis

Discussion

The figure depicts a posterior polar cataract, one of the more common types of visually symptomatic congenital cataracts. Posterior polar cataracts are dense, white opacities axially positioned on the posterior capsule. The central portion typically is circular and thick and has a characteristic concentric whorl-like appearance. Posterior capsular rupture is a particularly common complication when performing cataract surgery in these patients.[6] Ciliochoroidal detachments seen immediately following cataract surgery are common and are attributed to ocular hypotension. This type of postoperative choroidal detachment usually subsides within 3 weeks and requires no treatment. Late postoperative choroidal detachments occurring 7 to 21 days after surgery are frequently associated with a persistent wound leak, delayed wound healing, or rupture of an inadequately healed wound. As a rule, the first sign is some shallowing of the anterior chamber. Zonular dialysis may be associated with prior ocular trauma or the ectopia lentis syndromes. Postoperative uveitis is no more common with posterior polar cataracts than with any other type of cataract.

Preferred Response

c. intraoperative capsular rupture

C13

A 25-year-old patient with 6.00 D of preoperative spherical myopia in both eyes is 1 month post eight-incision radial keratotomy (RK) with a 3.0 mm optical zone in the right eye. Her current refractive error is OD −3.75 −2.00 × 175, OS −6.50 −1.00 × 5. Keratometry is 41.75 D/44.50 D × 90° in the right eye. Slit-lamp examination shows excellent depth for the 3 o'clock incision, and approximately 70% for the 9 o'clock incision. The incision depth is difficult to estimate for the other incisions.

The *most* appropriate step would be to

a. perform surgery on her left eye to relieve the anisometropia
b. add eight additional radial keratotomy incisions between the original eight in the right eye
c. obtain computerized video keratography
d. reduce the original optical zone to 2.5 mm with Russian-type out-to-in incisions

Discussion

Adding eight incisions with the same optical clear zone if the original incisions are of adequate depth rarely produces a significant benefit. Surgery on the opposite eye should be deferred until it can be determined whether the patient receives a satisfactory outcome in the first eye. If the original incisions are shallow, further deepening them and also extending the optical zone centrally runs the risk of an overcorrection and increases the risk of disabling glare caused by the smaller optical zone size.

Computerized video keratography can be a valuable aid to surgical planning by pinpointing areas of asymmetrical corneal flattening. Referring the patient to an excimer laser center would be appropriate if the patient showed symmetrical flattening by video keratography and slit-lamp evidence of proper depth for all incisions. Such a patient is most likely an "underresponder" and would be best served by a photorefractive keratectomy (PRK) in the left eye followed later by a PRK in the right eye for her residual myopia.

In this particular patient, the computerized video keratography (see the figure, part A, on page 82) demonstrated flattening over only one incision in the right eye (the 3 o'clock incision). Based on this map, it was elected to redeepen the other seven incisions from approximately a 7.0 mm optical zone into the original 3.0 mm optical zone and to add a single transverse incision at the 6.0 mm optical zone, 2 mm in length along the 90° meridian, between two previously made radial incisions. One month after this reoperation, uncorrected visual acuity was 20/20, the refraction was plano −0.25 × 180, and the video keratography showed symmetrical flattening of her cornea (see the figure, part B).

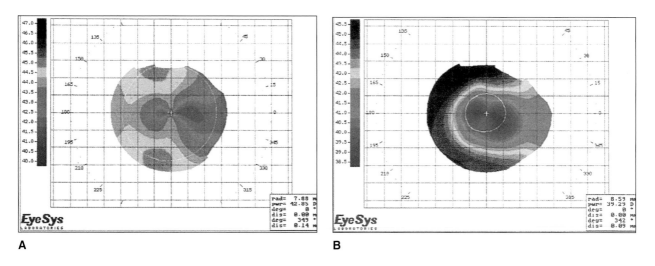

A   **B**

(A) Video keratograph demonstrating flattening only over the 3 o'clock incision following an eight-incision RK in the right eye. (B) Video keratograph demonstrating symmetrical corneal flattening following redeepening of the other seven incisions and a transverse incision at the 90° meridian.

Preferred Response   c. obtain computerized video keratography

C14

The *most* characteristic type of cataract in retinitis pigmentosa is

a. posterior subcapsular cataract
b. anterior polar cataract
c. nuclear sclerotic cataract
d. cortical spoke cataract

Discussion

Posterior subcapsular cataracts are a frequent complication of retinitis pigmentosa (RP) and may be the primary cause of poor central vision. The use of laser acuity meters or laser interferometry may help in differentiating the causes of acuity loss. If careful selection criteria are used, cataract extraction with intraocular lens insertion may improve vision. Unfortunately, in some patients, the retinal disease is too far advanced to warrant cataract surgery. The patient should be cautioned that the potential benefit is to central vision without improvement of the peripheral visual field. The other types of cataracts listed are not characteristic of RP.

Preferred Response   a. posterior subcapsular cataract

C15

Clear corneal cataract incisions can alter corneal curvature by

a. steepening in the meridian of the incision
b. flattening in the meridian of the incision
c. flattening 90° away from the incision
d. flattening the central cornea

Discussion   Clear corneal cataract incisions can function like arcuate incisions used to correct astigmatism. They flatten the cornea in the meridian of the incision and, by virtue of "coupling," steepen the cornea 90° away.[7] This is shown in the figure, part A, where the incision was made at axis 180°. The amount of effect is related to two variables: the size of the optical zone and the length of the incision. Because of these factors, some clear corneal cataract surgeons choose to make the incision on the steep meridian and will choose a PMMA lens rather than a foldable lens for cases of high preoperative cylinder. Temporal incisions under 3.5 mm (foldable IOLs) that are within 0.5 mm to 1.0 mm of the limbus can usually correct no more than 1.25 D. Adding a single matched peripheral arcuate incision 180° away can correct up to two or more diopters of astigmatism. Unsutured incisions of 5.0 mm and greater can correct up to 5.0 D of preexisting cylinder and can produce that much unwanted surgically induced astigmatism; see the figure, part B, where the incision was centered over the 120° axis and induced 3.0 D of flattening.

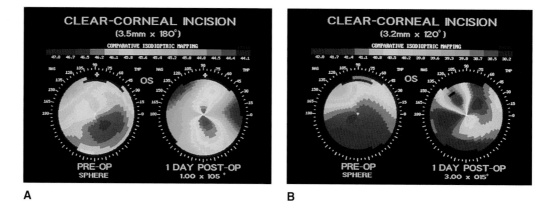

A   **B**

Preoperative and postoperative video keratographs. **(A)** "Coupling" (induced flattening over the clear corneal incision performed at 180° and steepening at 90°). **(B)** Unwanted flattening over a clear corneal incision at 120° with steepening at 15°.

Preferred Response   b. flattening in the meridian of the incision

Which statement is *most* correct regarding endothelial cell loss and phacoemulsification?

a. In-situ (within the lens capsule) phacoemulsification takes longer than nuclear tilt posterior chamber and anterior chamber phacoemulsification and, therefore, results in greater endothelial cell loss.

b. Scleral incisions have the same cell loss as corneal incisions.

c. In-situ phacoemulsification causes less cell loss than techniques involving emulsification of the nucleus anterior to the plane of the anterior capsule or iris.

d. Superior and temporal clear-corneal incisions have the same average cell loss.

Discussion

Studies of endothelial cell loss with phacoemulsification[8,9] have reported the following averages: anterior chamber, 20%; posterior chamber, 14%; in-situ, 7%; intercapsular, 4%. Extracapsular extraction was also reported to average 7% cell loss, approximately that of in-situ phacoemulsification. The reason most widely accepted to explain the decreased cell loss with in-situ phacoemulsification is that the damaging ultrasonic energy is farther away from the endothelium. It was also thought that in-situ phacoemulsification was so far away from the endothelium that the previously known linear relationship between ultrasound time and cell loss seen with both anterior and posterior chamber phacoemulsification no longer applied with in-situ techniques. Indeed, some cases of 15 and 20 minutes of ultrasound were anecdotally reported to have had no cell loss when all of the ultrasound energy was confined below the anterior capsule, such as in the chip-and-flip technique. Superior clear-corneal incisions have demonstrated more cell loss (15% average) than temporal incisions (7% average), theoretically because superior incisions are closer to the central endothelium than the more peripheral and more posterior temporal incisions (see the figure).

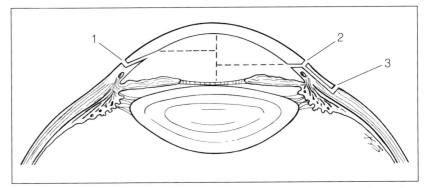

Diagram of corneal incisions demonstrating the more central location of superior vs temporal incisions due to the elliptical shape of the cornea. (1) Superior clear-corneal incision. (2) Temporal clear-corneal incision. (3) Scleral-pocket incision.

Preferred Response

c. In-situ phacoemulsification causes less cell loss than techniques involving emulsification of the nucleus anterior to the plane of the anterior capsule or iris.

Expected postoperative symptoms in the first week following radial keratotomy include all of the following *except*

a. visual fluctuation
b. starbursting
c. foreign-body sensation
d. metamorphopsia

Discussion

During the first few weeks following radial keratotomy (RK), some fluctuation of vision is expected. This is the result of resolving edema around the incision wounds. The edema contributes to increased midperipheral wound gaping; this is reflected topographically as increased midperipheral steepening and concomitant central flattening. The increased flattening, of course, refractively causes reduced convergence power. As the peri-incisional edema resolves, this artifactual flattening diminishes. Refractively, this results in reduced effect of the procedure. Fluctuation of vision may persist for many months due to the normal diurnal fluctuation of corneal edema from a closed-eye to open-eye state.

Both starbursting and halos are seen after RK. They appear to be the result of the (expected) prolonged time of corneal incision wound healing. Most patients experience these phenomena on the first day postoperatively along with a foreign-body sensation from the incisions. Usually, they will diminish significantly over a period of several weeks to months. Rarely, they may persist indefinitely. Metamorphopsia is an uncommon complication of radial keratotomy.

Preferred Response   d. metamorphopsia

You are asked to examine a 42-year-old engineer who does most of his work at near with a computer. He is a –6.50 D myope. You decide that he is a good candidate for radial keratotomy (RK). He is not worried about having to wear thin glasses but would like to be less dependent on glasses for his near work.

The *most* appropriate optical treatment for his needs would be to

a. fully correct him with RK for emmetropia
b. perform RK and tangential cuts (T-cuts) at 180° to induce with-the-rule cylinder and a multifocal cornea
c. undercorrect him by 1 D in both eyes
d. make him slightly hyperopic in one eye and myopic in the other

Discussion   This patient would be best served by undercorrecting him by a diopter in both eyes. This would be to his advantage for two reasons. First, it would minimize the effect of progressive hyperopic shift, such as occurred in 24% of patients in the Prospective Evaluation of Radial Keratotomy (PERK) study when measured from 6 months to 4 years postoperatively.[10] Eyes with larger amounts of preoperative myopia and smaller diameters of the clear zone were more likely to have an increasing effect of the surgery. The entire PERK study group on average had a 0.1 D shift per year. If this rate is held constant over a decade, all patients would have 1 D of hyperopic shift in a decade. For this reason, particularly in a high myope, it seems reasonable to deliberately undercorrect. The second advantage is that this patient prefers to be in better focus at near. Deliberately undercorrecting might eliminate his dependency on glasses for near work and would enhance patient satisfaction. T-cuts are not indicated because there is no preoperative astigmatism. Making him slightly hyperopic in one eye and myopic in the other would create anisometropia and would be poorly tolerated by this myopic patient.

Preferred Response   c. undercorrect him by 1 D in both eyes

At the conclusion of cataract extraction, an inferior zonular dialysis of approximately 90° is noted. The capsule is otherwise completely intact without a tear or rent. Which of the following statements concerning intraocular lens insertion in this situation is *most* correct?

a. The patient should receive no intraocular lens, since any lens is likely to dislocate.
b. Any appropriate intraocular lens may be inserted into the capsule, and the preferred orientation of the long axis of the implant is horizontal (perpendicular to the axis of the dialysis).
c. A single or multipiece PMMA IOL may be inserted into the ciliary sulcus, and the preferred orientation of the long axis of the implant is vertical (in the axis of the dialysis).
d. A single or multipiece PMMA IOL may be inserted into the ciliary sulcus, and the preferred orientation of the long axis of the implant is horizontal (perpendicular to the axis of the dialysis).

Discussion

In cases of a zonular dialysis that is equal to or less than 180° in extent, many patients will do well with intraocular lenses placed into the capsule. A longer, stiffer lens with a larger optic might be less prone to decentration or to visual symptomatology from mild degrees of decentration. Most surgeons recommend that the long axis of the implant be placed in the axis of the dialysis, ie, the haptics should be placed in the axis of the dialysis; this might prevent or minimize decentration by resisting contraction of the capsule. Placement of the implant into the ciliary sulcus is also possible. If this method of fixation is selected, however, the long axis of the implant should be placed perpendicular to the axis of the dialysis. If the implant is placed so the haptic(s) are in the region of the dialysis, decentration of the implant may occur, and this decentration will be in the direction of the dialysis.

Preferred Response

d. A single or multipiece PMMA IOL may be inserted into the ciliary sulcus, and the preferred orientation of the long axis of the implant is horizontal (perpendicular to the axis of the dialysis).

C20

Two years after uncomplicated phacoemulsification performed through a scleral corneal tunnel, the patient is noted to have the complication shown in the figure.

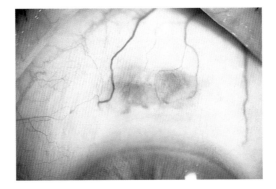

Scleral melting in area of previous superior scleral wound 2 years after uneventful cataract surgery.

The *most* appropriate course of action at this time would be

a. freehand graft with banked scleral tissue
b. diagnostic workup for a collagen vascular disease
c. suturing of the defect with 10-0 nylon sutures
d. placement of a hydrophilic bandage contact lens

Discussion   Scleral melting, or necrotizing scleritis, is a rare sequela to ocular surgery with potentially devastating consequences to the eye. O'Donoghue et al noted an associated underlying medical disorder in 63% of patients with postoperative scleral melting.[11] The most common among these was the group of collagen vascular disorders, especially rheumatoid arthritis. In most cases the onset of scleral necrosis is not in the immediate postoperative period but occurs months to years following surgery (usually cataract surgery but also strabismus, trabeculectomy, and retinal detachment surgery). Postsurgical necrotizing scleritis is believed to be due to an immunologic response. The treatment of choice is immediate high-dose corticosteroids and cytotoxic agents as necessary; the patient is usually co-managed with an internist familiar with these drugs and their side effects.[12] Surgical intervention is reserved for cases that progress despite adequate immunosuppressive therapy. In this patient, a workup for collagen vascular disease is the most appropriate course of action. Scleral patch grafting and resuturing of the wound should be undertaken only if the necrosis progresses despite adequate immunosuppression. In active necrotizing scleritis, suture closure and patch grafting are difficult due to the friable and necrotic tissue margins. A bandage contact lens has no role in limiting the necrosis.[11,12]

Preferred Response   b. diagnostic workup for a collagen vascular disease

Sunrise syndrome is shown in the figure.

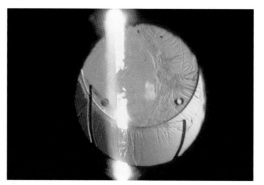

Sunrise syndrome with superior dislocation of the posterior chamber intraocular lens.

This syndrome is *most* likely caused by

a. an ovoid posterior capsulotomy
b. phacoemulsification of the lens nucleus
c. one lens haptic in the capsular bag and one lens haptic in the ciliary sulcus
d. reduced optic dimension

Discussion

Sunrise syndrome occurs when the IOL optic is displaced superiorly, out of the visual axis. One cause of this problem is placement of the inferior haptic within the bag and placement of the superior haptic within the sulcus. With contraction of the capsular bag, the inferior haptic is pushed upward, since there is no resistance from the capsule superiorly. Another cause of this problem is inferior zonular disinsertion with an in-the-bag placement of a flexible-haptic posterior chamber lens. The fibrosis of the capsule drags the optic superiorly, until the edge of the optic is in or above the visual axis. Finally, a disruption of the superior zonules when the inferior haptic is in the bag and the superior haptic is through the disinsertion will also cause a sunrise syndrome as contraction of the bag forces the superior haptic through the disinsertion.[1] The shape of a posterior capsulotomy does not affect capsular contraction dynamics or dislocations in an x or y axis. Phacoemulsification similarly does not affect IOL dislocations. A small-optic IOL may decenter slightly within an intact contracting capsule, but not to the degree seen in the figure.

Preferred Response

c. one lens haptic in the capsular bag and one lens haptic in the ciliary sulcus

C22

All of the following statements are true *except*

a. The cornea flattens directly over any sutured incision.
b. The central cornea steepens adjacent to tight limbal sutures.
c. The normal cornea steepens over any incision.
d. Tissue removal produces corneal flattening over the site of tissue removal, whether traumatic or surgically induced.

Discussion

The normal cornea flattens over any incision. This effect is attributable to gaping of the wound. A corneal incision slices through the corneal lamella, and intraocular pressure spreads the edges apart. This increases the radius of curvature of the cornea across the incision and flattens the cornea. The incision heals with a greater surface area, creating a microwedge addition. This concept provides the basis for incisional refractive surgery. Tight corneal sutures have the effect of flattening the cornea over the sutures but steepening the cornea central to the tight sutures. This insight is helpful in the modification of astigmatism by cutting (removing) overly tight sutures. Tissue removal acts as a large relaxing incision with increased gaping due to the loss of substance. Hence, the cornea will flatten over the site of the tissue removal.

Preferred Response

c. The normal cornea steepens over any incision.

C23

Which of the following statements regarding radial keratotomy (RK) and photorefractive keratectomy (PRK) and regression of effect is *most* accurate?

a. Regression of effect following refractive surgery for myopia implies that the refractive result shifts toward hyperopia. This finding is more profound after PRK.
b. Regression of effect following refractive surgery for myopia implies that the refractive result shifts toward hyperopia. This finding is more profound after RK.
c. Regression of effect following refractive surgery for myopia implies that the refractive result shifts toward myopia. This finding is more profound after PRK.
d. Regression of effect following refractive surgery for myopia implies that the refractive result shifts toward myopia. This finding is more profound after RK.

Discussion

Both RK and PRK can cause some regression of effect. In RK this is usually during the first week and is a result of edema around the incision wound. The edema contributes to increased midperipheral wound gaping, increased midperipheral steepening, and central flattening. As the edema resolves, this flattening is reduced, decreasing the overall effect and causing a shift toward myopia or away from hyperopia.

In PRK, the epithelium is replaced over the first month following the procedure. As the epithelial thickness is reestablished, the cornea steepens, thereby reducing the amount of corneal flattening and shifting the refraction toward myopia. This shift is much more profound in PRK than it is in RK and is particularly exaggerated when excess scarring occurs with subepithelial fibrosis, as seen in some PRK patients. Regression of effect in PRK has been noted as long as 12 to 18 months following the procedure.

Preferred Response

c. Regression of effect following refractive surgery for myopia implies that the refractive result shifts toward myopia. This finding is more profound after PRK.

C24

All of the following statements about the advantages of a continuous curvilinear capsulorhexis (CCC) are true *except*

a. It decreases posterior capsular opacification.
b. It makes removal of residual cortex by aspiration easier.
c. It eases and assures in-the-bag IOL implantation.
d. It allows hydrodissection of the nucleus without fear of anterior rim tear extension to the equator.

Discussion

Continuous curvilinear capsulorhexis (CCC) represents a major advance in small-incision cataract surgery.[13] An intact capsulorhexis allows hydrodissection of the nucleus and facilitates in-the-bag posterior chamber phacoemulsification. Removal of the cortex is facilitated because anterior capsular flaps are not continually caught in the aspirating port, and capsular tears that could extend to the equator are eliminated. CCC has no effect on posterior capsular opacification.

Preferred Response

a. It decreases posterior capsular opacification.

Which of the following statements regarding front-cutting and back-cutting diamond micrometer knives set at *identical* blade depths is true?

  a. The front-cutting knife (passed from the limbus toward the center optical zone, or uphill) will achieve a greater depth of cut centrally than the back-cutting knife (passed from the center optical zone to the limbus, or downhill).
  b. The back-cutting knife (passed from the center optical zone to the limbus, or downhill) will achieve a greater depth of cut centrally than the front-cutting knife (passed from the limbus toward the center optical zone, or uphill).
  c. The knives will achieve equal-depth cuts.
  d. Accidental invasion into the center optical zone is more frequent with a back-cutting knife (passed from the optical zone to the limbus) than a front-cutting knife (passed from the limbus toward the optical zone).

Discussion   Radically different vector forces are generated by the differing incision methods of a front-cutting (centripetal, Russian) incision as compared to a back-cutting (centrifugal, American) incision. In the front-cutting incision, the vertical diamond edge creates the incision. The vector of the resultant forces is parallel to the tissue plane, thus resulting in little or no resistance to or displacement of the knife blade relative to the tissue, enabling the tendency for uniformly deep incisions. In a back-cutting incision, the diamond's angled (downhill) margin creates the incisional cut. The forces exerted by the diamond upon the tissue as well as the equal and opposite forces exerted by the tissue upon the diamond are oriented at an oblique angle relative to the tissue plane. This oblique orientation serves to resist or displace the diamond blade, thus resulting in more shallow incisions (see the figures). Since the surgeon is moving away from the optical zone using a back-cutting knife, the chance of invasion into the optical zone is less than when working from the limbus toward the center with a front-cutting knife.

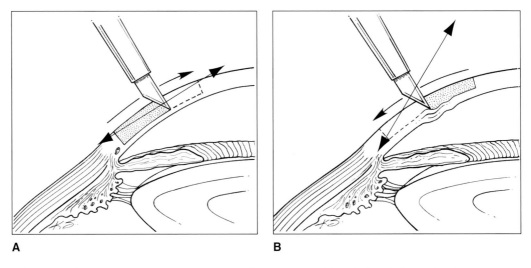

A   **B**

(A) Russian (front-cutting) incision showing no displacement of the blade relative to the tissue.
(B) American (back-cutting) incision showing displacement of the blade relative to the tissue and, hence, a more shallow incision.

Preferred Response

a. The front-cutting knife (passed from the limbus toward the center optical zone, or uphill) will achieve a greater depth of cut centrally than the back-cutting knife (passed from the center optical zone to the limbus, or downhill).

A 50-year-old man with 20/400 uncorrected visual acuity (VA) underwent refractive surgery for a −4.50 +0.75 × 96 refractive error. The surgical plan included a four-incision radial keratotomy with incisions performed at 12, 6, 9, and 3 o'clock and an optical zone of 3.75 mm. At 6 weeks postoperatively, his uncorrected VA was 20/60 with a refraction of −2.00 +0.75 × 85. His manifest VA was 20/15. He desired an enhancement to improve his uncorrected visual acuity. His postoperative corneal topography is shown in the figure.

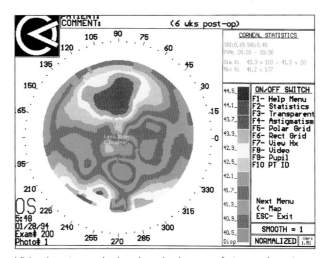

Video keratograph showing single area of steepening at 12 o'clock incision (red).

What is the enhancement procedure of choice?

a. The patient is undercorrected (spherical equivalent −1.75 OD) and needs all radial incisions lengthened to decrease the RK optical zone to 3.00 mm.

b. The astigmatism has not been corrected, and tangential cuts (T-cuts) need to be added.

c. The radial incision at 12 o'clock is less effective and needs to be redeepened.

d. The patient is undercorrected with persistent astigmatism and needs radial incisions redeepened and/or lengthened as well as a T-cut at 12 o'clock.

Discussion

The central aspect of the radial incision at 12 o'clock is probably short and shallow. This is demonstrated on the video keratograph in the figure where areas of flattening (blue) are seen over the incisions nasally, temporally, and inferiorly but steepening (red) is noted superiorly. Careful biomicroscopic examination confirmed this problem. Enhancement should be directed at redeepening the 12 o'clock incision and possibly lengthening this incision if it is felt to be short. Decreasing the optical zone to 3 mm would also reduce residual myopia but requires more surgery with the potential of increased complications (glare, perforation, invasion into the optical zone). Astigmatism of 1 D or less is usually well tolerated and, as the myopia (and spherical equivalent) is reduced, should not cause a significant reduction in visual acuity.

Preferred Response

c. The radial incision at 12 o'clock is less effective and needs to be redeepened.

C27

A 37-year-old contact-lens–intolerant patient who is actively involved in scuba diving and skiing and "hates wearing glasses" is interested in refractive surgery. The refractive error in his right eye is $-1.25 +2.50 \times 75$. The refraction in his other eye is similar. He is highly motivated to have his astigmatism corrected.

Which of the following is the most appropriate approach to this patient's needs?

a. Refer him to an excimer laser center.
b. Perform a four-incision radial keratotomy with a 4.0 mm optical zone and two transverse incisions along the 75° axis.
c. Determine the spherical equivalent before planning his surgery.
d. Perform two arcuate incisions in the 165° axis.

Discussion

Because the spherical equivalent is plano, radial keratotomy incisions would most likely induce hyperopia, which would be poorly tolerated in this prepresbyopic patient. It is therefore a mistake to consider him a –1.25 D myope, as neophyte refractive surgeons sometimes do when planning astigmatism surgery. The patient is *not* an appropriate candidate for an astigmatic excimer laser ablation, which might actually cause some flattening of both meridians, again possibly with a hyperopic result. This patient *is* an ideal candidate for an arcuate or transverse keratectomy. Tangential incisions of 3 mm to 4 mm in length and arcuate incisions of 30° to 45° not only flatten the meridian of the incision but also tend to produce steepening of the meridian 90° away. This phenomenon is called "coupling." The correct axis for the incisions is at 75°, not 165° (see the figure).

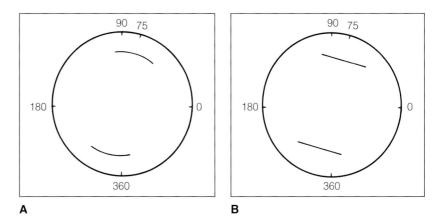

A   B

Paired arcuate incisions **(A)** and tangential incisions (T-cuts) **(B)** to correct astigmatism in the 75° meridian.

Preferred Response   c. Determine the spherical equivalent before planning his surgery.

All of the following factors have been shown to affect the outcome of radial keratotomy significantly *except*

a. patient age
b. number of incisions
c. keratometry
d. optical zone diameter

Discussion   The Prospective Evaluation of Radial Keratotomy (PERK) study and other studies have reported that incision depth, incision number, optical zone diameter, and patient age all significantly affect the outcome of radial keratotomy.[10] In fact, current radial keratotomy techniques take into account each of these factors (assuming consistently deep incisions at the optical zone border) in preoperative planning. These same studies demonstrated only minimal effect of scleral rigidity, intraocular pressure, keratometry, and corneal diameter on the procedure's outcome.

Preferred Response   c. keratometry

Phacoemulsification is performed after the creation of a continuous, circular capsulotomy. At the completion of nucleus and cortex removal, a radial anterior capsular tear is noted at 6 o'clock, and the posterior capsule appears to be intact.

In this situation, which of the following statements is *least* correct?

a. A multipiece foldable IOL can be placed in the capsular bag.
b. A single-piece (plate) foldable IOL can be placed in the capsular bag.
c. A three-piece or one-piece polymethylmethacrylate (PMMA) IOL can be placed in the capsular bag.
d. A three-piece or one-piece PMMA IOL can be placed in the ciliary sulcus.

Discussion   A multipiece foldable IOL can be placed in the capsular bag. Since these lenses do not rotate after insertion, they will not escape into the ciliary sulcus. Placement of a multipiece foldable (silicone) IOL into the ciliary sulcus is also possible, but no data exist to substantiate safety. Single-piece (plate) foldable IOLs should not be implanted in patients who do not have an intact, continuous, circular capsulotomy, as these lenses may migrate and escape into the ciliary sulcus. These lenses should not be placed into the ciliary sulcus, because pseudophacodonesis will occur with current designs, and pigment release and/or recurrent iritis may ensue. A one-piece or three-piece PMMA IOL may be placed into the capsular sac or ciliary sulcus. If inserted into the sulcus, horizontal positioning in this patient would be preferable because the radial anterior capsular tear may have extended into the peripheral (unseen) posterior capsule and vertical placement of the IOL within the sulcus could result in the postoperative development of a sunset syndrome.

Preferred Response   b. A single-piece (plate) foldable IOL can be placed in the capsular bag.

A patient presents with a decrease in vision. As you shake hands with him, you note that his hands have prominent knuckles and short, stubby fingers (see the figure, part A). On ocular examination, you note a mildly cataractous lens shortened in its horizontal and vertical dimensions and slightly increased in its anteroposterior dimension (see the figure, part B). Additionally, the lens is slightly dislocated inferiorly.

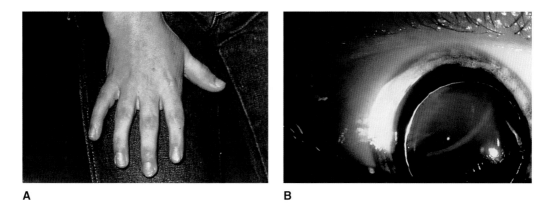

A   B

(A) Hand demonstrating short, stubby fingers with prominent knuckles in a patient with Weill-Marchesani syndrome. **(B)** Spherophakia and lens dislocation in a patient with Weill-Marchesani syndrome.

The *most* likely diagnosis is

a. osteogenesis imperfecta
b. Weill-Marchesani syndrome
c. Marfan syndrome
d. homocystinuria

Discussion

The Weill-Marchesani syndrome (spherophakia-brachymorphia syndrome) occurs as an autosomal recessive trait and ranks third behind Marfan syndrome and homocystinuria as a cause for dislocated lenses on a hereditary basis. The musculoskeletal system shows characteristic brachymorphia characterized by short stature, short hands with spade-like, stubby fingers, prominent knuckles, and knobby interphalangeal joints (see the figure, part A). The ocular findings are the most prominent and disabling part of the disease. The lens approaches sphericity (see the figure, part B). The small, round lens commonly dislocates and may move either up, down, anteriorly, or posteriorly. Cataract formation is common, and the zonules are elongated and irregular. Lens extraction often becomes necessary because of cataract formation or pupillary-block glaucoma due to lens dislocation. Surgical complications are common due to laxity and loss of the zonules. Homocystinuria and Marfan syndrome are both associated with ectopia lentis but affected patients have long and slender musculoskeletal findings, in contrast to patients with Weill-Marchesani syndrome. Cardiovascular problems (heart block) are also seen in Marfan patients. The triad of brittle bones, blue scleras, and deafness makes up the syndrome of osteogenesis imperfecta.

Preferred Response

b. Weill-Marchesani syndrome

Six weeks after phacoemulsification with implantation of a 12.0 mm overall length single-piece (plate) silicone foldable posterior chamber lens implant, an Nd:YAG laser posterior capsulotomy was performed. Shortly thereafter vision decreased, and the condition shown in the figure was noted on examination.

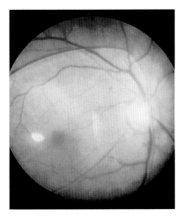

Dislocation of a single-piece silicone IOL into the vitreous.

All of the following factors contributed to this finding *except*

a. implant design
b. implant size
c. timing of the capsulotomy
d. intraocular pressure

Discussion

It has been proposed that the placement of a single-piece silicone intraocular lens in the capsular bag in conjunction with a capsulorhexis provides a snug environment for the lens because of the small anterior opening with a smooth edge, which is more resistant to radial tears than a can-opener capsulotomy. This effect is enhanced by capsular-bag contraction following surgery. Since the single-piece silicone intraocular lens is designed to maximize contact with the posterior capsule, it will have a tendency to redistribute any applied forces posteriorly against the capsule. Unlike the smooth edge created by a capsulorhexis in the anterior capsule, an Nd:YAG laser posterior capsulotomy creates a jagged and irregular opening. If an implant of this design is oversized, significant force will be exerted against the posterior capsule, and posterior radial tears can easily occur. Since the posterior capsule is the main support for this type of implant, the lens is free to dislodge into the vitreous. The implant design, size, and capsulorhexis are then intimately tied to the loss of the lens through a posterior capsular opening. It has been suggested that a longer time period (3 to 6 months) from implantation is necessary before Nd:YAG laser capsulotomy is performed, to allow for complete capsular contraction to occur, minimizing the "expression" of the lens through the posterior capsular opening due to further capsular contraction.[14] Intraocular pressure has no effect on posterior capsular contraction.

Preferred Response

d. intraocular pressure

The change shown in the figure was noted during preoperative evaluation for cataract extraction.

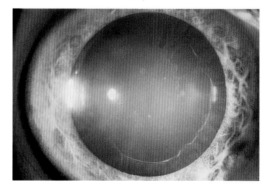

Exfoliation syndrome. Note exfoliative material on the anterior lens capsule.

All of the following statements are true *except*

a. The patient is at risk for spontaneous corneal edema following cataract extraction.
b. The patient is at risk for intraoperative zonular dialysis.
c. This condition is associated with an increased incidence of narrow angles.
d. This condition is associated with open-angle glaucoma.

Discussion

Exfoliation syndrome is characterized by the presence of gray or white flakes on the pupillary margin and anterior lens capsule, increased trabecular meshwork pigmentation, and an association with open-angle glaucoma.[15] Narrow anterior chamber angles may also be seen in this condition. Spontaneous and intraoperative lens dislocation is a less commonly recognized feature of this syndrome and is probably due to weakness of the lens zonules or their attachments to the ciliary processes. Preoperative phacodonesis, asymmetric anterior chamber depth, and excessive lens movement during the anterior capsulotomy should alert the surgeon to the potential for intraoperative zonular dialysis. Patients with exfoliation syndrome are not at particular risk for postoperative corneal edema.

Preferred Response

a. The patient is at risk for spontaneous corneal edema following cataract extraction.

A patient presents with the condition shown in the figure. Following your examination, you decide that the cataract will be removed using a phacoemulsification technique.

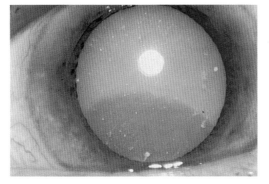

Morgagnian cataract showing liquefied cortex and inferiorly displaced nucleus.

Which of the following steps in the procedure will be the easiest to perform?

a. anterior capsulorhexis
b. nuclear cracking
c. nucleus emulsification
d. aspiration of cortex

Discussion

In a morgagnian cataract (see the figure), the cortex is liquefied and often opaque. Capsulorhexis is difficult because visualization is poor, and there is little underlying support to provide appropriate countertraction for gentle, controlled capsular tearing. The nucleus is often hard and therefore difficult to emulsify. The nucleus is also very mobile because of inadequate surrounding cortical support. Typically, little direct cortical aspiration is required because the liquefied cortex is removed during the early phases of the emulsification.

Preferred Response

d. aspiration of cortex

For chemical preparation of the eye prior to ophthalmic surgery, which of the following is *most* effective in decreasing the bacterial flora of the conjunctiva without causing ocular surface toxicity?

a. a mild silver protein solution (Argyrol)
b. 5% (half-strength) povidone-iodine (Betadine) solution
c. 5% (half-strength) povidone-iodine (Betadine) solution followed by irrigation of the conjunctival fornix with saline
d. 5% povidone-iodine (Betadine) scrub/soap

Discussion

Half-strength povidone-iodine (Betadine) solution has been proven to be the most effective chemical preparation for the eye prior to ophthalmic surgery.[16] Povidone-iodine scrub/soap, on the other hand, is toxic to the epithelial surface and causes a mild chemical burn. Irrigation of the fornix with saline increases bacterial flora counts of the conjunctiva by liberating organisms from the conjunctival folds within the fornix. Argyrol solution does not have a significant antibacterial effect on the conjunctiva. Chlorhexidine (Hibiclens) soap, commonly used as a hand-washing scrub prior to surgical procedures, is also toxic to the ocular surface and should not be used in the chemical preparation of the eye prior to surgery.

Preferred Response

b. 5% (half-strength) povidone-iodine (Betadine) solution

C35

The two posterior chamber intraocular lenses shown in the figure have optics and haptics made of polymethylmethacrylate (PMMA). They are of equal overall length (13.0 mm) and identical power (21.0 D). The only difference between the two lenses is that the optic of the left lens is 5 mm × 6 mm in diameter (oval) and the optic of the right lens is 7.0 mm in diameter (round).

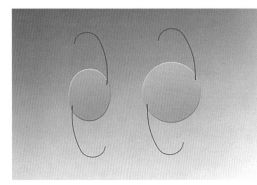

A 5 mm x 6 mm oval optic PMMA IOL (left) and a 7.0 mm round optic PMMA IOL (right).

All of the following statements are true *except*

a. The refractive index of these two lens optics is identical.
b. The center thickness of the round lens is greater than that of the oval lens.
c. The center thickness of the oval lens is less than the center thickness of a 6 mm round PMMA optic of the same dioptric power.
d. Both of these lenses will fit into the capsular bag.

Discussion

A 5 mm × 6 mm oval intraocular lens has the same thickness as a 6 mm round intraocular lens. An oval lens can be best thought of as a round lens with two of the sides cut off to make an oval. The diameter determines the overall thickness of the lens. A larger diameter lens will be thicker than a lens of identical power but smaller diameter. This is shown in the figure below, a scanning electron micrograph of two lenses of identical power. The top lens is an oval optic 5 mm × 6 mm in diameter and the bottom lens is a 5.5 mm round optic. It is clear that the overall thickness of the 5 mm × 6 mm oval is greater than the 5.5 mm round lens even though there is only one-half millimeter difference in the optic diameter. The refractive index of any material is identical regardless of differences in optic size and configuration.

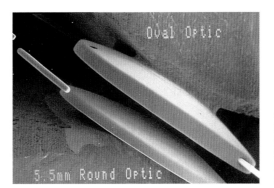

A scanning electron micrograph showing the difference in thickness of a 5.5 mm round optic IOL (bottom) and 5 mm x 6 mm oval optic IOL.

Preferred Response

c. The center thickness of the oval lens is less than the center thickness of a 6 mm round PMMA optic of the same dioptric power.

C36

All of the following statements about extracapsular cataract extraction in a patient with diabetes mellitus are true *except*

a. Cataract extraction is highly associated with progression of nonproliferative retinopathy in the operated eye.
b. Patients with preexisting nonproliferative diabetic retinopathy have a worse visual prognosis than those without retinopathy.
c. Overweight women with diabetes have a significantly worse visual outcome than patients with normal body weight and diabetes.
d. The cataract procedure of choice in diabetic patients is a small-incision phacoemulsification in which a 5.0 mm optic IOL is placed through a similarly sized capsulorhexis opening into the capsular bag.

Discussion

Patients with symmetric nonproliferative retinopathy who underwent extracapsular cataract extraction and intraocular lens implantation were followed postoperatively to determine the incidence of progression of diabetic retinopathy, visual acuity, and factors predictive of progression of retinopathy in final visual acuity.[17] Progression of retinopathy, defined as development of clinically significant macular edema and an increase in intraretinal hemorrhages or hard exudate, was assessed. Cataract extraction was highly associated with asymmetric progression of nonproliferative retinopathy; progression occurred only in the operated eye in 7 of 19 patients (37%), but in no patients did progression occur in the fellow eye alone. Women had a significantly increased risk of progression, and overweight women had a significantly worse visual outcome than those patients with normal body weight.

Because of the increase in diabetic retinopathy following cataract extraction and intraocular lens implantation, large-optic intraocular lenses should be placed at the time of surgery with large capsulorhexis openings to allow adequate peripheral visualization for panretinal photocoagulation, which may be necessary months to years following the procedure.

Preferred Response

d. The cataract procedure of choice in diabetic patients is a small-incision phacoemulsification in which a 5.0 mm optic IOL is placed through a similarly sized capsulorhexis opening into the capsular bag.

Phacolytic glaucoma is characterized by all of the following *except*

a. a visible break in the lens capsule with inflammation around the lens material
b. a unilateral red eye with diffuse corneal edema
c. an elevated intraocular pressure in the presence of a mature or hypermature cataract
d. a deep anterior chamber with circulating large, white, clumped cells

Discussion

Phacolytic glaucoma presents with a unilateral red eye, diffuse corneal edema, and elevated intraocular pressure in the presence of a mature or hypermature cataract. Lens protein leaks from a mature or hypermature cataract without a break in the lens capsule.[18] The circulating large, white cells seen in phacolytic glaucoma represent foamy macrophages that have ingested the leaking lens protein. Phacoanaphylactic endophthalmitis is a unilateral zonal, granulomatous inflammation around lens material and is dependent on a ruptured lens capsule for its development.

Preferred Response

a. a visible break in the lens capsule with inflammation around the lens material

C38

All of the following statements regarding peribulbar anesthesia are true *except*

a. Globe perforation with peribulbar anesthesia is not possible.
b. Peribulbar anesthesia can be performed with needles that are shorter than those that are required for retrobulbar anesthesia.
c. Supplemental anesthesia may be required.
d. Subdural injection is less common with a peribulbar technique than with a retrobulbar technique.

Discussion

Peribulbar anesthesia has fewer serious complications than retrobulbar anesthesia and usually does not cause a profound loss of vision. Because the needle does not enter the muscle cone, subdural injection is virtually impossible. Because the peribulbar injection can be made in any of the four quadrants, perforation of the globe is possible and has been anecdotally reported. A shorter needle is utilized to avoid a conal injection, and adequate anesthesia and akinesia is achieved in most instances. Supplemental anesthesia by repeat peribulbar or retrobulbar injection is required in some cases.[19–21]

Preferred Response

a. Globe perforation with peribulbar anesthesia is not possible.

C39

Indications for small-incision phacoemulsification surgery through a temporal clear-corneal incision under topical anesthesia include all of the following *except*

a. a patient on warfarin (Coumadin) therapy for valvular heart disease
b. an uncooperative patient with a history of psychosis
c. a monocular patient with glaucoma and a functioning superior filtering bleb
d. a patient with recurrent but now quiescent cicatricial ocular pemphigoid

Discussion

Temporal clear-corneal incisions under topical anesthesia minimize the chance of any bleeding complications, including retrobulbar hemorrhage during a retrobulbar block and periocular ecchymoses during a peribulbar block. In addition, conjunctival and scleral bleeding is avoided. Similarly, anesthesia risks are minimized in a monocular patient if topical anesthesia is utilized, and manipulation of the sclera and conjunctiva is avoided with a clear-corneal incision in the presence of a functioning filtering bleb. Inflammation is also minimized using a clear-corneal approach, which reduces postoperative exacerbations of cicatricial ocular pemphigoid following cataract extraction. An uncooperative patient is a contraindication to topical anesthesia because unwanted eye movement at inappropriate times may lead to serious complications. In general, most cataract procedures can be done through a scleral tunnel incision; however, under certain circumstances clear-corneal incisions can be advantageous.

Preferred Response

b. an uncooperative patient with a history of psychosis

C40

All of the following are risk factors in developing an expulsive suprachoroidal hemorrhage *except*

a. axial length greater than or equal to 26.0 mm
b. a history of glaucoma
c. intraoperative pulse greater than or equal to 85 beats per minute
d. an isolated traumatic cataract after remote trauma

Discussion

Intraoperative suprachoroidal hemorrhage is an uncommon event with a reported incidence of 0.05% to 0.8%. Statistically significant risk factors for suprachoroidal expulsive hemorrhage in one age-adjusted analysis included glaucoma, increased axial length, elevated intraocular pressure, generalized atherosclerosis, and elevated intraoperative pulse.[22] Attention to multiple preoperative and intraoperative ocular and systemic variables may allow identification of patients at risk for suprachoroidal expulsive hemorrhage so that appropriate preventive measures may be instituted.

Preferred Response

d. an isolated traumatic cataract after remote trauma

Which of the following is *least* likely to be a complication of the procedure shown in the figure?

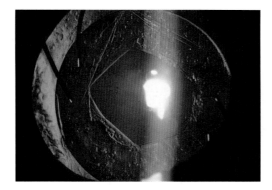

Central posterior capsular opening following an Nd:YAG posterior capsulotomy.

a. increased intraocular pressure
b. acute angle-closure glaucoma
c. retinal detachment
d. cystoid macular edema

Discussion

Opacification of the posterior capsule is a consequence of extracapsular cataract surgery. As the opacification increases, the patient begins to notice a decrease in visual function that can lead to functional impairment. The time of onset of opacification after cataract surgery is quite variable. Based on current literature, the rate in the first 2 years after surgery appears to be less than 25%.[23] The major complications of Nd:YAG laser posterior capsulotomy include elevated intraocular pressure, rupture of the hyaloid face, retinal detachment, cystoid macular edema, damage to the intraocular lens, hyphema, dislocation of the intraocular lens, and corneal edema.[24,25]

Preferred Response

b. acute angle-closure glaucoma

Which of the following statements regarding preoperative testing in a patient with biomicroscopic evidence of cataract is *most* accurate?

a. Contrast sensitivity will help differentiate between visual loss due to the cataract and visual loss from a macular problem.
b. In a patient with good Snellen acuity and complaints of glare, glare testing should be performed as part of the preoperative evaluation.
c. In eyes with opaque media and vision of 20/200 or worse, potential visual acuity testing with interferometry provides an accurate estimate of visual outcome and should be performed.
d. Patients at risk for corneal decompensation from surgery are often difficult to identify through history and clinical examination. Specular microscopy should be routinely performed in patients anticipating cataract extraction by phacoemulsification.

Discussion

It is reasonable to perform a glare test as part of the evaluation of patients who complain of glare, have symptoms potentially attributable to glare, or who have a cataract (particularly a posterior subcapsular cataract) and good Snellen acuity. However, glare testing should not be required by utilization review or quality assessment organizations (eg, peer review organizations) as objective documentation of visual disability sufficient to justify the potential benefit of surgery. Glare testing is not useful in patients with cataract who do not complain of symptoms potentially attributable to glare regardless of their visual acuity. Contrast sensitivity testing does not differentiate between visual loss due to cataract and visual loss from other causes. Also, in eyes with opaque media and vision of 20/200 or worse, none of the tests of potential vision provide an accurate estimate of visual outcome after uncomplicated cataract surgery. Electrophysiologic tests may, however, be useful in determining whether light signals are being received by the retina or brain. Evidence is also lacking in the published literature that potential vision measurement increases the accuracy of the predicted outcome beyond that based on history and ocular examination alone. There is currently no evidence in the published literature and no compelling rationale to support routine use of specular microscopy in patients for whom cataract surgery is being considered. Most patients at risk of corneal decompensation can be identified through history and clinical examination.[23]

Preferred Response

b. In a patient with good Snellen acuity and complaints of glare, glare testing should be performed as part of the preoperative evaluation.

C43

Three months following transscleral fixation of a secondary posterior chamber intraocular lens, the patient returns to your office complaining of foreign-body sensation in the operative eye. Slit-lamp examination reveals the condition shown in the figure on page 104.

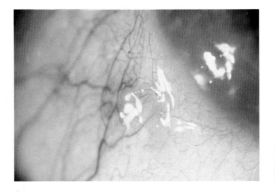

Exposure of a transscleral polypropylene suture barb through the conjunctiva.

All of the following statements are true *except*

a. This complication could have been avoided if the polypropylene knot and loop had been buried under a scleral flap.
b. This patient is at risk for endophthalmitis.
c. The suture should not be cut and removed, since IOL dislocation would be likely.
d. A return to the operating room is often necessary to rebury the exposed knot or barb.

Discussion

Transscleral fixation of a posterior chamber intraocular lens has a number of theoretical advantages over anterior chamber intraocular lenses. These include avoiding contact of the intraocular lens with the corneal endothelium and trabecular meshwork. Iris contact is minimized, and the procedure is more applicable in cases of distorted pupils, sector iridectomies, and disrupted anterior segments. Disadvantages include intraocular lens dislocation by suture slippage off of the haptics, technical difficulty, and erosion of the polypropylene suture through scleral and conjunctival flaps.

In a recent series, scleral flaps were performed at the time of surgery to bury polypropylene sutures holding the posterior chamber intraocular lens in place. All (100%) of these sutures had eroded through the scleral flap at one year.[26] Exposure of a polypropylene knot through the conjunctiva predisposes the patient to endophthalmitis, since the suture can act as a wick for bacteria to enter the inner eye from the external environment.[27] When an exposed knot is noted clinically, it should be repaired. Thermal cautery can often be used to melt the polypropylene, which will retract beneath the conjunctiva. If this is unsuccessful, it is often necessary to bring the patient to the operating room to dissect the suture free from the conjunctiva and rebury it. Occasionally, a piece of donor cornea is used to cover the exposed knot, assuring that erosion will not occur again.[28] Cutting the polypropylene suture and removing it will most likely cause the intraocular lens to dislocate, since very little fibrosis occurs, especially in the first 3 months postoperatively.

Preferred Response

a. This complication could have been avoided if the polypropylene knot and loop had been buried under a scleral flap.

In the early postoperative period, superior corneal edema near the incision and the complication shown in the figure are noted during slit-lamp examination.

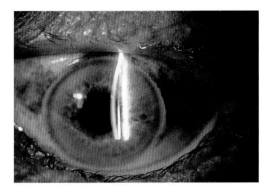

Superior Descemet's detachment.

Which of the following is *least* likely to be a cause of this complication?

a. improper introduction of the phacoemulsification tip
b. faulty or difficult insertion of the intraocular lens
c. poor wound closure
d. improper introduction of the irrigation/aspiration tip

Discussion

The figure shows a stripped Descemet's membrane. Improper introduction of any surgical instrument or cannula into the eye may catch Descemet's membrane at the incision site and strip it downward. This is frequently seen with the silastic sleeves on irrigation/aspiration (I/A) or phacoemulsification needles. Faulty intraocular lens implantation may also cause stripping of Descemet's membrane as the leading edge of the implant comes into contact with the internal wound.

Preferred Response

c. poor wound closure

Which of the following statements about refractive surgery is true?

a. Excimer photorefractive keratectomy is effective only for the reduction of myopia.
b. The effect of radial keratotomy decreases with increasing patient age.
c. Keratomileusis in situ (automated lamellar keratectomy, or ALK) can effectively reduce myopia and hyperopia.
d. Astigmatic arcuate incisions cause an overall flattening of the cornea and hence reduce not only astigmatism but also myopia.

Discussion

Keratomileusis in situ (automated lamellar keratectomy, or ALK) is a lamellar refractive surgical procedure developed in Colombia. It involves the use of a microkeratome to make a planar, lamellar resection of corneal stroma. Refractive changes can be effected in two ways. For myopia, a two-step procedure is used. First, a relatively large diameter, shallow resection is performed. This first lenticule (as it is called) is saved or a hinge is created. The second step involves a second resection of smaller diameter (also shallow). This second lenticule is discarded. The first lenticule is replaced and secured by drying or sutures. The result is a thinner central area, thus, a flatter central curvature and decreased convergence power (decreased myopia). For hyperopia, a single deep resection is performed. The lenticule is then replaced. The refractive effect is achieved because the deep resection results in steepening of the thin remaining central stroma. The replaced lenticule, secured only by air drying, conforms to this steep curvature. Thus, the central anterior corneal curvature is steepened and the hyperopia is reduced. Radial keratotomy flattens the central curvature and thus is not effective for hyperopia. Additionally, the effect of this procedure increases with increasing patient age. Excimer photorefractive keratectomy can be effectively performed for both myopia and astigmatism; its efficacy in hyperopia has yet to be established. Arcuate incisions flatten in the meridian of the incision and steepen an equal amount in the meridian 90° away. Overall, there is no net change in the spherical equivalent.

Preferred Response   c. Keratomileusis in situ (automated lamellar keratectomy, or ALK) can effectively reduce myopia and hyperopia.

During phacoemulsification a capsular break is noted with vitreous in the anterior chamber. Nucleus removal is incomplete. All of the following steps should be taken *except*

a. continue gentle phacoemulsification, since the phacoemulsification instrument efficiently cuts vitreous
b. inject viscoelastic beneath the nuclear remnant to keep it elevated
c. consider conversion to an extracapsular procedure with utilization of a lens loop to remove the nuclear fragment
d. remove all vitreous from the anterior chamber using an automated vitrector and low inflow

Discussion   When a capsular break is noted during phacoemulsification and nucleus removal is incomplete, strategies must be undertaken to remove the nuclear fragment(s) and avoid the potential for a "dropped" nucleus. Visualization of the limits of the break, or dehiscence, must be made. If the break is enlarging, it is best to stop and convert to an extracapsular procedure. The wound should be enlarged and viscoelastic should be injected beneath the nuclear remnant to keep it elevated. The nuclear fragment can be "tire-ironed" up with a cyclodialysis spatula, and a lens loop can be inserted to remove the nuclear fragment(s). Expression-type techniques should be avoided, since these will increase vitreous pressure. All vitreous can then be removed from the anterior chamber using low-inflow vitrectomy to minimize extension of the rent.

If the capsular break is not enlarging, the surgeon should check for external pressure on the lid and globe by the speculum. The bottle should be lowered to minimize inflow and, hence, extension of the break. The anterior chamber should be swept with a cyclodialysis spatula to check for the presence of vitreous. Inefficient aspiration either in the irrigation/aspiration or phacoemulsification mode indicates that vitreous is present in the anterior chamber. Careful phacoemulsification can proceed if the extent of the rent is visualized, and a second instrument can be used to prevent nuclear fragments from migrating through the capsular opening. Some surgeons advocate the use of a Sheets glide (a small piece of plastic) that is slid under the nucleus and over the capsular opening, thus protecting against loss of nuclear material through the rent as phacoemulsification proceeds.

Following removal of the nucleus, retained cortex can be removed by pulling the cortical material toward the break rather than away from the break, which can extend the rent. During cortical removal, a second irrigating port can be utilized to minimize inflow. A "dry technique" cortical removal can also be used, in which the anterior chamber is filled with viscoelastic and a manual aspirating cannula is used to remove residual cortical material. Importantly, the phacoemulsification tip is not a vitreous cutter and should never be used to remove vitreous.

Preferred Response

a. continue gentle phacoemulsification, since the phacoemulsification instrument efficiently cuts vitreous

C47

All of the following are signs of a posterior capsular rupture during phacoemulsification *except*

a. constriction of the pupil
b. slight deepening of the anterior chamber
c. the appearance of vitreous in the anterior chamber
d. an area of the posterior capsule that appears "too clear" compared to adjacent areas

Discussion

Deepening of the anterior chamber and vitreous in the anterior chamber are both early signs of a posterior capsular rupture. Additionally, the equatorial lens capsule may come into view if there is a zonular dehiscence. If an area of the capsule appears "too clear," one must also be suspicious of an opening in the capsule, with the clear area representing the open capsule. Constriction of the pupil is not typically associated with posterior capsular rupture.

Preferred Response

a. constriction of the pupil

A scleral-pocket incision and closure (which enters the anterior chamber anterior to Schwalbe's line) is shown in the figure.

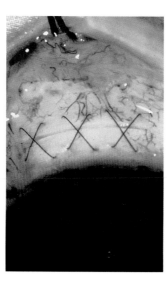

Scleral-pocket incision with nylon X-suture closure.

This technique would be expected to produce

a. transient keratometric steepening in the surgical meridian
b. transient keratometric flattening in the surgical meridian
c. transient keratometric steepening 90° away from the surgical meridian
d. emmetropia

Discussion

Phacoemulsification has allowed the wound to be reduced in size. Scleral-pocket incisions and closure techniques have been developed to afford control of astigmatism while providing a stable, watertight wound. This enables the cataractous patient virtually full activity in the immediate postoperative period. Studies have demonstrated that small posteriorly placed scleral incisions retain, to a large extent, presurgical astigmatism after complete healing of the wound.[29] However, during the early postoperative period, there is an induced with-the-rule astigmatic change that wanes with time and healing of the wound. The type of incision demonstrated is a scleral-pocket 2-plane (mortised) incision, which enters the anterior chamber anterior to Schwalbe's line but does not enter into clear cornea, as the no-stitch type valve incisions do. By reducing this initial astigmatic shift with the use of tunnel incisions that enter the anterior chamber through clear cornea just in front of the vascular arcade, the patient benefits by earlier visual rehabilitation during the early postoperative period.

Preferred Response

a. transient keratometric steepening in the surgical meridian

C49

All of the following are components of one or more of the commercially available viscoelastic materials *except*

a. sodium hyaluronate
b. chondroitin sulfate
c. hydroxypropylmethylcellulose
d. keratan sulfate

Discussion

Sodium hyaluronate, a mucopolysaccharide found in connective tissues, possesses a high viscosity and high molecular weight. It is the exclusive component in Healon, AmviscPlus, Vitrax, and ProVisc. Chondroitin sulfate, one of the mucopolysaccharides of the cornea, possesses medium molecular weight and medium viscosity. Chondroitin sulfate is a component of Viscoat along with sodium hyaluronate. Hydroxypropylmethylcellulose is a cellulose polymer not naturally occurring in animals. It is a structural substance in plant fibers and possesses a low molecular weight and low viscosity. It is the major component of OcuCoat. Keratan sulfate, a mucopolysaccharide found in the cornea, is not a component of any currently available viscoelastic material.

Preferred Response

d. keratan sulfate

C50

When comparing radial keratotomy (RK) to excimer laser photorefractive keratectomy (PRK), which of the following statements is *most* accurate?

a. PRK is more predictable than RK in the −1 D to −4 D myopic range.
b. PRK flattens the central cornea and RK steepens the central cornea.
c. Reading glasses are needed less often in presbyopic patients undergoing PRK as compared to RK.
d. Early postoperative vision is worse and pain more significant following PRK as compared to RK.

Discussion

Both RK and PRK flatten the central cornea. This is accomplished by central flattening through the removal of tissue in PRK and by a central flattening due to midperipheral steepening caused by the radial incisions of RK. With current radial keratotomy nomograms and enhancement techniques, correction in the low myopia range (−1 D to −6 D) appears equally predictable at this time. Studies indicate that more than 90% achieve 20/40 or better visual acuity in this low-myopia group for both procedures.[10,30,31]

Because of the large epithelial defect that occurs following PRK, vision is often quite limited for the first several days to weeks. Similarly, because of the large ablated area, the eye is often uncomfortable for a number of days until complete epithelialization is achieved.[32] Early postoperative vision is often quite good following RK, and discomfort is minimal. The overall effect of PRK and RK is corneal flattening and the reduction of myopia. Therefore, regardless of the procedure, prepresbyopes will find an increased dependency on glasses for near vision.

Preferred Response

d. Early postoperative vision is worse and pain more significant following PRK as compared to RK.

References

1. Davison JA: Capsule contraction syndrome. *J Cataract Refract Surg* 1993;19: 582–589.

2. Masket S: Pseudophakic posterior iris chafing syndrome. *J Cataract Refract Surg* 1986;12:252–256.

3. Johnson SH, Kratz RP, Olson PF: Iris transillumination defect and microhyphema syndrome. *J Am Intraocul Implant Soc* 1984;10:425–428.

4. Koch DD, Liu JF, Hyde LL, et al: Refractive complications of cataract surgery after radial keratotomy. *Am J Ophthalmol* 1989;108:676–682.

5. Carpel EF: Pupillary dilation in eyes with pseudoexfoliation syndrome. *Am J Ophthalmol* 1988;105:692–694.

6. Osher RH, Wu BC, Koch DD: Posterior polar cataracts: a predisposition to intraoperative posterior capsular rupture. *J Cataract Refract Surg* 1990;16:157–162.

7. Thornton SP: Astigmatic keratotomy: a review of basic concepts with case reports. *J Cataract Refract Surg* 1990;16:430–435.

8. Kraff MC, Sanders DR, Lieberman HL: Serial corneal endothelial cell loss with lathe-cut and injection-molded posterior chamber intraocular lenses. *J Am Intraoc Implant Soc* 1983;9:301–305.

9. Koch DD, Liu JF, Glasser DB, et al: A comparison of corneal endothelial changes after use of Healon or Viscoat during phacoemulsification. *Am J Ophthalmol* 1993; 115:188–201.

10. Waring GO, Linn MJ, Strahlman ER, et al: Stability of refraction four years after radial keratotomy in the Prospective Evaluation of Radial Keratotomy study. *Am J Ophthalmol* 1991;111:133–144.

11. O'Donoghue E, Lightman S, Tuft S, et al: Surgically induced necrotising sclerokeratitis (SINS): precipitating factors and response to treatment. *Br J Ophthalmol* 1992;76:17–21.

12. Consultation Section: *J Cataract Refract Surg* 1993;19:662–665.

13. Gimbel HV, Neuhann T: Development, advantages, and methods of the continuous circular capsulorhexis technique. *J Cataract Refract Surg* 1990;16:31–37.

14. Levy JH, Pisacano AM, Anello RD: Displacement of bag-placed hydrogel lenses into the vitreous following neodymium:YAG laser capsulotomy. *J Cataract Refract Surg* 1990;16:563–566.

15. Skuta GL, Parrish RK II, Hodapp E, et al: Zonular dialysis during extracapsular cataract extraction in pseudoexfoliation syndrome. *Arch Ophthalmol* 1987;105: 632–634.

16. Apt L, Isenberg S, Yoshimora R, et al: Chemical preparation of the eye in ophthalmic surgery. III. Effect of povidone-iodine on the conjunctiva. *Arch Ophthalmol* 1984;102:728–729.

17. Jaffe GJ, Burton TC, Kuhn E, et al: Progression of nonproliferative diabetic retinopathy and visual outcome after extracapsular cataract extraction and intraocular lens implantation. *Am J Ophthalmol* 1992;114:448–456.

18. Lane SS, Kopietz LA, Lindquist TD, et al: Treatment of phacolytic glaucoma with extracapsular cataract extraction. *Ophthalmology* 1988;95:749–753.

19. Weiss JL, Deichman CB: A comparison of retrobulbar and periocular anesthesia for cataract surgery. *Arch Ophthal* 1989;107:96–98.

20. Davis DB II, Mandel MR: Posterior peribulbar anesthesia: an alternative to retrobulbar anesthesia. *J Cataract Refract Surg* 1986;12:182–184.

21. Agrawal V, Athanikar NS: Single injection, low volume periocular anesthesia in 1,000 cases. *J Cataract Refract Surg* 1994;20:61–63.

22. Speaker MG, Guerriero PN, Met JA, et al: A case-control study of risk factors for intraoperative suprachoroidal expulsive hemorrhage. *Ophthalmology* 1991;98: 202–210.

23. *Cataract in Adults: Management of Functional Impairment.* Clinical practice guideline #4, US Department of Health and Human Services. Rockville, Maryland. AHCPRPUB #93–0542, February 1993.

24. Rickman-Barger L, Florine CW, Larson RS, et al: Retinal detachment after neodymium:YAG laser posterior capsulotomy. *Am J Ophthalmol* 1989;107:531–536.

25. Koch DD, Liu JF, Gill EP, et al: Axial myopia increases the risk of retinal complications after neodymium:YAG laser posterior capsulotomy. *Arch Ophthalmol* 1989; 107:986–990.

26. Solomon K, Gussler JR, Gussler C, et al: Incidence and management of complications of transsclerally sutured posterior chamber lenses. *J Cataract Refract Surg* 1993;19:488–493.

27. Schechter RJ: Suture-wick endophthalmitis with sutured posterior chamber intraocular lenses. *J Cataract Refract Surg* 1990;16:755–756.

28. Bucci FA Jr, Holland EJ, Lindstrom RL: Corneal autografts for external knots in transsclerally sutured posterior chamber lenses. *Am J Ophthalmol* 1991;112: 353–354.

29. Masket S: Astigmatic analysis of the scleral pocket incision and closure technique for cataract surgery. *CLAO J* 1985;11:206–209.

30. Salz JJ, Maguen E, Nesburn AB, et al: A two-year experience with excimer laser photorefractive keratectomy of myopia. *Ophthalmology* 1993;100:873–882.

31. Werblin TP, Stafford GM: The Casebeer system for predictable keratorefractive surgery: one-year evaluation of 205 consecutive eyes. *Ophthalmology* 1993;100: 1095–1102.

32. Sher NA, Frantz JM, Talley A, et al: Topical diclofenac in the treatment of ocular pain after excimer photorefractive keratectomy. *Refract Corneal Surg* 1993;9: 425–436.

Additional Resources From the AAO

Academy Statements

Cataract Surgery in the Otherwise Healthy Adult Second Eye. Policy Statement. 1991.

Choosing a Cataract Surgeon. Information About Eye Care. 1992.

Complications of Closed Loop Flexible and Semi-flexible Anterior Chamber Intraocular Lenses. Clinical Alert. 1987.

Intraocular Irrigating Solutions (Precautions Regarding Use in Eye Surgery). Clinical Alert. 1987.

Keratophakia and Keratomileusis: Safety and Effectiveness. Ophthalmic Procedures Assessment. 1992. (Item No. 112005)

Photo-Refractive Keratectomy. Information Statement. 1990.

Potentially Deceptive Advertisements Concerning (1) "Laser Cataract Surgery" and (2) "Free Surgery." Advisory Opinion. 1992.

Radial Keratotomy for Myopia. Ophthalmic Procedures Assessment. 1992. (Item No. 112010)

Basic and Clinical Science Course

Glaucoma. Section 10. Updated annually.

Lens and Cataract. Section 11. Updated annually.

Optics, Refraction, and Contact Lenses. Section 3. Updated annually.

Focal Points

Foster CS: *Cataract Surgery in the Patient With Uveitis.* Vol XII, Module 4. 1994. (Item No. 029012)

Hoyt CS: *Management of Congenital Cataracts.* Vol I, Module 6. 1983. (Item No. 029001)

Johnson SH: *Phacoemulsification.* Vol XII, Module 6. 1994. (Item No. 029012)

Koch DD: *The Role of Glare Testing in Managing the Cataract Patient.* Vol VI, Module 4. 1988. (Item No. 029006)

Lembach RG: *Aphakic and Myopic Extended-Wear Contact Lenses.* Vol II, Module 6. 1984. (Item No. 029002).

McDonald MB, Kaufman HE: *Refractive Corneal Surgery.* Vol II, Module 11. 1984. (Item No. 029002)

Mandelbaum S, Forster RK: *Infectious Endophthalmitis.* Vol I, Module 9. 1983. (Item No. 029001)

Meisler DM: *Intraocular Inflammation and Extracapsular Cataract Surgery.* Vol VIII, Module 7. 1990. (Out of print)

Rowsey JJ, Hays JC: *Corneal Astigmatism: Topographic and Surgical Insights.* Vol V, Module 4. 1987. (Out of print)

Stern WH, O'Donnell FE: *Vitrectomy Techniques for the Anterior Segment.* Vol V, Module 11. 1987. (Out of print)

Waring GO III: *Radial Keratotomy for Myopia.* Vol X, Module 5. 1992. (Item No. 029010)

Wilkinson CP: *Retinal Complications Following Cataract Surgery.* Vol X, Module 12. 1992. (Item No. 029010)

Yannuzzi LA: *Cystoid Macular Edema Following Cataract Surgery.* Vol III, Module 10. 1985. (Out of print)

Monographs and Manuals   Michels RG: *Vitreous Surgery.* 1982. (Item No. 0210132)

Stamper RL, Sugar A, Ripkin DJ: *Intraocular Lenses: Basics and Clinical Applications.* Ophthalmology Monograph 7. 1993. (Item No. 0210152)

Videotapes   Byrne SF: *A-scan Biometry.* Clinical Skills Series. 1988. (Item No. 0250733)

Chen CJ: *Management of Suprachoroidal Hemorrhage With Perfluorophenanthrene.* Annual Meeting Series. 1994. (Item No. 0252033)

Cobo ML: *Intraocular Lens Removal: Indications and Technique.* Clinical Short Subjects Series. 1988. (Item No. 0251043)

Connor CS: *The Radial Flap Incision;* Solomon KD, Auffarth GU, Wesendahl TA, et al: *Fixation of Posterior Chamber Lenses in the Absence of Capsular Support.* Annual Meeting Series. 1994. (Item No. 0252053)

Feder RS, Mandel M, Krachmer JH: *Technique and Complications of Penetrating Keratoplasty.* Classic Series. 1985. (Item No. 0250663)

Gelender H, Mandelbaum SH: *Postoperative Astigmatism: Prevention and Management.* Clinical Short Subjects Series. 1987. (Item No. 0251083)

Guyton D: *Aphakic Spectacles in Perspective.* Classic Series. 1980. (Item No. 0250303)

Singer JA: *Phaco at 500;* Klaas DW: *The One-Hand Phacofracture Technique.* Annual Meeting Series. 1994. (Item No. 0252043)

Steinert RF, Wright PL: *Making the Transition to Phacoemulsification.* Clinical Skills Series. 1992. (Item No. 0250933)

Wasson PJ: *Introduction to First Assisting in Cataract Surgery.* Clinical Skills Series. 1989. (Item No. 0250823)

Weiss JL, Deichman CB: *A Comparison of Retrobulbar and Periocular Anesthesia.* Classic Series. 1987. (Item No. 0251023)

Wilson RP: *Management of Combined Cataract and Glaucoma.* Classic Series. 1989. (Item No. 0250843)

NEURO-OPHTHALMOLOGY

N1

A 65-year-old woman presents with acute visual loss OD and periocular ache. The results of her examination are as follows:

Best-corrected acuity: 20/40 OD, 20/20 OS

Ishihara color plates: 9/10 correct OD, 10/10 correct OS

Pupils: 5 mm OU and round, + RAPD OD

Motility: Normal, no proptosis

Visual fields: OD shown in the figure; OS normal

Fundi: Optic disc swollen OD, normal OS

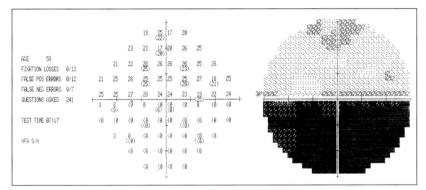

Automated threshold visual field, central 30°, right eye. Left eye is normal.

What is the *most* appropriate diagnostic test to perform *immediately?*

a. CT scan of the orbits (axial and coronal, with 1 mm to 2 mm sections, with contrast)
b. fluorescein angiography
c. MRI of the head with gadolinium and of the orbits with fat suppression
d. erythrocyte sedimentation rate

Discussion

Taken in isolation, the clinical picture is consistent with many kinds of optic neuropathy, be it anterior ischemic optic neuropathy, optic neuritis, orbital pseudotumor, or infiltrative optic neuropathies such as malignant carcinomatosis. All of these conditions might cause a swollen disc in the setting of acute visual loss. However, in an optic neuropathy in the appropriate age group, temporal arteritis must always be ruled out, as failure to diagnose may lead to contralateral blindness in a significant number of cases, as well as further ipsilateral visual loss.[1] At age 65, this patient is in a typical age group for temporal arteritis. The condition is rare below the age of 55; 95% of cases occur in those over 50 years of age. The reported incidence rises with the age of the studied population.

Pain may be a feature of ischemic optic neuropathy, optic neuritis, and orbital pseudotumor. In typical ischemic optic neuropathy or optic neuritis, CT scan is usually not necessary. In the patient in whom optic neuritis is suspected (this patient is old for the classic case of optic neuritis), MRI is indicated; however, obtaining MRI is less emergent than obtaining the sedimentation rate, which must be done immediately to rule out temporal arteritis and avoid its risk of blindness in the fellow eye. Fluorescein angiography, which may demonstrate delayed choroidal filling in the arteritic form,[2,3] may be useful in selected cases, but it is not necessary in all cases.

Preferred Response   d. erythrocyte sedimentation rate

In a patient who has acute optic neuritis in the right eye, which of the following is true?

a. There must be a relative afferent pupillary defect present in the right eye.

b. There cannot be a better pupillary response in the right eye than in the left.

c. It would be rare for the patient to have a new visual field defect on automated perimetry in the left eye.

d. With the information given, the results of the relative afferent pupillary defect test cannot be predicted.

Discussion   Optic neuritis frequently is a sign of multiple sclerosis. Many patients with optic neuritis have a prior history of contralateral optic neuritis. If this patient had had a prior optic neuritis in the left eye, a relative afferent pupillary defect (RAPD) might not be present when acute optic neuritis occurred in the right eye. Indeed, if optic nerve function were worse in the left eye than in the right at the time of examination, the RAPD might be in the left eye and the pupil might respond better in the right eye. In the case described, therefore, with no information about the contralateral eye, the results of the RAPD testing cannot be predicted. At the time of acute optic neuritis, contralateral asymptomatic visual field defects are commonly seen.[4]

Preferred Response   d. With the information given, the results of the relative afferent pupillary defect test cannot be predicted.

An emergent consultation is requested on a comatose man with significant periocular trauma to the right eye. A CT scan of the head is essentially normal. The patient's pupils are 8 mm OD, 4 mm OS; the right pupil does not react to direct light. The right eye is exodeviated and has complete ptosis, and oculocephalic maneuver indicates that the right eye does not cross the midline in the field of action of the right medial rectus muscle. There is no enophthalmos or proptosis. Intraocular pressures are 19 mm Hg OD and 12 mm Hg OS. Both fundi are unremarkable.

For the purpose of guiding emergent treatment, which of the following is the *most* appropriate test to perform?

a. a CT scan of the orbits
b. forced duction of the right eye
c. examination of the relative magnitude of the pupillary response of the left eye when the left and then the right eye is illuminated
d. a pattern visual evoked response

Discussion

In the trauma patient, determination of the status of the optic nerves is of paramount importance. In this comatose patient with an apparent traumatic right pupil–involving oculomotor palsy, the direct response of the right pupil cannot be used to evaluate right optic nerve function. However, a constrictive response of the left pupil when the light is swung from the right eye to the left eye, and a dilation of the right pupil when the light is swung back to the right eye, would indicate that the right optic nerve is carrying less afferent information than the left optic nerve. This is the only immediately available bedside method of assessing the right optic nerve function.

Preferred Response

c. examination of the relative magnitude of the pupillary response of the left eye when the left and then the right eye is illuminated

A 20-year-old woman presents with pupils of unequal size. The examination is normal but for the pupillary examination, which reveals:

Dim light: 8 mm OD, 4 mm OS

Bright light: 8 mm OD, 2 mm OS

Near fixation: 8 mm OD, 1.5 mm OS

What is the *most* appropriate sequence of pharmacologic testing to perform on the patient?

a. 1% pilocarpine, 2.5% methacholine (Mecholyl)
b. 0.05% pilocarpine, 1% pilocarpine
c. 5% cocaine, 1% hydroxyamphetamine (Paredrine)
d. 1% hydroxyamphetamine (Paredrine), 0.5% phenylephrine

Discussion

The patient has a pupil that does not respond either to light or at near. Here, the first consideration is whether the patient has an Adie's tonic pupil. In Adie's tonic pupil, the pupil will not seem to respond at near; however, if near fixation is continued, the pupils will gradually show miosis. In this disorder, the postganglionic efferent nerve in the parasympathetic pathway is affected, and the end organ (iris sphincter) develops denervation supersensitivity. This supersensitivity develops only when there is postganglionic involvement. While a normal pupil will constrict to 1% pilocarpine, only a pupil with denervation supersensitivity will constrict to a concentration as dilute as 0.05%, demonstrating postganglionic involvement and confirming the tonic pupil.[5,6] In Adie's pupil, segmental paresis manifesting as vermiform movements of the pupils is a useful sign seen at the slit lamp, but its absence does not rule out the diagnosis of Adie's pupil.

If the pupil does not respond to dilute pilocarpine, then 1% pilocarpine is used to see if the pupil is capable of constricting to that dose. Traumatic or mechanical disruption of the pupil or pharmacologic dilation (as with atropine) might cause failure to dilate to this normal strength of pilocarpine. Methacholine is an appropriate substitute for 0.05% pilocarpine in this test, but it is infrequently used because of its instability. Cocaine 5%, hydroxyamphetamine 1%, and phenylephrine 0.5% are agents used to evaluate sympathetically denervated pupils.[7,8]

Preferred Response   b. 0.05% pilocarpine, 1% pilocarpine

A 22-year-old woman exhibits a dilated right pupil that you clinically suspect is an Adie's tonic pupil. The pupils are 8 mm OD, 5 mm OS in dim light, and 8 mm OD, 2 mm OS in bright light. The motility is normal, and there is no ptosis. While preparing the appropriate pharmacologic solutions, you take a more detailed history.

Which of the following historical points would be of the *least* significance in a patient who demonstrates a large pupil that does not constrict?

a. The patient is an ICU nurse who runs cardiac resuscitation codes.
b. The patient is aware of an inability to read with the right eye only.
c. The patient says that the right eye with the larger pupil has always had a lighter colored iris than the left eye.
d. The patient has a history of motion sickness and has just returned from a cruise.

Discussion   The question is, What in the history is consistent with having an ipsilateral *dilated pupil*? That the patient is an ICU nurse is relevant because during cardiac resuscitation, ampules of atropine are used in haste, and a resuscitation team member might become subject to atropinization by inadvertent hand–eye contact. Inability to read due to loss of ipsilateral accommodation is a symptom of Adie's tonic pupil. The most effective pharmacologic treatment of motion sickness is transdermal scopolamine, which may cause ipsilateral pupillary dilation by direct inoculation from the fingers. A lighter iris in the affected eye is insignificant for two reasons: pupils in Horner's syndrome do respond to light; furthermore, even if this patient had a congenital Horner's syndrome, the lighter iris would be ipsilateral to the smaller pupil.[5–8]

Preferred Response   c. The patient says that the right eye with the larger pupil has always had a lighter colored iris than the left eye.

An 8-year-old girl is brought in by her mother because of difficulty reading. The mother mentions that the child has a chronic "cold in the eye" because both eyes are always red (see the figures). The vision is 20/20 OU at near and at distance; the pupils and fundi are normal. You also notice that the child has difficulty moving her eyes in the horizontal plane, and that this paresis is overcome by the oculocephalic maneuver.

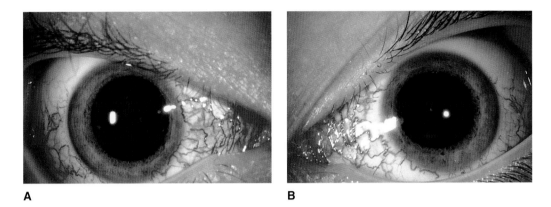

A   **B**

Conjunctival signs of ataxia telangiectasia (Louis-Bar syndrome) in an 8-year-old child. **(A)** Right eye. **(B)** Left eye.

Based upon the presentation and the external eye appearance, what is the *most* appropriate course of action?

a. Prescribe a trial of topical sulfa-corticosteroid combination for 2 weeks.
b. Inquire if the child has missed her early developmental milestones.
c. Inquire if the child is often sick and is more clumsy lately.
d. Prescribe a course of oral trimethoprim-sulfamethoxazole (Bactrim) for 3 weeks.

Discussion

The clinical description is that of ataxia telangiectasia, or Louis-Bar syndrome. This autosomal recessive neurocutaneous disorder is characterized by normal early development, followed by progressive onset of truncal ataxia and athetoid movements, and sometimes early graying of the hair. The conjunctival telangiectasia is usually present by age 3. Affected children have thymic hypoplasia, decreased serum IgA with subsequent propensity to frequent infections, and a high incidence of lymphoma and leukemia. They have reduced volitional eye movements and an intact oculocephalic maneuver, ie, a supranuclear ophthalmoplegia.[9,10]

Preferred Response

c. Inquire if the child is often sick and is more clumsy lately.

A man presents after having fallen off a scaffold 20 feet from the ground. He had loss of consciousness for an hour and is still lethargic. He has an orbital roof fracture on the right and a temporal bone fracture on the left. Because of lethargy, the patient's acuity cannot adequately be assessed. His pupils are 6 mm OU, round, reactive to light, with a trace relative afferent pupillary defect OD. The motility shows a 2+ underaction of the right lateral rectus, right medial rectus, inferior rectus, and inferior oblique muscles. There is 2 mm ptosis OD. The right eye's external appearance is shown in the figure; the left eye is normal externally. The right fundus shows venous distention but is otherwise normal.

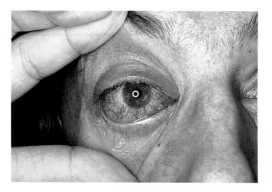

Engorged, arterialized conjunctival vessels in a patient with a traumatic carotid-cavernous fistula.

All of the following would be consistent with the clinical presentation *except*

a. 4 mm of proptosis of the right eye
b. intraocular pressures of 14 mm Hg OD and 24 mm Hg OS
c. ocular bruit OD
d. depressed corneal reflex OD

Discussion

This is a classic description of a traumatic carotid-cavernous fistula. The figure shows the engorged, arterialized conjunctival vessels. Engorgement of the veins in the fundus may accompany this. Increased blood flow in the superior ophthalmic vein and consequent orbital engorgement lead to the ipsilateral elevated intraocular pressure, ocular bruit, and proptosis that are typical in this disorder. Cranial nerves III, IV, and VI may be affected, resulting in motility disorders. Involvement of the trigeminal nerve, especially the first (corneal reflex) and second divisions, also occurs from compression in the cavernous sinus.[11] Whereas contralateral raised intraocular pressure may occur due to flow through venous channels interconnecting the two cavernous sinuses, the contralateral eye would not typically have a higher pressure without other signs of congestion.

Preferred Response

b. intraocular pressures of 14 mm Hg OD and 24 mm Hg OS

A 65-year-old woman presents with double vision, which has been present for 3 weeks. She has had good general health until she recently developed an arrhythmia. Although her internist placed her on oral procainamide for this arrhythmia 3 months ago, she has continued to feel weak and tired; the internist, who has already obtained a negative MRI of the head with gadolinium, has referred her to you. Her ocular and neurologic examinations are normal except for her horizontal eye movements, which are shown in the figures. She thinks that her right eye becomes "more droopy" in the evening.

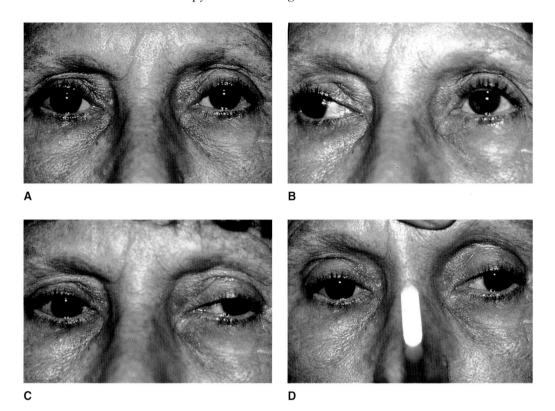

Ocular rotations of a 65-year-old woman with bilateral adduction deficits. **(A)** Primary gaze. **(B)** Right gaze. **(C)** Left gaze. **(D)** Near fixation.

Which of the following points is *most* relevant in arriving at the patient's ultimate diagnosis and a treatment plan?

a. She has taken 50,000 units of vitamin A daily for 6 weeks.
b. Discuss with the internist whether another agent is available for her arrhythmia therapy.
c. The diplopia is more noticeable when she reads than when she performs distance tasks.
d. She is allergic to penicillin.

Discussion

The eye movements are consistent with bilateral adduction defects, or "pseudo-internuclear ophthalmoplegia." The differential diagnosis of this includes bilateral internuclear ophthalmoplegia due to demyelinating disease (usually presenting in younger patients), and infarction. With the history of the onset of ptosis with diurnal variation, myasthenia and myasthenic-like syndromes causing a bilateral "pseudo-internuclear ophthalmoplegia" must also be considered.

Many drugs are known to cause a myasthenic-like syndrome. These include the polymyxin and aminoglycoside classes of antibiotics, tetracycline, d-penicillamine, and the anticonvulsant phenytoin (Dilantin). In a patient with an arrhythmia, however, one must inquire whether the patient is on procainamide, which may worsen preexisting undiagnosed myasthenia.[12,13] Discontinuation of the agent may be curative.

In causing pseudotumor cerebri, vitamin A intoxication might result in sixth-nerve palsies, but not *ad*duction deficits. The increased difficulty with reading is inherent in the nature of the movement deficit and does not help with the diagnosis. The allergy to penicillin is irrelevant.

Preferred Response

b. Discuss with the internist whether another agent is available for her arrhythmia therapy.

A patient is brought to the emergency room comatose with a head injury from a motor vehicle accident. He has no other medical problems. In your initial evaluation, the pupillary responses are normal, and there is no relative afferent pupillary defect (RAPD). One hour later, after the neurosurgery service finishes its evaluation and you reevaluate the patient, the pupils are 4 mm OU, and a 4+ RAPD is seen in the left eye. The intraocular pressure is 16 mm Hg OD, and 42 mm Hg OS. The external examination reveals mild chemosis and 4 mm of proptosis OS. The neurosurgeon asks you not to dilate the pupils because the patient is comatose and she wishes to observe the pupils for dilation indicative of cerebral herniation. The right fundus is normal; the left cannot be visualized. The orbital CT scan is shown in the figure.

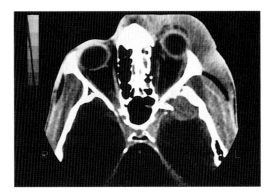

Orbital CT scan showing anterior soft-tissue damage and a lateral orbital fracture compromising the optic canal.

All of the following are a part of an appropriate treatment plan *except*

a. performing a right lateral canthotomy
b. administering intravenous megadose corticosteroids (at least 1 g of methylprednisolone or equivalent daily)
c. planning with the orbital surgeon and neurosurgeon for possible optic canal and optic nerve sheath exploration and/or decompression if the neuro-ophthalmic examination shows no improvement and the patient is cleared for the operating room
d. starting no therapy and reevaluating the patient in 48 hours with a dilated fundus examination

Discussion

In addition to the anterior soft-tissue damage, the CT scan shows a lateral orbital fracture compromising the optic canal (medial fracture is actually more common). Traumatic optic neuropathy is an emergency requiring prompt evaluation and possible treatment; however, this treatment must not threaten the patient's life. Canthotomy at the bedside is indicated by the raised intraocular pressure and the soft-tissue injury. The currently recommended potential therapies for traumatic optic neuropathy include megadose corticosteroid therapy and optic canal and optic nerve sheath decompression.[14] The development of an afferent pupillary defect that was not present on the initial examination is similar to the "lucid interval" in an alert patient with traumatic optic neuropathy, where the patient states that the visual loss was not initially present but developed over time. This raises the possibility of the presence of an optic nerve sheath hematoma, which would be an indication for surgical exploration if the initial therapeutic measures yielded no response. In the setting of a clearly evolving optic neuropathy, waiting 48 hours is not indicated, because therapy, at least a canthotomy, aimed at lowering the intraocular pressure, is emergent.

Preferred Response

d. starting no therapy and reevaluating the patient in 48 hours with a dilated fundus examination

Based on the data generated by the Optic Neuritis Treatment Trial, which of the following is true about the management of patients with acute unilateral optic neuritis?

a. Patients should be treated with intravenous corticosteroids because they demonstrated significantly better visual acuity performance at 1 year than did patients treated with placebo therapy.
b. All patients with an acute optic neuritis should be treated with intravenous corticosteroids.
c. MRI should be performed on a patient with acute unilateral optic neuritis with no history of prior neurologic disease.
d. Patients with acute unilateral optic neuritis should be treated with oral prednisone to diminish the frequency of subsequent attacks of optic neuritis.

Discussion

The data from the Optic Neuritis Treatment Trial (ONTT) showed that there was no significant difference in the visual acuity at 1 year between the placebo group and the group treated with intravenous corticosteroid (methylprednisolone sodium succinate [Solumedrol]). A key finding was that patients who had MRI at study entry with two or more plaques, when treated with intravenous corticosteroids, had a significantly lower rate of developing multiple sclerosis in the next 2 years. This was not true of patients with normal MRI results. Thus, the data do not support treating patients with normal MRIs to prevent the development of multiple sclerosis. Oral prednisone therapy for acute optic neuritis was associated with a significantly increased risk of further attacks of optic neuritis.[15–17]

Preferred Response

c. MRI should be performed on a patient with acute unilateral optic neuritis with no history of prior neurologic disease.

N11

A 22-year-old woman presents with acute optic neuritis OS of 1 day's duration. Her past medical history and neurologic examination are normal. The results of her ophthalmic examination are as follows:

Best-corrected acuity: 20/20 OD, 20/40 OS

Ishihara color plates: 10/10 correct OD, 3/10 correct OS

Pupils: 7 mm OU, round and reactive; 3+ RAPD OS

Motility: Normal

Slit lamp: Normal

Intraocular pressures: Normal

Visual fields: Normal OD, 10° central scotoma OS

Fundi: Normal OD, trace hyperemic swelling OS, no hemorrhages or exudates

Which of the following is the *most* appropriate sequence of management steps in this patient?

a. Obtain a chest x-ray, treat with 250 mg q6h methylprednisolone sodium succinate (Solumedrol) IV for 3 days, followed by 11 days of oral prednisone.
b. Obtain antinuclear antibody (ANA) and a chest x-ray; if ANA is positive, treat with oral prednisone, 80 mg/day for 2 weeks.
c. Obtain MRI the next morning, and see the patient in the afternoon after the scan is completed.
d. Begin the patient on 80 mg/day of prednisone while awaiting results of MRI.

Discussion

MRI should be obtained as soon as possible. If MRI demonstrates a significant number of plaques, prompt treatment with intravenous Solumedrol may be indicated to delay or decrease the chance of development of multiple sclerosis.

In the Optic Neuritis Treatment Trial, the intravenous therapy arm received 250 mg q6h Solumedrol for 3 days, followed by 11 days of oral prednisone (1 mg/kg/day). When data were analyzed for results at 1 year after the acute optic neuritis, patients treated with this regimen did not demonstrate better visual outcomes, although they did recover earlier. Intravenous Solumedrol had much less of an effect of hastening recovery in those with better visual function at time of onset. A positive ANA in this group of patients without collagen vascular disease did not alter the visual outcome; therefore, it did not alter the therapeutic recommendations. Oral prednisone is not indicated as the sole initial therapy in optic neuritis because it does not offer better visual outcome and actually increases the risk of further attacks.[15–17]

Preferred Response

c. Obtain MRI the next morning, and see the patient in the afternoon after the scan is completed.

A patient presents with gradual visual loss in both eyes over 3 weeks. The results of the examination are as follows:

Best corrected acuity: 20/20 OU

Pupils: 5 mm OU, round and reactive; 1+ RAPD OD

Motility: Normal

Slit lamp: Normal

Intraocular pressures: 12 mm Hg OD, 14 mm Hg OS

Visual fields: Shown in the figures

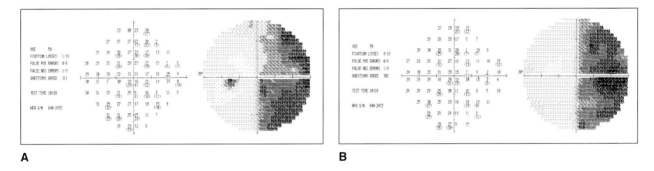

A   **B**

Visual fields showing right homonymous hemianopsia due to a lesion in the left optic tract. **(A)** Left eye. **(B)** Right eye.

Which of the following statements is true?

a. Two lesions are required to cause this presentation.
b. A lesion in the left anterior-most occipital lobe could cause this presentation.
c. If followed over time, this patient will not develop any optic atrophy.
d. The lesion is in the left optic tract.

Discussion

These findings, with a noncongruous right homonymous hemianopsia and a right RAPD, localize the lesion to the left optic tract.[18] Patients with such lesions often develop "bow-tie" optic atrophy over time. A lesion in the left anterior occipital lobe might cause a monocular field defect in the right eye, the so-called monocular temporal crescent.

Preferred Response

d. The lesion is in the left optic tract.

A 10-year-old boy is examined for bilateral progressive visual loss that has occurred over 1 month. He has polyuria and polydipsia and is found to have diabetes insipidus.

Which of the following is the *most* likely associated visual field deficit?

a. a unilateral nasal step
b. a bilateral nasal defect respecting the midline
c. a complete left homonymous hemianopsia
d. a bilateral temporal defect respecting the midline, denser in the inferior quadrants

Discussion

The onset of diabetes insipidus in a child with bilateral visual loss should make one suspect a lesion *superior* to the chiasm, in the hypothalamic region. Lesions here may press on the chiasm from above, giving the bilateral inferotemporal scotoma.[19]

Preferred Response

d. a bilateral temporal defect respecting the midline, denser in the inferior quadrants

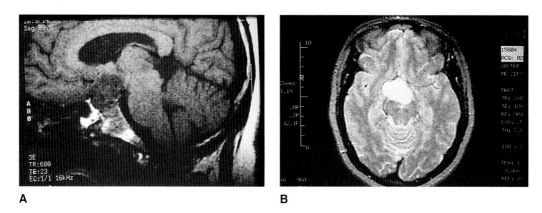

The figures show the MRI results of a child with the same histologic lesion as the child in Question N13 but in another location.

A   **B**

(A) T1-weighted MRI, sagittal projection, without gadolinium. **(B)** T2-weighted MRI, axial projection.

What is the *most* likely pathology of the lesion shown?

a. pituitary adenoma
b. meningioma
c. craniopharyngioma
d. anterior communicating artery aneurysm

Discussion

With MRI, T1 images can normally be recognized by the dark appearance of cerebrospinal fluid and vitreous, while on T2 images they appear bright. Orbital fat appears bright on T1 and dark on T2. These MRIs show an intrasellar mass displacing the chiasm upward, which is not bright on T1 (see the figure, part A) and is extremely bright on T2 (see the figure, part B), indicating mobile proteins in the fluid-filled proteinaceous cyst. This, taken with the history, makes the diagnosis of a cystic craniopharyngioma most likely, although the intrasellar location is less frequently encountered than the suprasellar location. A pituitary adenoma would be seen as a mass arising out of the sella below the chiasm, but it would not be this bright on a T2 image. Meningiomas are often isointense to brain on nonenhanced T1 and T2 images; they may intensely enhance with gadolinium. Aneurysms will have different appearances depending on whether flow, thrombosis, or hemorrhage is present, but they would not be so bright on T2.[20]

Preferred Response

c. craniopharyngioma

A 17-year-old boy receives an ophthalmic examination before beginning driver's education. The results of the examination are as follows:

Uncorrected acuity: 20/20 OU

Pupils: 5 mm OU, round and reactive; mild RAPD OD

Motility: Normal

Slit lamp: Normal

Intraocular pressures: 16 mm Hg OD, 18 mm Hg OS

Visual fields: Inferior altitudinal defect OD, normal OS

All of the following points in the history or examination, if elicited, would aid in arriving at a diagnosis *except*

a. He has optic nerve hypoplasia OD, and his mother has insulin-dependent (juvenile-onset) diabetes mellitus.
b. A cilioretinal artery is present OD only.
c. The patient had an episode of marked acute visual loss OD with pain on ocular rotation 2 years before, with partial recovery.
d. A superior hemiretinal detachment is present OD.

Discussion

Offspring of mothers with insulin-dependent (juvenile-onset) diabetes mellitus may have optic nerve head hypoplasia with an associated congenital altitudinal scotoma.[21] Optic neuritis and a hemiretinal detachment could also cause an altitudinal scotoma. The finding of a cilioretinal artery has no bearing on the presence of the altitudinal field defect.

Preferred Response   b. A cilioretinal artery is present OD only.

All of the following statements about optokinetic response testing are true *except*

a. Absence of response with the tape moving to the patient's left may indicate a left frontal lobe lesion.
b. Absence of response with the tape moving to the patient's right may indicate a right parietal lesion.
c. Presence of optokinetic nystagmus response to an optokinetic drum at a test distance of 3 feet indicates a visual acuity of 20/60 or better.
d. In a patient with a complete right adduction deficit, ability to cause the right eye to fully adduct in response to an optokinetic drum indicates that the ophthalmoparesis is not infranuclear in origin.

Discussion   The optokinetic response may be thought of as a pursuit movement in the direction of the movement of the drum or tape, and a refixational saccadic movement in the direction away from the movement of the drum or tape. In the case of a drum moving to the patient's *right*, the following pursuit movement toward the right is mediated by the *right* parietal lobe. The refixational *leftward* saccade is mediated by the *right* frontal lobe. Thus, optokinetic response testing may be thought of as testing the saccade and pursuit initiation in the frontal and parietal lobes on the side toward which the tape or drum is moving.[22] As with caloric or oculocephalic maneuvers, optokinetic response testing may be used to demonstrate that the final common pathway from the nucleus to nerve to extraocular muscle is intact, or that the ocular rotation defect is supranuclear in origin. An optokinetic drum may also be used to estimate visual acuity (as in cases of functional visual loss), but the minimum acuity requisite to obtain a response to a drum at 3 feet is only counting fingers at 3 to 5 feet.

Preferred Response   c. Presence of optokinetic nystagmus response to an optokinetic drum at a test distance of 3 feet indicates a visual acuity of 20/60 or better.

N17   A patient involved in a motor vehicle accident had loss of consciousness for 10 minutes. She has an abduction deficit of the right eye, with only about 10% of normal amplitude of abduction beyond the midline remaining. The anterior examination is normal; exophthalmometry readings are symmetric.

Which of the following would be consistent with the presence of a right sixth-nerve palsy *without* an entrapped medial rectus?

a. restriction of the right eye on forced abduction, no force generated with attempted abduction on forced generation test
b. ability to induce full abduction OD with oculocephalic maneuver
c. no restriction on forced abduction OD, diminished force generated with attempted abduction on forced generation test
d. exodeviation on right gaze

Discussion   In significant head trauma, it is possible to see both a neurogenic sixth-nerve palsy from the closed head injury and medial rectus entrapment from an orbital fracture. In the setting of a medial orbital fracture *with* medial rectus entrapment and *without* sixth-nerve dysfunction, the forced duction would demonstrate resistance opposite to the field of action of the restricted muscle. In a nearly complete sixth-nerve paresis, one would not be able to completely overcome the abduction deficit with oculo-cephalic maneuver. Also, in an isolated acute right sixth-nerve paresis, there would be an *eso*deviation in all fields of gaze. In an acute sixth-nerve paresis without entrapment, there would be no resistance to forced ductions, but there would be either no force or reduced force imparted to the right globe in right abduction, because the right lateral rectus is not receiving normal neural input to induce its contraction.

Preferred Response   c. no restriction on forced abduction OD, diminished force generated with attempted abduction on forced generation test

A 68-year-old man complains only of recent onset of "trouble reading." There is no past medical history. The results of the patient's examination are as follows:

Best-corrected acuity: Distance—20/25 OU; near—20/20 OU

Pupils: 3 mm OU, round and reactive; no RAPD

Lid fissures: 10 mm OU

Motility: Horizontal eye movements normal, volitional down gaze severely and symmetrically limited, up gaze mildly limited. Oculo-cephalic maneuver completely overcomes the vertical eye movement deficiency.

Slit lamp: Normal

Intraocular pressures: Normal

Visual fields: Normal

Fundi: Normal

The *most* likely diagnosis is

a. botulism
b. myasthenia gravis
c. congenital fibrosis syndrome
d. progressive supranuclear palsy (Steele-Richardson-Olszewski syndrome)

Discussion   The onset of a supranuclear gaze paresis in the vertical plane, especially if worse on down gaze, should alert the ophthalmologist to the possibility of progressive supranuclear palsy (PSP). This disorder often impairs down gaze first, and at first the gaze dysfunction may be overcome by oculocephalic and caloric maneuvers. Although myasthenia gravis could present with a significant symmetric down gaze weakness, it would not be completely overcome by oculocephalics. Botulism may present with an ophthalmoparesis, but the pupils are most often affected, and this presynaptic blockade would not be overcome by the oculocephalic maneuver. The pupils are typically dilated and poorly responsive to light in this disorder, which has a more acute onset than the case described. In congenital fibrosis syndrome, there is usually marked horizontal restriction as well as vertical impairment, and the rotational deficit would not be overcome by the oculocephalic maneuver.

Preferred Response   d. progressive supranuclear palsy (Steele-Richardson-Olszewski syndrome)

N19

Which of the following would be *most* inconsistent with the diagnosis of the patient in Question N18?

a. extensor neck rigidity
b. dementia
c. pigmentary retinopathy
d. square wave jerks

Discussion   Progressive dementia, square wave jerks (small amplitude saccadic jerky movements away from fixation), ataxia, and axial rigidity are all typical in the course of progressive supranuclear palsy.[23] Pigmentary retinopathy is a feature of the Kearns-Sayre syndrome, which is in the differential of a progressive symmetric ophthalmoparesis, but would not have late onset and would not be likely to respond to the oculocephalic maneuver.

Preferred Response   c. pigmentary retinopathy

N20

A 3-year-old girl is brought in by her mother for evaluation of a mass that is medial and superior to the left medial canthus and that has been present since birth. The mother is not sure if it has been growing. The examination is normal except for nystagmus OU. You have difficulty visualizing the fundus. The child is short for her age; otherwise, she is doing well.

Appropriate management at this point includes all of the following *except*

a. examination under anesthesia
b. neuroimaging
c. pediatric endocrinologic consultation
d. needle biopsy of the mass, followed by neuroimaging if not inflammatory

Discussion   Septo-optic dysplasia (de Morsier's syndrome) consists of a triad of growth failure, optic nerve hypoplasia, and nystagmus. Neuroimaging serves two purposes. First, it will demonstrate the classic finding of an absent septum pellucidum (the so-called upside-down Liberty Bell sign). Second, as these dysplasias may be associated with basal encephaloceles and other midline abnormalities, neuroimaging will be needed to demonstrate that the mass is not an encephalocele before any biopsy is performed.[24] In a child with unexplained nystagmus where the fundus cannot be well visualized in the examination room, examination under anesthesia is a reasonable part of the ophthalmologist's evaluation. Because patients with septo-optic dysplasia may have hypothalamic dysfunction (including deficiencies of growth hormone, adrenocorticotropic hormone, and antidiuretic hormone), endocrinologic evaluation is part of their assessment.

Preferred Response   d. needle biopsy of the mass, followed by neuroimaging if not inflammatory

Which of the following conditions is the *most* likely explanation for the visual fields shown in the figures?

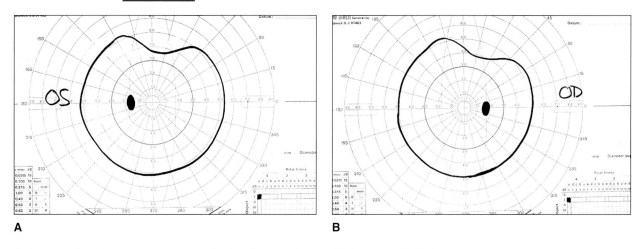

A   **B**

Goldmann visual fields demonstrating tilted optic nerve heads. **(A)** Left eye. **(B)** Right eye.

a. pituitary adenoma
b. tilted optic nerve heads
c. bilateral optic nerve pits
d. craniopharyngioma

Discussion   The figures show a bitemporal visual field defect that does not respect the midline. Pituitary adenomas present with superotemporal defects that respect the midline. Depending on whether they are infrachiasmal or suprachiasmal, craniopharyngiomas present with either superotemporal or inferotemporal field defects that respect the midline. Optic nerve pits may be associated with serous macular detachments, and thus cause field defects that are usually central or cecocentral. With tilted optic nerve heads, the inferonasal portions of the discs are often more posterior with associated crescents, producing superotemporal defects that do not respect the midline.

Preferred Response   b. tilted optic nerve heads

A 335-pound 25-year-old woman comes in on a Monday for evaluation of bilateral synchronous visual obscurations lasting 15 seconds. These have been occurring for 3 weeks. She has no other medical history and is on no medications. Her examination is normal except for enlarged blind spots on visual field testing and marked bilateral papilledema.

What is the *most* reasonable next step in her management?

a. Obtain an MRI that day; if it is negative, begin her on acetazolamide 500 mg q6h and see her in 3 days to determine whether the papilledema has improved.

b. Obtain an MRI on her that day; if it is negative, arrange for a spinal tap shortly thereafter.

c. Start her on acetazolamide 500 mg q6h, and refer her to a neurologist on Thursday.

d. Put her on a weight-reduction and salt-restriction diet, start her on acetazolamide 500 mg q6h, and see her in 4 days to determine whether the papilledema has improved and to reassess the visual function.

Discussion

Even in the patient whose presentation is classic for pseudotumor cerebri, two critical steps must be taken before the diagnosis can be made.[25] First, it is imperative to rule out the presence of an intracranial mass, which can be a neurosurgical emergency and can certainly occur in the obese patient. MRI is the imaging method of choice; it also serves to establish that the pseudotumor cerebri is not secondary to dural sinus thrombosis. If there is no mass, the second requisite for establishing the diagnosis of pseudotumor cerebri is that the spinal tap show raised intracranial pressure with normal chemical and cellular composition of the spinal fluid (eg, no evidence of inflammation or infection). Only after these steps are taken is it appropriate to begin therapy for pseudotumor cerebri.

Preferred Response

b. Obtain an MRI on her that day; if it is negative, arrange for a spinal tap shortly thereafter.

Which of the following is true about Leber's hereditary optic neuropathy?

a. It is purely a clinical diagnosis, based on the family inheritance pattern.

b. Females may develop Leber's hereditary optic neuropathy.

c. It is rare for affected patients to have no family history of visual loss.

d. The onset in the two eyes is always simultaneous.

Discussion

Although males are most often affected (80% to 90% of cases in Caucasians, 60% of cases in Japanese), females are affected more often than was previously reported. Males at genetic risk have a higher chance of developing visual loss than do females at genetic risk for Leber's hereditary optic neuropathy (LHON). We now know that LHON is a phenotypic expression of several different mitochondrial genetic alterations.

These mitochondrial genetic sequences can now be established, allowing for laboratory confirmation in nearly all cases. Worldwide, the 11778 point mutation accounts for about 50% of all LHON cases. The 3460 point mutation accounts for 8% to 25% of LHON cases. A third point mutation at locus 14484 may cause 10% of LHON. Many LHON patients have a negative family history. The interval between the involvement of the first and the second eye is usually days to weeks, but it may extend to months or years in some cases.[26–28]

Preferred Response   b. Females may develop Leber's hereditary optic neuropathy.

A 70-year-old man presents with a 7-day history of diplopia, having just been discharged from the hospital by his neurologist. He is referred to you to see if prism glasses are indicated. He has a complete right pupil-involving third-nerve palsy. The neurologist tells you that his examination is otherwise normal. The patient says that since he has had the double vision, he has also had a headache with loss of appetite. The results of the evaluation performed by the neurologist are as follows:

MRI with gadolinium: Normal

Lumbar puncture: Normal

Cerebral angiography: Normal

Edrophonium (Tensilon) test: Normal

Acetylcholine receptor antibody: Normal

Glucose tolerance test: Normal

Syphilis and Lyme serologies: Normal

Blood count, ANA, rheumatoid factor: Normal

The results of your examination of the patient are as follows:

Best-corrected acuity: 20/40 OD, 20/30 OS

Ishihara color plates: Normal OU

Pupils: Dim—8 mm OD, 7 mm OS; light—8 mm OD, 2 mm OS; near—8 mm OD, 2 mm OS

Lid fissures: 0 mm OD, 10 mm OS

Motility: 4+ underaction of right inferior oblique, inferior rectus, superior rectus, and medial rectus muscles; lateral rectus muscle intact, incyclotorsion present. Motility of left eye normal. No aberrant regeneration is seen.

Prism cover test: At distance, exotropia = 25 prism diopters; at near, exotropia = 35 prism diopters

Slit lamp: Normal

Intraocular pressures: Normal

Media: 2+ nuclear sclerotic cataract OD, 1+ nuclear sclerotic cataract OS

Fundi: Normal

Which of the following is the *most* important and appropriate immediate step in the management of this patient?

a. Repeat the edrophonium (Tensilon) test with a prism cover test.
b. Obtain an erythrocyte sedimentation rate.
c. Give him 10 base-in ground-in prism in front of the OD for distance, and give him a 25 prism diopter Fresnel prism base-in for near.
d. Give him a patch to use as needed.

Discussion

Any patient in the age group in which temporal arteritis is in the differential diagnosis who presents with one of the common ocular signs of temporal arteritis (anterior ischemic optic neuropathy, amaurosis fugax, or diplopia) must have a sedimentation rate promptly. Failure to diagnose temporal arteritis may be followed by infarction of the optic nerve. Diplopia, which may be the presenting sign of temporal arteritis in about 12% of cases,[1] may be due to either ischemia of the extraocular muscles themselves or ischemia of the vessels supplying the third, fourth, and sixth cranial nerves.[29] In two series, 50% to 58% of those with diplopia progressed to blindness.[30, 31] Although a pupil-involving third-nerve palsy would be a rare presentation of temporal arteritis, this man also has constitutional signs consistent with temporal arteritis, namely, headache and anorexia, which should raise suspicion. Repeating the edrophonium (Tensilon) test is not necessary, as the pupil findings preclude myasthenia. The symptomatic therapy is indicated after temporal arteritis is excluded.

Preferred Response

b. Obtain an erythrocyte sedimentation rate.

A 9-year-old girl is brought in by her father, a pediatrician. She has had six episodes that are extremely similar, one every 4 weeks; he took pictures of the last episode (see the figures). She becomes cranky and lethargic, and 1 day later, gets the ophthalmoparesis shown in the figures. Her pupils are 6 mm OU in dim light, 3 mm in bright light, round and reactive to light, with no RAPD. There are no other neurologic signs. As soon as the ophthalmoparesis begins, she feels better. The ophthalmoparesis lasts 1 week. Once it resolves, her examination results return to normal. The father has already obtained MRI and a high-resolution magnetic resonance angiogram, which are both normal.

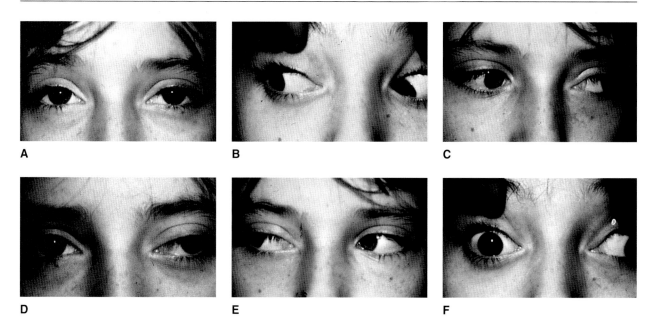

Eye movements of a 9-year-old girl. Before episode: **(A)** Primary gaze; **(B)** right gaze; **(C)** left gaze. During episode: **(D)** Primary gaze; **(E)** right gaze; **(F)** left gaze.

Which of the following is the *most* appropriate management step?

a. Perform a neostigmine (Prostigmin) test.
b. Obtain a spinal tap.
c. Start her on pyridostigmine bromide (Mestinon), 30 mg q4–6h.
d. Begin a trial of propranolol (Inderal) or amitriptyline (Elavil) determined as appropriate for her age and size by her pediatrician father.

Discussion   The syndrome described is classic for ophthalmoplegic migraine.[32] The repetitive course of lethargy, irritability, photophobia, and perhaps headache, followed by ophthalmoplegia (90% of the time, the oculomotor nerve), is typical. Usually, at the moment the ophthalmoparesis begins, the other symptoms abate. The key to management is recognition of the syndrome. Aneurysms would not cause this stereotypical repetitive pattern, and their occurrence as a cause of third-nerve palsies in children is rare. Ocular myasthenia would not be so stereotypical, nor would it have the prodromal symptoms. While pupillary dilation may be a feature of migraine, it is not seen in myasthenia. If the frequency of the attacks warrants, a trial of an appropriate antimigraine prophylactic agent should be prescribed.

Preferred Response   d. Begin a trial of propranolol (Inderal) or amitriptyline (Elavil) determined as appropriate for her age and size by her pediatrician father.

A 45-year-old right-handed male executive who is an avid golfer presents with the complaint that for the past year, whenever he addresses a golf ball, it appears to be shimmering up and down, with perhaps a rotatory component to it. Sometimes the ball looks double to him in the vertical plane. The patient, a good observer, says that the image moves and is double only when viewed with the right eye. The results of his examination are normal.

Which of the following is the *most* appropriate action to take?

a. Start the patient on carbamazepine (Tegretol).
b. Obtain a psychiatric consultation.
c. Start the patient on phenytoin (Dilantin).
d. Perform an edrophonium (Tensilon) test.

Discussion

The patient has given a classic description of superior oblique myokymia.[33] In this disorder, there is an intermittent rapid oscillopsia, which is largely a cyclorotatory phenomenon, with intorsional movements. These episodes may be triggered by moving the eye into the field of action of the affected superior oblique muscle. When a right-handed golfer addresses a golf ball, the eye moves into a depressed and adducted position, which can trigger these attacks. Carbamazepine (Tegretol) seems to help most patients with this condition, although some report that the beneficial effect is transitory.

Preferred Response

a. Start the patient on carbamazepine (Tegretol).

A 67-year-old Asian man consulted you 3 months ago with an isolated right sixth-nerve palsy that had been present for 3 months. His CT scan with contrast of the head, edrophonium (Tensilon) test, glucose tolerance test, sedimentation rate, and serologies for Lyme disease and syphilis were normal. He now presents with a left sixth-nerve palsy to accompany the persistent right sixth-nerve palsy. The results of the rest of the examination remain normal. There is no proptosis. A spinal tap performed by his neurologist 1 day earlier was normal.

The *most* likely location of the pathologic process is

a. bilateral abducens nucleus
b. both orbital apices
c. genu of right facial nerve around abducens nucleus
d. clivus

Discussion

Both sixth nerves come together to ascend the clivus. The sequential involvement of both abducens nerves should alert the ophthalmologist to consider a mass lesion in this location. Although a process involving both orbital apices could theoretically cause bilateral sixth-nerve palsies, proptosis and other signs of orbital involvement would be expected. A lesion of the genu of the right facial nerve might give an ipsilateral sixth- and seventh-nerve paresis, but not bilateral sixth-nerve palsies. Bilateral nuclear sixth-nerve palsies would give the patient bilateral gaze paresis.

Preferred Response   d. clivus

In the patient in Question N27, which of the following is the *least* important in terms of his management plan?

a. Obtain MRI of the base of the brain.
b. Obtain an otolaryngology consult.
c. Perform another spinal tap in a few days.
d. Obtain cervical carotid ultrasonography.

Discussion   In an Asian male presenting with bilateral sixth-nerve palsies, nasopharyngeal carcinoma is a concern, as the ophthalmoparesis may be the presenting sign from tumor extension along the clivus.[34] Otolaryngologic consultation is thus indicated. Multiple spinal taps may be required to detect carcinomatous meningitis; thus, repeat spinal tap is appropriate. As the CT scan of the head may not image the base of the brain well, MRI is indicated. Carotid atherosclerotic disease would not present in this manner.

Preferred Response   d. Obtain cervical carotid ultrasonography.

A 56-year-old woman presents with a history of 12 months of double vision and 6 months of ptosis OS. She says that her vision is normal in each eye, and that she has no pain. Her past medical history is normal. The results of her examination are as follows:

Best-corrected acuity: 20/20 OU

Ishihara color plates: Normal OU

Pupils: 5 mm OU, round and reactive; no RAPD

Lid fissures: 10 mm OD, 7 mm OS

Corneal reflex: Depressed OS; rest of trigeminal function remarkable for decreased cutaneous sensation in the distribution of the left maxillary nerve.

Motility: Normal OD; OS 3+ underaction of lateral rectus muscle; 1+ underaction of left medial, superior, and inferior rectus muscles; trace underaction of left inferior oblique muscle; superior oblique muscle normal.

Exophthalmometry: Base 103 mm, OD 18 mm, OS 20 mm

Slit lamp: Mild superficial punctate staining OS, otherwise normal

Intraocular pressures: 14 mm Hg OU, normal pulse pressure

Visual fields: Normal

Fundi: Normal

The *most* likely location of the lesion is

a. limited to the left cavernous sinus, sparing the chiasm
b. involving the left cavernous sinus and the chiasm
c. limited to the left orbital apex
d. left maxillary sinus

Discussion   The key here is evidence of the left third, fifth (first and second divisions), and sixth cranial nerve involvement, with 2 mm of proptosis and sparing of the optic nerve. A lesion contained in the orbital apex would not involve the maxillary nerve, nor would it be as likely to spare the optic nerve. Proptosis greater than 2 mm would be more common in an orbital apex lesion than with a cavernous sinus lesion. As in this case, lesions of the cavernous sinus that spare the chiasm may involve the third, fourth, fifth, and sixth cranial nerves. Although lesions of the sphenoid sinus could cause combined involvement of the second, third, fifth, and sixth cranial nerves, lesions of the maxillary sinus would ordinarily not do so.

Preferred Response   a. limited to the left cavernous sinus, sparing the chiasm

   With the presentation and the MRI scans (shown below) from the patient in Question N29, what is the likely underlying pathophysiology?

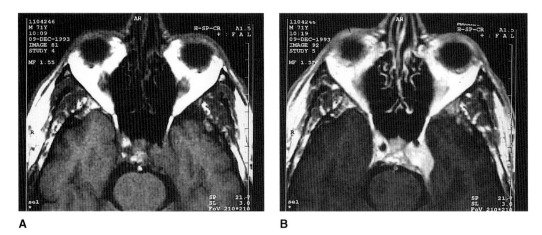

A   **B**

MRI scans. **(A)** T1, without gadolinium. **(B)** T1, with gadolinium.

a. meningioma
b. Tolosa-Hunt syndrome
c. dysthyroid ophthalmopathy
d. pituitary apoplexy

Discussion   This presentation in a female of this age group should raise the suspicion of meningioma. In this case, we see that the lesion is nearly isointense to brain on T1 without gadolinium (part A), and enhances intensely with gadolinium (part B), features typical of the highly vascular nature of the meningioma.[35] The case is not typical of Tolosa-Hunt syndrome, as the patient does not have pain. In dysthyroid ophthalmopathy or the myositic forms of orbital pseudotumor, one would see enlarged muscles. In pituitary apoplexy, which can cause involvement of the second, third, fourth, fifth, and sixth cranial nerves, one would not see a mass that enhances so intensely with contrast.

Preferred Response   a. meningioma

A 57-year-old woman comes for a routine periodic examination to have her reading glasses changed. She has no complaints. Your screening protocol includes a visual field examination that shows a normal field OS and an inferior field defect OD (see the figures). The results of the rest of the examination are as follows:

Best-corrected acuity: 20/20 OU

Ishihara color plates: Normal OU

Pupils: 4 mm OU, round and reactive; 1+ RAPD OD

Motility: Normal

Exophthalmometry: Base 98 mm, OD 19 mm, OS 18 mm

Slit lamp: Normal

Intraocular pressures: Normal

Fundi: Mild disc edema OD, normal OS

The patient denies pain. Because of the findings, you elect to obtain an imaging study. What is the *most* appropriate study to request?

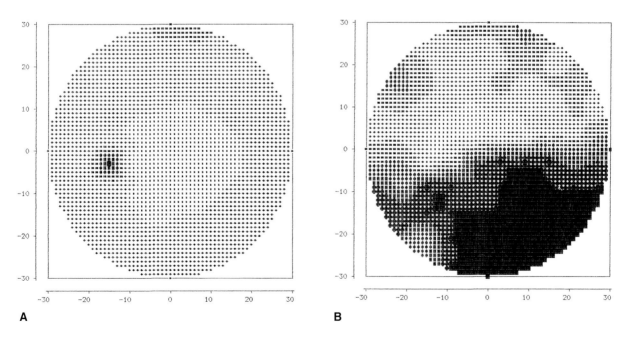

A   **B**

Automated visual fields of a patient with unilateral (right) optic neuropathy. **(A)** Left eye. **(B)** Right eye.

a. CT scan of the orbit, without contrast
b. MRI of the brain, with gadolinium
c. CT scan of the head, with contrast
d. MRI of the orbit/optic nerves, with gadolinium and fat-suppression sequences

Discussion

The clinical presentation is that of a unilateral optic neuropathy. A CT scan of the orbit, if selected, should be done with contrast to look for vascular masses. A CT scan of the head would probably not image the optic nerve well, as is the case with MRI of the *brain*. The ideal method of imaging the optic nerve is with MRI, concentrating on the optic nerve with fat-suppression sequences. This will help delineate the optic nerve in stark contrast to the orbital fat, which looks black on this technique. In such a case, one should make sure that the optic nerve is well imaged back to the chiasm.

Preferred Response

d. MRI of the orbit/optic nerves, with gadolinium and fat-suppression sequences

N32

The figures show the MRI results for the patient in Question N31. Part A is a T1 weighted image without contrast; part B is a T1, fat-suppressed, gadolinium-enhanced image.

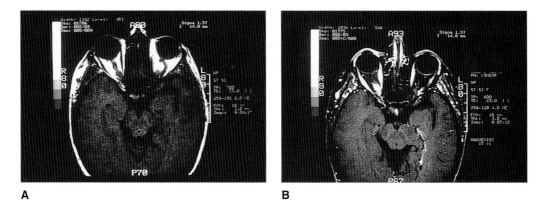

A   **B**

MRI results of a patient with optic nerve meningioma. **(A)** T1 without contrast. **(B)** T1 with fat suppression and gadolinium.

Given the presentation and the MRI results, what is now the *most* appropriate management of this patient?

a. Perform a biopsy of the optic nerve.
b. Perform a CT scan of the optic nerve with contrast.
c. Do nothing now and reexamine the patient in 2 months; if still stable, see again in a few months, with a repeat MRI at 6 months.
d. Give a diagnostic and therapeutic course of corticosteroids.

Discussion

In terms of both its presentation and imaging, the lesion is typical of an optic nerve meningioma. Given that the patient has no clinical symptoms, it would be most appropriate to follow the patient, as in many of these cases progression either does not occur or is extremely slow. Resection of the lesion would blind the eye; it is likely that biopsy would cause significant worsening. A CT scan probably would not add any information that would alter the management of the case. The lesion does not appear inflammatory (also, the patient has no pain); thus, a diagnostic/therapeutic trial of corticosteroids, such as for inflammatory orbital pseudotumor, is not indicated.

Preferred Response

c. Do nothing now and reexamine the patient in 2 months; if still stable, see again in a few months, with a repeat MRI at 6 months.

The patient in Question N31 returns for her 6-month followup. At the previous visit, her examination was unchanged from the initial evaluation. Her visual acuity OD has now dropped to 20/60; the color plates are now 4/10 correct OD; the afferent pupillary defect is more apparent; and an optociliary shunt vessel is now seen on the right disc. The visual field defect is also worse, with a central scotoma breaking out into the old inferior scotoma.

What is the *most* appropriate next course of action?

a. Repeat the MRI; if no change, see the patient again in 4 months.
b. Repeat the MRI; if no growth, resect the lesion.
c. Repeat the MRI; irradiate the lesion.
d. Obtain a CT scan of the optic nerves to see if any calcifications have developed.

Discussion

Anterior visual pathway meningiomas may respond to irradiation.[36] When the patient has very mild disease (as was the case at the first visit), the risks of irradiation (eg, radiation optic neuropathy) do not justify its use. However, with clear progression to significant optic neuropathy, the possible benefits outweigh the risks. Optic neuropathy may progress without MRI evidence of growth, but the MRI is still obtained to define treatment ports. It is not appropriate just to follow the patient in the setting of relatively rapid visual loss. Resection of the lesion would blind the eye. With a presumably benign lesion, trying irradiation first to preserve vision is more appropriate. Evidence of calcifications on a CT scan would not change the management in this case.

Preferred Response

c. Repeat the MRI; irradiate the lesion.

N34

Which of the following historical points or physical findings would *most* call for MRI in a patient who is having an eleventh bout of a classic migraine syndrome?

a. The patient is 17 years old.
b. The patient is a male.
c. Hemianopia is always on the same side.
d. The visual phenomena are homonymous.

Discussion

Migraine is not uncommon at age 17, and although migraine headaches are more common in females, they are not unusual in males. In classic migraine, the visual phenomenon (scintillating scotoma) is typically homonymous. Although these episodes may be rather stereotypical, and they most often may be on one particular side of the head, *always* having the symptoms on one side raises the question of a fixed lesion causing the migrainous phenomenon, such as an arteriovenous malformation.[37]

Preferred Response

c. Hemianopia is always on the same side.

N35

A patient presents with optic neuropathy and uveitis with mutton-fat keratic precipitates. The patient is noted to have bilateral large, nodular lacrimal glands and a white raised lesion on the involved optic nerve head.

Which of the following test results would be *most* likely to exclude the diagnosis of sarcoidosis in this patient?

a. a normal chest x-ray
b. a normal ACE (angiotensin converting enzyme)
c. a normal conjunctival biopsy
d. a positive PPD (purified protein derivative), with the rest of the anergy panel negative (normal cutaneous response was present to mumps)

Discussion

A patient may have ocular involvement of sarcoidosis without having an abnormal chest x-ray. Similarly, the ACE is typically not elevated unless there is pulmonary disease. Positive conjunctival biopsies are useful in making the diagnosis, as they provide histologic confirmation of the diagnosis, which is preferred when one needs to institute systemic therapy for sarcoidosis. However, many patients with systemic sarcoidosis will have normal conjunctival biopsies, particularly if no lesion is clinically visible. Patients with tuberculosis may, on occasion, have an elevated ACE and certainly would have an abnormal chest x-ray. They may also have optic nerve involvement and uveitis. Patients with sarcoidosis usually show lack of response (anergy) on the anergy panel, whereas tuberculosis patients will typically have positive response to cutaneous testing with PPD. A patient with this presentation and a positive PPD must be considered to have tuberculosis and not sarcoidosis.[38]

Preferred Response

d. a positive PPD (purified protein derivative), with the rest of the anergy panel negative (normal cutaneous response was present to mumps)

N36

All of the following syndromes with neuro-ophthalmic signs are associated with the endocrinopathy mentioned *except*

a. chiasmal trauma/diabetes insipidus
b. de Morsier's syndrome/growth failure
c. angiomatosis retinae (von Hippel-Lindau disease)/pheochromocytoma
d. chiasmal sarcoidosis/Cushing's disease

Discussion

Due to concomitant trauma to the hypothalamic-pituitary axis, chiasmal trauma is often associated with diabetes insipidus. Septo-optic dysplasia, or de Morsier's syndrome, consists of agenesis of the septum pellucidum, optic nerve hypoplasia, and growth failure.[24] Angiomatosis retinae may have several extraocular manifestations, including hemangioblastoma of the central nervous system; renal, pancreatic, hepatic, or epididymal cysts; and pheochromocytoma.[39] Sarcoidosis of the chiasm is often accompanied by diabetes insipidus, not Cushing's disease, due to the attendant hypothalamic infiltration and dysfunction.[40]

Preferred Response

d. chiasmal sarcoidosis/Cushing's disease

N37

A 37-year-old woman presents with ptosis and ophthalmoplegia. She first noted ptosis at age 12, and noted trouble moving her eyes 3 years later. It has been progressive over the years; she never had any diplopia, and she believes that her vision, once her eyelids are raised, is normal. There is no family history. She denies other medical problems, and she has not seen a physician for 10 years. The results of her examination are as follows:

Uncorrected acuity: 20/20 OU

Ishihara color plates: Normal OU

Pupils: 4 mm OU, round and reactive; no RAPD

Lid fissures: 2 mm OU

Orbicularis tone: Mild symmetric weakness

Ocular rotations: Complete ophthalmoplegia, not overcome by oculocephalic (doll's head) maneuver or Bell's phenomenon

Neck: No rigidity

Fundi: Discs sharp and pink, questionable slight "salt and pepper" appearance to peripheral retinal pigment epithelium OU

The *most* likely diagnosis is

a. Usher's syndrome
b. progressive supranuclear palsy (Steele-Richardson-Olszewski syndrome)
c. ocular myasthenia
d. Kearns-Sayre syndrome

Discussion

The presentation of bilateral symmetric and progressive ophthalmoparesis and ptosis in a young patient who has never had diplopia suggests chronic progressive external ophthalmoplegia (CPEO). Neither progressive supranuclear palsy nor myasthenia would demonstrate a pigmentary retinopathy; the former also typically shows neck rigidity as a sign.[23] Usher's syndrome causes retinitis pigmentosa and hearing loss, and even ataxia, but not ophthalmoparesis. A subset of CPEO, the Kearns-Sayre syndrome has several other features, including early onset (before age 20), and pigmentary retinopathy.[41,42]

Preferred Response   d. Kearns-Sayre syndrome

Regarding the patient in Question N37, all of the following could be appropriate actions to take at the initial visit *except*

a. perform edrophonium (Tensilon) test
b. schedule muscle biopsy
c. send off mitochondrial genetic analysis
d. schedule cardiac evaluation

Discussion   Besides ophthalmoplegia and retinopathy, patients with Kearns-Sayre syndrome should also have at least one of the following other three manifestations for the clinical diagnosis to be made: cardiac conduction abnormalities (ie, heart block), elevated cerebrospinal fluid protein, or cerebellar dysfunction. The clinical diagnosis is supported by muscle biopsy demonstrating "ragged red fibers." Mitochondrial genetic analysis shows gene deletions in many cases, confirming the diagnosis. Spinal fluid analysis is also useful, because elevated cerebrospinal fluid protein is a criterion for diagnosis.[43] Because cardiac conduction abnormalities (including heart block, which may cause sudden death) may be a feature of Kearns-Sayre syndrome, insertion of a pacemaker is often part of the management of these cases. Thus, edrophonium (which may cause bradycardia) should not be given to a patient in whom Kearns-Sayre syndrome is in the differential diagnosis until the patient has had a cardiac evaluation.

Preferred Response   a. perform edrophonium (Tensilon) test

A 26-year-old woman presents with progressive visual loss that has occurred over 6 years. Best-corrected visual acuity is 20/80 in each eye. The results of visual field testing are shown in the figure.

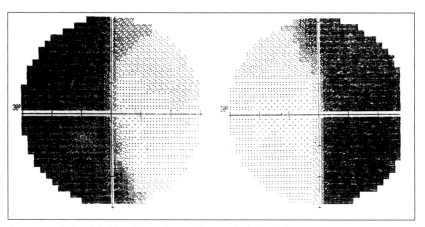

Automated visual fields of a patient with a probable pituitary tumor.

Given the visual fields, which of the following statements is *most* inconsistent with the rest of the evaluation?

a. She has missed a few menstrual cycles over the past year.
b. She is infertile.
c. She has a 3+ to 4+ RAPD OS.
d. She has sparing of the nerve fiber layer along the temporal arcades of both eyes.

Discussion

The visual field defect localizes to the optic chiasm, and a pituitary tumor is a likely cause. With pupillary testing in the setting of symmetric visual loss, there is rarely enough disparity to give a significant *relative* afferent pupillary defect, because each optic nerve's afferent dysfunction is essentially the same. Endocrinopathy, as manifested by menstrual irregularities and infertility, is not uncommon in this setting. With temporal field loss and nasal field sparing, the preserved nerve fiber layer, corresponding to the spared nasal field, would be the temporal nerve fiber layer.

Preferred Response

c. She has a 3+ to 4+ RAPD OS.

A 7-year-old boy is referred by a pediatrician for evaluation of his visual status. The child is said to be slow in school and is being placed in special education. The pediatrician wishes to ensure that a refractive error is not contributing to the poor performance. The child has had three seizures, and a raised papular rash in a butterfly distribution has been noted on his cheeks. Some patchy hypopigmented areas are also seen on the trunk. The child is otherwise well.

The *most* likely diagnosis is

a. tuberous sclerosis (Bourneville's disease)
b. encephalotrigeminal angiomatosis (Sturge-Weber syndrome)
c. juvenile-onset systemic lupus erythematosus with cerebritis
d. neurofibromatosis type I (von Recklinghausen's disease)

Discussion

All of the entities listed are capable of causing fundus abnormalities and seizures with cutaneous findings. However, the triad of mental retardation, seizures, and the rash described in a butterfly distribution (adenoma sebaceum, actually angiofibromas) is most consistent with the diagnosis of tuberous sclerosis, or Bourneville's disease. This autosomal dominant disorder also has a typical CT scan finding of calcifications from intracerebral astrocytic hamartomas. Periungual fibromas may be seen, as well as cutaneous hypopigmented "ash-leaf" spots. Sturge-Weber syndrome has a different cutaneous manifestation, the typical nevus flammeus. Lupus erythematosus can cause seizures from cerebritis, but other clinical signs would probably be seen; in addition, the rash is different and would not include "ash-leaf" spots. Neurofibromatosis would not have a raised rash, and the rash would not be in this distribution.

Preferred Response

a. tuberous sclerosis (Bourneville's disease)

N41

If a fundus abnormality were encountered in the patient in Question N40, which of the following would it *most* likely be?

a. choroidal hemangioma
b. branch retinal artery occlusion
c. retinal astrocytic hamartoma (mulberry astrocytic hamartoma)
d. racemose angioma

Discussion

The typical fundus manifestation in this disorder (see the figure) is the astrocytic (mulberry) hamartoma of the optic nerve.[44] Choroidal hemangioma is the typical fundus manifestation of Sturge-Weber syndrome. Many retinal manifestations may occur in systemic lupus erythematosus, and retinal vascular occlusive disease is not unusual. Racemose angioma is the characteristic fundus finding in Wyburn-Mason's syndrome.

Astrocytic (mulberry) hamartoma of the optic nerve.

Preferred Response

c. retinal astrocytic hamartoma (mulberry astrocytic hamartoma)

N42

A 30-year-old woman whom you have examined several times in the past for a refractive error consults you as an emergency. In the past, aside from mild myopia, her examinations have always been normal. Specifically, you are sure that there has been no anisocoria or ptosis. The patient complains of a 1-day history of headache and severe pain in the left jaw and left upper neck, with local neck tenderness, and the new onset of ptosis. She tells you that she has taken up karate and had an especially vigorous workout yesterday evening. The results of her examination are as follows:

Best-corrected acuity: 20/20 OU

Pupils: Dim—8 mm OD, 3 mm OS; light—3 mm OD, 2.5 mm OS

Lid fissures: 10 mm OD, 8 mm OS

Motility: Normal

Exophthalmometry: Base 102 mm, OD 18 mm, OS 18 mm

Slit lamp: Normal, no injection of globes

Intraocular pressures: 12 mm Hg OD, 14 mm Hg OS

Fundi: Normal

With this history, the lesion of concern is *most* likely located in the

a. left brain stem
b. left cervical carotid artery
c. left cavernous sinus
d. left orbit

Discussion

The acute onset of a Horner's syndrome with ipsilateral jaw pain, particularly in the setting of neck trauma, should make the examiner suspicious of a traumatic carotid dissection.[45] Severe rotational or flexion extension injuries may cause this syndrome; a karate blow to the neck is a recognized cause. Severe jaw and neck pain with local tenderness would be unlikely features of orbital, cavernous sinus, or brain stem disease.

Preferred Response

b. left cervical carotid artery

A patient's routine examination is normal except for his pupils. The right pupil is 2.5 mm, the left pupil is 2.0 mm, neither reacts well to light, and both appear to react briskly to near.

Which of the following statements is true?

a. If the patient is a diabetic, no workup is needed.
b. If the fluorescent treponemal antibody (FTA), Lyme titer, and micro- hemagglutination test (MHA-TP) are positive, the patient should be treated for early Lyme disease, with no spinal tap being performed.
c. If the VDRL is negative, no spinal tap is needed.
d. If the FTA is positive, a spinal tap is needed.

Discussion

The clinical demonstration of a light-near dissociated pupil requires consideration of neurosyphilis until proven otherwise. Although patients with diabetes mellitus may have pupils that react poorly to light and better to near, the diabetic is not immune to syphilis, and one must proceed with the appropriate workup, which includes a serum VDRL and FTA.[46] The light-near dissociated pupil due to tertiary neurosyphilis has been termed the Argyll Robertson pupil. In Lyme disease, the MHA-TP, which is specific for syphilis, is typically negative. In tertiary neurosyphilis, the VDRL may revert to normal, but the FTA remains positive. Thus, if either the VDRL or the FTA is positive, a spinal tap will be needed to look for cerebrospinal fluid abnormalities and serology. The results of the spinal tap will dictate the therapy the patient receives.

Preferred Response

d. If the FTA is positive, a spinal tap is needed.

A 23-year-old woman presents with typical optic neuritis OD. She has no history of a prior episode of visual loss in either eye, nor any past history or physical finding to suggest neurologic disease outside of the visual system. The results of the examination are as follows:

Best-corrected acuity: 20/40 OD, 20/20 OS

Ishihara color plates: 6/10 correct OD, 10/10 correct OS

Visual fields: Shown in the figure, parts A and B

The representative MRI is shown in the figure, parts C and D. All images not shown are normal.

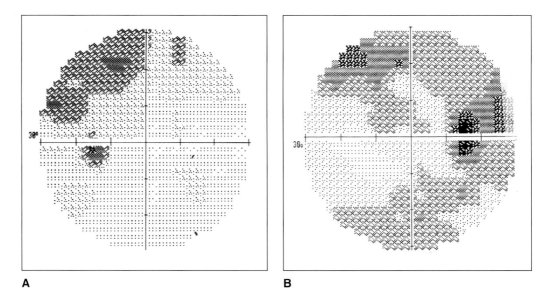

A   B

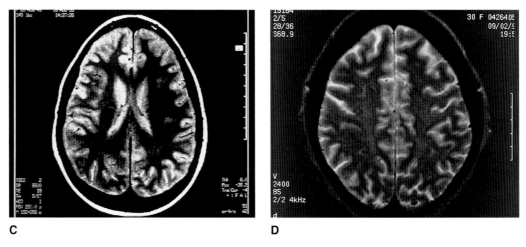

C   D

(A, B) Left and right visual fields of a 23-year-old woman with typical optic neuritis OD. **(C, D)** Normal MRIs of the same patient.

Which of the following statements is true?

a. The patient has the criteria for the diagnosis of multiple sclerosis at this time.
b. The patient may not have had a *prior* optic neuritis OS.
c. The patient should be treated with oral corticosteroids.
d. The patient has at least a 25% chance of developing multiple sclerosis in the next 2 years.

Discussion

Visual field changes not noted by the patient in the eye contralateral to the eye with acute optic neuritis were a frequent finding in the Optic Neuritis Treatment Trial. As the time course of their resolution followed that of the clinically involved eye, such a finding is not considered a second neurologic event.[4] Multiple sclerosis remains a clinical diagnosis, generally requiring evidence of two areas of involvement of the nervous system at two points in time. Here, there is no past history of disease, and the examination does not suggest other neurologic foci. Thus, as the subclinical simultaneous visual field change is not considered a second event, there is not enough evidence to support the diagnosis of multiple sclerosis. Oral corticosteroids as the sole treatment have no role in the therapy of optic neuritis, as they do not favorably affect the final visual outcome, and they increase the risk of further episodes of optic neuritis. Patients with isolated optic neuritis, no prior neurologic history, and a negative MRI have a very low risk of developing multiple sclerosis in the next 2 years.[15–17]

Preferred Response

b. The patient may not have had a *prior* optic neuritis OS.

Which of the following findings would be unusual in a patient presenting for an examination before craniotomy for a large pineal tumor?

a. light-near dissociation of the pupils
b. skew deviation
c. convergence-retraction nystagmus only on attempted saccades downward
d. lid retraction

Discussion

In Parinaud's syndrome (also known as dorsal midbrain syndrome, or sylvian aqueduct syndrome), the pupils may not react to light, but will react to near fixation. These pupils tend to be midsize or large, of greater size than those seen with syphilis. Lid retraction (Collier's sign) is typical, and skew deviation may be part of the findings. In this disorder, there is a selective involvement of *up* gaze, and, early on, saccades may be affected more than pursuit. Attempts at upward saccades may induce convergence-retraction nystagmus. Isolated convergence-retraction nystagmus on attempted *down* gaze is not a feature of this syndrome.

Preferred Response

c. convergence-retraction nystagmus only on attempted saccades downward

A 37-year-old man's examination is normal, but his history is striking. He has had, in the past few weeks, several bouts of severe right periocular pain associated with the right eye tearing. His nose runs, but only from the right nostril. His wife thinks that the right eye gets red during the episodes of pain. She knows when his pain occurs, because it always awakens him, and thus her, 2 hours before her alarm clock is set to go off.

The *most* likely diagnosis is

a. cluster headache
b. left frontal sinusitis
c. ophthalmoplegic migraine
d. left cervical carotid dissection

Discussion

This syndrome of stereotypical severe headache associated with unilateral rhinorrhea, lacrimation, ocular injection, and a definite periodicity is typical of cluster headache. Ingestion of alcohol incites attacks in many patients with cluster headache. Cluster headache is a distinct headache syndrome and is treated with drugs such as prednisone, nifedipine, verapamil, lithium, and cyproheptadine. Inhalation of 100% oxygen breaks many attacks. Frontal sinusitis can give a headache that is positional, but the other features would be unusual. Ophthalmoplegic migraine involves ophthalmoparesis, which is not present here. Cervical carotid dissection could produce an ipsilateral Horner's syndrome.

Preferred Response   a. cluster headache

A 16-year-old girl is referred to you for a further opinion. She has had three bouts of orbital pseudotumor. She is well except for what has clinically been diagnosed as asthma. She has had three needle biopsies of the orbit performed. The cytopathologist does not feel that a final diagnosis can be made, as all three demonstrated a mixed polyclonal inflammatory response. She responds to high doses of prednisone, but whenever she is tapered below 20 mg, she seems to flare again with ocular pain and proptosis. In examining her, you notice that the bridge of her nose seems too small for the rest of her nose. She confirms that the bridge is getting smaller, but blames it on the side effects of the prednisone.

Which of the following would be the *least* appropriate next step in her management?

a. Obtain a serum ANCA (antineutrophilic cytoplasmic antibody).
b. Obtain a chest x-ray and urinalysis.
c. Put her on 1 mg/kg of prednisone, do not taper for 1 year, then slowly wean.
d. Perform a biopsy via orbitotomy.

Discussion

The constellation of "recurrent orbital pseudotumor" with a loss of the bridge of the nose (saddle nose deformity) should raise the suspicion of an underlying systemic disorder. The differential of a saddle nose deformity includes Wegener's granulomatosis; malignant lymphoma; malignant polymorphic reticulosis (lymphomatoid granulomatosis) and idiopathic midline destructive disease, which may be forms of the same entity; chronic infection (eg, tuberculosis, syphilis, leprosy); nasal carcinoma; and relapsing polychondritis.[47] Among these, lymphomatoid granulomatosis and Wegener's granulomatosis would have a predilection for the orbit in this age group.[48–49] The serum ANCA is positive in about 95% of cases of Wegener's granulomatosis and is nearly diagnostic, although pathologic confirmation is always preferred.[50] As Wegener's granulomatosis typically involves the lungs (nearly 100% of cases) and the kidneys (81% of cases), chest x-ray and urinalysis are part of the workup. To be confident of starting more specific immunosuppressive therapy, such as cytotoxic agents, one would want definitive tissue diagnosis, hence the need for orbitotomy. Treating for a full year with corticosteroids would not be appropriate unless the diagnosis was definitive.

Preferred Response

c. Put her on 1 mg/kg of prednisone, do not taper for 1 year, then slowly wean.

N48

Two patients present with bilateral internuclear ophthalmoplegia. One is 20 years old, and the other is 65. The younger patient has no other medical history, and the 65-year-old has always been well but for recently diagnosed hypertension. Their examinations are otherwise normal.

All of the following statements are true *except*

a. The most likely problem in the younger patient is demyelinating disease.
b. The older patient should be treated with 1 g of methylprednisolone sodium succinate (Solumedrol) daily for 3 days.
c. The older patient probably has a vasculopathic process.
d. The problem in both patients localizes to the pons.

Discussion

Bilateral internuclear ophthalmoplegia localizes to the pons. In the young, a common cause is multiple sclerosis.[51] In the older age group, where atherosclerotic lesions are common, the etiology is often vasculopathic.[52] For a 65-year-old to have this presentation as an isolated first sign of demyelination would be distinctly unusual, and further evidence for demyelination would need to be found before embarking on a trial of corticosteroids.

Preferred Response

b. The older patient should be treated with 1 g of methylprednisolone sodium succinate (Solumedrol) daily for 3 days.

A patient presents with complete bilateral ophthalmoplegia that has lasted 1 week. The lid fissures are 3 mm OU. The pupils are 3 mm OU, round, reactive to light, and without RAPD. The afferent visual system is unaffected, and the patient can read with either eye without difficulty. The patient had a viral episode with diarrhea, nausea, and vomiting 2 days before the onset of the ocular symptoms. Despite having one eye patched, she is ataxic and areflexic. The rest of the examination is normal.

All of the following statements are true *except*

a. The patient probably does not have botulism.
b. The patient should undergo spinal tap.
c. The patient might have Miller Fisher syndrome.
d. The patient probably has myasthenia.

Discussion

This is another classic neuro-ophthalmic triad, that is, ophthalmoplegia, areflexia, and ataxia. This defines the Miller Fisher variant of Guillain-Barré syndrome.[53] Botulism is an unlikely diagnosis without either pupillary involvement or blurred vision at near.[54] Myasthenia would not cause areflexia or ataxia. The spinal fluid findings of a marked rise in protein without cellular infiltrate (pleocytosis) help confirm the clinical diagnosis of Miller Fisher syndrome.

Preferred Response

d. The patient probably has myasthenia.

All of the following are true about neuro-ophthalmic disease and child-bearing *except*

a. Although pseudotumor cerebri may be seen early in pregnancy, pregnancy may not be a definite risk factor for its development; when seen, pseudotumor cerebri is often self-limited and abates by the fifth month.
b. Preexisting meningiomas do not get worse during pregnancy.
c. Preexisting pituitary tumors may grow during pregnancy and encroach upon the chiasm, causing visual loss, even in the absence of overt apoplexy.
d. Multiple sclerosis may relapse during the postpartum period.

Discussion

All of the statements are true except for that regarding meningiomas, which are known to accelerate their growth in pregnancy. Pregnancy may not be a definite risk factor for pseudotumor cerebri but may simply reflect diagnosis in a population at risk due to its sex and age.[55,56] The incidence of relapses of multiple sclerosis is not higher *during* pregnancy, but there appears to be an increase in the first 3 months postdelivery.[57]

Preferred Response

b. Preexisting meningiomas do not get worse during pregnancy.

References

1. Goodman BW Jr: Temporal arteritis. *Am J Med* 1979;67:839–852.
2. Quillen DA, Cantore WA, Schwartz SR, et al: Choroidal nonperfusion in giant cell arteritis. *Am J Ophthalmol* 1993;116:171–175.
3. Siatkowski RM, Gass JD, Glaser JS, et al: Fluorescein angiography in the diagnosis of giant cell arteritis. *Am J Ophthalmol* 1993;115:57–63.
4. Beck RW, Kupersmith MJ, Cleary PA, et al: Fellow eye abnormalities in acute unilateral optic neuritis: experience of the Optic Neuritis Treatment Trial. *Ophthalmology* 1993;100:691–698.
5. Thompson HS: Adie's syndrome: some new observations. *Trans Am Ophthalmol Soc* 1977;75:587–626.
6. Thompson HS, ed: *Topics in Neuro-Ophthalmology*. Baltimore: Williams & Wilkins; 1979:95–96.
7. Thompson HS, Mensher JH: Hydroxyamphetamine test in Horner's syndrome. *Am J Ophthalmol* 1975;79:523–526.
8. Thompson HS: Diagnosing Horner's syndrome. *Trans Am Acad Ophthalmol Otolaryngol* 1977;83:840–842.
9. Smith JL, Cogan DG: Ataxia-telangiectasia. *Arch Ophthalmol* 1959;62:364–369.
10. Baloh RW, Yee RD, Boder E: Eye movements in ataxia-telangiectasia. *Neurology* 1978;28:1099–1104.
11. Kupersmith MJ, Berenstein A, Flamm E, et al: Neuroophthalmologic abnormalities and intravascular therapy of traumatic carotid cavernous fistulas. *Ophthalmology* 1986;93:906–912.
12. Argov Z, Mastiglia FL: Drug-induced neuromuscular disorders in man. In: Walton J, ed: *Disorders of Voluntary Muscle*. 5th ed. Edinburgh: Churchill Livingstone; 1988:981–1005.
13. Drachman DB, Skom JH: Procainamide—a hazard in myasthenia gravis. *Arch Neurol* 1965;13:316–320.
14. Mauriello J, Schulder M, Krieger A, et al: Management of traumatic optic neuropathy—a study of 23 patients. *Br J Ophthalmol* 1992;76:349–352.
15. Beck RW, Cleary PA, Anderson M Jr, et al: A randomized, controlled trial of corticosteroids in the treatment of acute optic neuritis. *N Eng J Med* 1992;326:581–588.
16. Beck RW, Cleary PA, Trobe JD, et al: The effect of corticosteroids for acute optic neuritis on the subsequent development of multiple sclerosis. *N Engl J Med* 1993;329:1764–1769.
17. Beck RW, Cleary PA: Optic Neuritis Treatment Trial: one-year follow-up results. *Arch Ophthalmol* 1993;111:773–775.
18. Newman SA, Miller NR: Optic tract syndrome: neuro-ophthalmologic considerations. *Arch Ophthalmol* 1983;101:1241–1250.
19. Bartlett JR: Craniopharyngiomas—a summary of 85 cases. *J Neurol Neurosurg Psychiatry* 1971;34:37–41.
20. Freeman MP, Kessler RM, Allen JH, et al: Craniopharyngioma: CT and MR imaging in nine cases. *J Comput Assist Tomogr* 1987;11:810–814.
21. Peterson RA, Walton DS: Optic nerve hypoplasia with good visual acuity and visual field defects: a study of children of diabetic mothers. *Arch Ophthalmol* 1977;95:254–258.

22. Smith JL, Cogan DG: Optokinetic nystagmus: a test for parietal lobe lesions. *Am J Ophthalmol* 1959;48:187–193.

23. Steele JC, Richardson JC, Olszewski J: Progressive supranuclear palsy. *Arch Neurol* 1968;10:333–359.

24. Margalith D, Tze WJ, Jan JE: Congenital optic nerve hypoplasia with hypothalamic-pituitary dysplasia: a review of 16 cases. *Am J Dis Child* 1985;139:361-366.

25. Corbett JJ: Diagnosis and management of idiopathic intracranial hypertension (pseudotumor cerebri). *Focal Points*. Vol VII, Module 3. San Francisco: American Academy of Ophthalmology; 1989.

26. Newman NJ: Leber's hereditary optic neuropathy: new genetic considerations. *Arch Neurol* 1993;50:540–548.

27. Weiner NC, Newman NJ, Lessell S, et al: Atypical Leber's hereditary optic neuropathy with molecular confirmation. *Arch Neurol* 1993;50:470–473.

28. Johns DR, Smith KH, Miller NR: Leber's hereditary optic neuropathy: clinical manifestations of the 3460 mutation. *Arch Ophthalmol* 1992;110:1557–1581.

29. Barricks ME, Traviesa DB, Glaser JS, et al: Ophthalmoplegia in cranial arteritis. *Brain* 1977;100:209–221.

30. Hollenhorst RW, Brown JR, Wagner HP, et al: Neurologic aspects of temporal arteritis. *Neurology* 1960;10:490–498.

31. Whitfield AGW, Bateman M, Cooke WT: Temporal arteritis. *Br J Ophthalmol* 1963;47:555–566.

32. Bailey TD, O'Connor PS, Tredici TJ, et al: Ophthalmoplegic migraine. *J Clin Neuroophthalmol* 1984;4:225–228.

33. Rosenberg ML, Glaser JS: Superior oblique myokymia. *Ann Neurol* 1983:13:667–669.

34. Smith JL, Wheliss JA. Ocular manifestations of nasopharyngeal tumors. *Trans Am Acad Ophthalmol Otolaryngol* 1962:66:659–664.

35. Yeakley JW, Kulkarni MV, McArdle CB, et al: High-resolution MR imaging of juxtasellar meningiomas with CT and angiographic correlation. *Am J Neuroradiol* 1988;9:279–285.

36. Kupersmith MJ, Warren FA, Newall J, et al: Irradiation of meningiomas of the intracranial anterior visual pathway. *Ann Neurol* 1987;21:131–137.

37. Troost BT, Newton TH: Occipital lobe arteriovenous malformations: clinical and radiologic features in 26 cases with comments on the differentiation from migraine. *Arch Ophthalmol* 1975;93:250–256.

38. Klintworth GW: Sarcoidosis. In: Gold DH, Weingeist TA, eds. *The Eye in Systemic Disease*. Philadelphia: JB Lippincott Co; 1990:289–293.

39. *Neuro-Ophthalmology*. Section 5 of Basic and Clinical Science Course. San Francisco: American Academy of Ophthalmology; 1994:153.

40. Tang RA, Grotta JC, Lee KF, et al: Chiasmal syndrome in sarcoidosis. *Arch Ophthalmol* 1983;101:1069–1073.

41. Mullie MA, Harding AE, Petty RK, et al: The retinal manifestations of mitochondrial myopathy: a study of 22 cases. *Arch Ophthalmol* 1985;103:1825–1830.

42. Kearns TP: External ophthalmoplegia, pigmentary degeneration of the retina, and cardiomyopathy: a newly recognized syndrome. *Trans Am Ophthalmol Soc* 1965;63:559–625.

43. Moraes CT, DiMauro S, Zeviani M, et al: Mitochondrial DNA deletions in progressive external ophthalmoplegia and Kearns-Sayre syndrome. *N Engl J Med* 1989;320:1293–1299.

44. Waziri M: Tuberous sclerosis. In: Gold DH, Weingeist TA, eds. *The Eye in Systemic Disease*. Philadelphia: JB Lippincott Co; 1990:450–452.

45. Kline LB, Viteck JJ, Raymon BC: Painful Horner's syndrome due to spontaneous carotid artery dissection. *Ophthalmology* 1987;94:226–230.

46. Loewenfeld IE: The Argyll Robertson pupil, 1869–1969: a critical survey of the literature. *Surv Ophthalmol* 1969;14:199–299.

47. Frohman L, Bielory L: Ocular manifestations of vasculitic and autoimmune disorders. In: Burde RM, Slamovits TL: *Advances in Clinical Ophthalmology.* 2nd ed. St Louis: CV Mosby Co; 1995.

48. Bullen CL, Liesegang TJ, McDonald TJ, et al: Ocular complications of Wegener's granulomatosis. *Ophthalmology* 1983;90:279–290.

49. Parelhoff ES, Chavis RM, Friendly DS: Wegener's granulomatosis presenting as orbital pseudotumor in children. *J Pediatr Ophthalmol Strab* 1985;22:100–104.

50. Pulido JS, Goeken JA, Nerad JA, et al: Ocular manifestations of patients with circulating antineutrophil cytoplasmic antibodies. *Arch Ophthalmol* 1990;108: 845–850.

51. Muri RM, Meienberg O: The clinical spectrum of internuclear ophthalmoplegia in multiple sclerosis. *Arch Neurol* 1985;42:851–855.

52. Gonyea EF: Bilateral internuclear ophthalmoplegia: association with occlusive cerebrovascular disease. *Arch Neurol* 1974;31:168–173.

53. Fisher M: An unusual variant of acute idiopathic polyneuritis (syndrome of ophthalmoplegia, ataxia, and areflexia). *N Engl J Med* 1956;255:57–65.

54. Miller NR, Moses H: Ocular involvement in wound botulism. *Arch Ophthalmol* 1977;95:1788–1789.

55. Greer M: Benign intracranial hypertension. III. Pregnancy. *Neurology* 1963;13: 670–672.

56. Digre KB, Varner MW, Corbett JJ: Pseudotumor cerebri and pregnancy. *Neurology* 1984;34:721–729.

57. Korn-Lubetzki I, Kahana E, Cooper G, et al: Activity of multiple sclerosis during pregnancy and puerperium. *Ann Neurol* 1984;16:229–231.

Additional Resources From the AAO

Basic and Clinical Science Course

Neuro-Ophthalmology. Section 5. Updated annually.

Focal Points

Beck RW: *Anterior Ischemic Optic Neuropathy.* Vol IV, Module 3. 1986. (Item No. 029004)

Corbett JJ: *Diagnosis and Management of Idiopathic Intracranial Hypertension (Pseudotumor Cerebri).* Vol VII, Module 3. 1989. (Item No. 029007)

Drake MV: *A Primer on Automated Perimetry.* Vol XI, Module 8. 1993. (Item No. 029011)

Goodwin JA: *Temporal Arteritis.* Vol X, Module 2. 1992. (Item No. 029010)

Katz B: *Myasthenia Gravis.* Vol VII, Module 7. 1989. (Item No. 029007)

Newman SA: *Diagnosis and Treatment of Chiasmal Lesions.* Vol V, Module 1. 1987. (Out of print)

Thompson HS: *Clinical Importance of Pupillary Inequality.* Vol X, Module 10. 1992. (Item No. 029010)

Trobe JD: *Managing Optic Neuritis: Results of the Optic Neuritis Treatment Trial.* Vol XII, Module 2. 1994. (Item No. 029012)

LEO Clinical Topic Update Friedman DI: *Neuro-Ophthalmology.* 1995. (Item No. 0212220)

Monographs Walsh TJ, ed: *Visual Fields: Examination and Interpretation.* Ophthalmology Monograph 3. 1990. (Item No. 0210090)

Wirtschafter JD, Berman EL, McDonald CS: *Magnetic Resonance Imaging and Computed Tomography: Clinical Neuro-Orbital Anatomy.* Ophthalmology Monograph 6. 1992. (Item No. 0210211)

Videotape Behrens M: *Neuro-Ophthalmic Motility Disorders.* Classic Series. 1975. (Item No. 0250053)

ORBIT AND OPHTHALMIC PLASTIC SURGERY

O1

A 10-year-old boy sustained a right upper eyelid laceration after falling from his bicycle. The laceration measures 15 mm and extends from the eyelid margin to above the eyelid crease. There is an avulsed avascular section of the laceration superiorly. The results of his ocular examination are normal except for marked swelling of the eyelid.

The *least* appropriate action in the management of this case is to

a. check the tetanus status
b. repair the eyelid margin
c. discard the avulsed tissue
d. check the status of the levator muscle

Discussion

Eyelid lacerations often appear more destructive than they actually are. Proper cleaning of the laceration is important. A complete eye examination is required to detect ocular injuries, which are often associated with eyelid lacerations. The tetanus status is important, especially if the exact history of the injury is unknown. Repair of eyelid lacerations requires a good working knowledge of eyelid anatomy, since repair of deeper structures, such as a dysfunctional levator muscle, is often required. In deep lacerations, foreign bodies should be searched for and removed if present. Eyelid margin repair is critical, since it will affect the eyelid contour and appearance. In general, it is best to avoid discarding tissue, since the facial region has a good blood supply and the survival rate of reimplanted tissue is excellent.

Preferred Response

c. discard the avulsed tissue

All of the following will prevent a notch of the eyelid margin after a laceration repair *except*

a. reapproximating the tarsus
b. inverting sutures at the eyelid margin
c. everting sutures at the eyelid margin
d. reapproximating the eyelid skin edges

Discussion   Proper alignment is important for eyelid margin repair. The cut edges of the laceration should be pulled together to ensure that the tension on the wound is not tight. The tarsus is reapproximated with interrupted 5-0 polyglactin 910 (Vicryl) suture. This reapproximation should place the eyelid margin in proper orientation. A 6-0 or 7-0 silk suture is placed at the level of the meibomian gland orifices and the anterior lash line in a vertical mattress fashion (see the figure). These sutures will evert the wound edge, allowing for contraction of the wound during healing and preventing an eyelid notch. The silk sutures are left long and are incorporated into the closure of the skin to avoid ocular irritation. Suturing the eyelid margin in a fashion that will invert the wound edges will precipitate eyelid notch formation during wound contraction.[1]

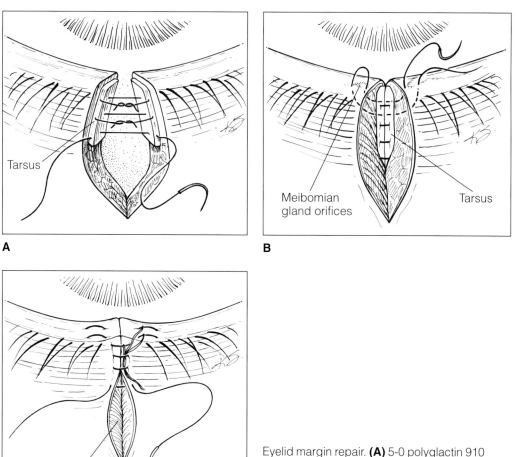

A

B

C

Eyelid margin repair. **(A)** 5-0 polyglactin 910 (Vicryl) suture reapproximates the tarsus. **(B)** Vertical mattress 6-0 silk suture everts the eyelid margin. **(C)** Skin is closed with 7-0 Vicryl suture.

Preferred Response   b. inverting sutures at the eyelid margin

A patient presents with the condition shown in the figure.

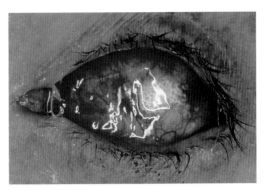

Exposed anterior surface of a hydroxyapatite implant.

The *least* appropriate treatment for this condition is

a. topical antibiotics
b. scleral patch graft
c. direct closure of the conjunctiva
d. removal of the implant

Discussion

Hydroxyapatite and other porous implants are now often used for rehabilitation of the anophthalmic socket. These implants have the potential for orbital tissue integration and improved motility. Exposure of this implant (see the figure) is a complication that is being seen more frequently with increased use of these implants. Proper identification and treatment of this problem may allow for the retention of these implants. Treatment options for an exposed implant include conjunctival closure, scleral patch or mucous membrane grafts, topical antibiotics, and observation. Implant removal is generally reserved for recalcitrant cases or cases associated with cellulitis.[2,3]

Preferred Response

d. removal of the implant

A 27-year-old man presents with the mass shown in the figure. This mass has been present all his life but now is a cosmetic concern for the patient.

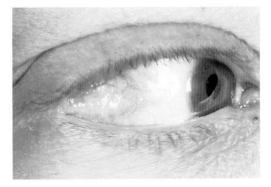

Dermolipoma. Note the whitish yellow appearance.

The *most* likely diagnosis is

a. prolapsed lacrimal gland
b. dermolipoma
c. prolapsed orbital fat
d. lymphangioma

Discussion

The appearance of this subconjunctival lesion (see the figure on page 157) is typical for a dermolipoma. Located on the temporal aspect of the eye, dermolipomas are usually whitish yellow and are composed of a mixture of fat and fibrous tissue. This mixture of tissue distinguishes this tumor from prolapsed orbital fat, which is purely fat beneath the conjunctiva (see the figure below). Prolapse of the lacrimal gland is usually located in the superior aspect of the lateral canthal space. Examination will show glandular tissue and a minimal amount of fat. Lymphangiomas are cystic infiltrative tumors that may involve the eyelids, ocular adnexa, and orbital structures. The appearance is typically that of a clear, multiloculated cystic lesion, except when bleeding into the tumor occurs. Both dermolipomas and lymphangiomas occur most commonly in the first decade of life, whereas prolapsed orbital fat and prolapsed lacrimal glands typically occur later.

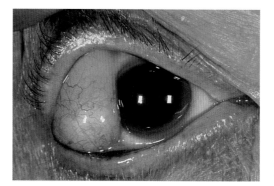

Prolapsed orbital fat in the same location as in the photograph above. Note the color difference between the two conditions.

Preferred Response   b. dermolipoma

The patient in Question O4 desires that his lesion be removed for cosmetic purposes. The *most* appropriate management is

a. fixation in the lacrimal gland fossa
b. laser ablation
c. complete excision
d. partial excision

Discussion

Dermolipomas usually do not require treatment unless they become a cosmetic problem or cause functional problems. If excision is done, only the anterior portion should be removed. A useful technique is to mark the conjunctiva at the level that will remove all visible tumor. The excision should be limited to this point. Care is taken not to damage extraocular muscles or the lacrimal gland and its ductules.[4] Complete excision is risky due to extension of the lesion into the orbit. Fixation of the tumor in the lacrimal gland fossa would be inappropriate and difficult. Laser ablation has no role in the management of this lesion.

Preferred Response   d. partial excision

The *least* likely ocular complication from endoscopic sinus surgery is

a. tearing
b. blindness
c. diplopia
d. ptosis

Discussion   Functional endoscopic sinus surgery is becoming increasingly popular. The availability of endoscopic instruments has made this surgery useful in the diagnosis and treatment of sinus disease. The close proximity of the paranasal sinuses and the orbit has led to a number of complications with the use of these endoscopes. Damage to the nasolacrimal duct may occur in attempting to enlarge the natural ostium into the maxillary sinus.[5] Blindness may occur after inadvertent entry into the orbit and resultant orbital hemorrhage or direct optic nerve damage. Orbital entry may also lead to damage of the extraocular muscles, such as the medial rectus muscle, and diplopia. The location of the levator muscle in the superior orbit makes ptosis from this surgical technique unlikely.

Preferred Response   d. ptosis

A 56-year-old man complains of an aching sensation around his left eye that has lasted for 6 weeks. The discomfort increases on up gaze. One week ago, he noted blurred vision in the left eye and a low-grade fever. His visual acuity is 20/20 OD and 20/40 OS. The patient has 3 mm of proptosis in the left eye and mild erythema and tenderness around the left eyelid. Results of biomicroscopy and dilated fundus examination are normal.

The *most* helpful diagnostic test for this patient is

a. complete blood count
b. skull films
c. CT scan of the orbits
d. thyroid function tests

Discussion   In this case, the most helpful tool for evaluating proptosis and motility abnormalities would be a CT scan. The differential diagnosis can be rapidly narrowed to orbital tumor, orbital cellulitis, orbital pseudotumor, and thyroid-related orbitopathy. A complete blood count is useful in evaluating the patient's fever. Orbital cellulitis or an orbital abscess may result in an elevated white blood cell count. Orbital pseudotumor may occasionally be associated with an increased eosinophil count, but affected patients usually have a normal complete blood count. Unilateral proptosis and a motility abnormality in any patient should raise the concern of thyroid disease, especially in the presence of eyelid abnormalities such as lid retraction or lid lag. In evaluating an orbital process, skull films are unlikely to provide useful information that would not immediately require confirmation and further detail from a CT scan or magnetic resonance imaging (MRI).

Preferred Response   c. CT scan of the orbits

A CT scan of the patient in Question O7 shows clear sinus structures, proptosis, and infiltration of the orbital fat in the left orbit (see the figure).

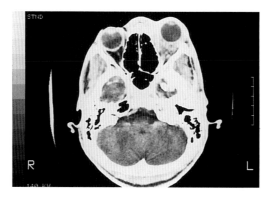

Axial CT scan showing diffuse infiltration of left orbital tissue. Note the location of the lateral orbital rim behind the equator of the globe, evidence of proptosis. The ethmoid sinuses are clear.

The *most* appropriate initial intervention should include

a. intravenous antibiotics
b. oral corticosteroids
c. orbital irradiation
d. propylthiouracil

Discussion   The most conservative therapy would involve antibiotics. The risk of orbital and ocular complications from orbital cellulitis warrants immediate therapy with antibiotics. Although antibiotics carry some risk of untoward side effects and possible allergic response, they are generally a conservative treatment over a period of 24 to 48 hours. Initial therapy could be with a penicillinase-resistant synthetic penicillin, such as nafcillin 1 to 2 g IV every 4 hours. Oral corticosteroids are useful in treating both orbital pseudotumor and acute-onset thyroid-related orbitopathy, but they could obviously exacerbate any bacterial or fungal infection in the orbit. Propylthiouracil is used in the treatment of systemic hyperthyroidism but is not useful in the treatment of thyroid-related orbitopathy.

Preferred Response   a. intravenous antibiotics

O9

The blood tests of the patient in Question O7 show a normal white blood cell count. The patient has received 48 hours of intravenous antibiotics. The patient's symptoms and signs have not improved. Echography of the orbit fails to show evidence of an orbital abscess. The next therapeutic intervention should include

a. intravenous antibiotics
b. oral corticosteroids
c. orbital irradiation
d. ethmoidectomy

Discussion

Most patients with orbital cellulitis should respond to broad-spectrum intravenous antibiotics over a 48-hour period. The lack of effect in this patient could be due to an inappropriate choice of antibiotic or the subsequent development of an orbital abscess that would require surgical drainage. However, since the echography examination has ruled out an orbital abscess and the white blood cell count is normal, the possibility of orbital pseudotumor should now be considered. A trial of corticosteroids is appropriate. The initial dose of prednisone can range from 60 mg to 100 mg daily. The duration and amount of corticosteroid is based on the clinical symptoms, clinical response, and occurrence of adverse side effects.

Preferred Response

b. oral corticosteroids

O10

The symptoms of the patient in Question O7 disappear after 48 hours of prednisone 80 mg daily. The *most* likely diagnosis is

a. orbital cellulitis
b. thyroid-related orbitopathy
c. orbital pseudotumor
d. orbital mucocele

Discussion

A rapid response to oral corticosteroids (prednisone) in this patient suggests a diagnosis of orbital pseudotumor, a collective term that has more recently been described as idiopathic orbital inflammation. Although a similar response could be seen in the treatment of thyroid-related orbitopathy, the CT findings make thyroid-related orbitopathy an unlikely diagnosis. Recurrence of signs and symptoms during the corticosteroid tapering is not unusual. In such cases, an orbital biopsy to confirm the diagnosis of orbital pseudotumor should be considered. Providing the patient with a definite histopathologic diagnosis is useful before continuing a long course of corticosteroid therapy with its potential side effects. Orbital cellulitis or mucocele usually would worsen or be unaffected by oral corticosteroid therapy.

Preferred Response

c. orbital pseudotumor

O11

All of the following orbital diseases may improve with corticosteroids *except*

a. orbital lymphoma
b. thyroid-related orbitopathy
c. orbital mucocele
d. orbital pseudotumor

Discussion

It is important to recognize that many orbital processes can respond initially to oral or intravenous corticosteroids. These include lymphomatous or inflammatory processes such as thyroid-related orbitopathy and orbital pseudotumor. Although pseudotumor has been described as the most likely diagnosis in this scenario, the physician should remain concerned about the possibility of these other diagnoses. An orbital mucocele is related to chronic inspissation of the sinus from blockage of its normal drainage ostium. A diagnosis of mucocele is suspected by findings on CT scan. Mucoceles usually do not respond to corticosteroids but would require surgical drainage.

Preferred Response

c. orbital mucocele

O12

A 75-year-old woman complains of restriction of her upper field of vision and difficulty reading when looking down. She denies any discomfort, epiphora, or diplopia. Her vision is J1+ OU through her well-positioned bifocal segments. A basic tear secretion test is normal. Examination shows an eyelid malposition.

The *most* likely diagnosis is

a. ectropion
b. entropion
c. involutional ptosis
d. dermatochalasis

Discussion

Involutional ptosis results from a dehiscence or disinsertion of the levator aponeurosis. This ptosis is accentuated on down gaze in many patients, resulting in further closure of the ptotic eyelid. These patients not only lose the superior visual field in primary gaze but also note visual field impairment in down gaze, since the eyelid rests in a lower position.[6] Some patients with normal palpebral fissures in primary gaze have ptosis with down gaze.[7] Entropion could conceivably cause difficulty in reading; however, ocular discomfort or pooling of tears would be expected. Ectropion and dermatochalasis, unless excessive, are unlikely to cause problems with reading.

Preferred Response

c. involutional ptosis

Which of the following is *least* useful in the evaluation of a patient with acquired ptosis?

a. margin-reflex distance
b. interpalpebral fissures
c. levator muscle function
d. frontalis muscle excursion

Discussion

The evaluation of a patient with ptosis is very important in determining proper management of the condition. The interpalpebral fissure is the distance between the upper and lower eyelid margins. The margin-reflex distance (MRD) is the distance between the upper eyelid margin and the corneal light reflex in primary gaze. This allows for an accurate measurement of ptosis when the lower eyelid margin is not in its normal position at the limbus. A positive MRD is the number of millimeters *above* the light reflex, whereas a negative MRD would be the number of millimeters *below* the corneal light reflex. Ptosis is present when the MRD is 2 mm or less. The MRD allows for comparison of the position of each upper eyelid and the amount of ptosis in unilateral cases. The levator function is an important measurement in determining the type of ptosis surgery to be performed. This is done by measuring the distance the upper eyelid moves between extreme down gaze and extreme up gaze. Acquired ptosis usually has normal levator function (12 mm or more), whereas congenital ptosis will demonstrate a diminished levator function. The eyelid crease is usually higher than normal in acquired ptosis and absent or faint in congenital ptosis. The influence of the frontalis muscle is eliminated during ptosis evaluation by immobilizing this muscle with the examiner's thumb on the brow while measuring the levator function. Frontalis muscle contraction is commonly seen as a compensatory mechanism in patients with ptosis. The degree of frontalis muscle excursion is of limited value, however, in the assessment of patients with acquired ptosis.[8]

Preferred Response

d. frontalis muscle excursion

The patient shown in the figure on page 164 has complained of a droopy left upper eyelid. The results of the eye examination are as follows.

	Right Eye	Left Eye	Normal
Margin-reflex distance	+4 mm	+1.5 mm	+4–5 mm
Levator function	14 mm	15 mm	15 mm
Fissures	10 mm	7.5 mm	10 mm
Eyelid crease	8 mm	12 mm	8–10 mm
Schirmer's test	10 mm	10 mm	

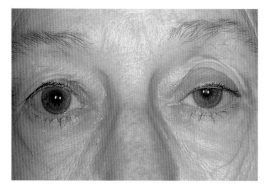

Involutional ptosis of the left upper eyelid. The eyelid creases are asymmetric, with the left crease higher than the right.

Which of the following is the *most* appropriate surgical management?

a. levator aponeurosis advancement
b. blepharoplasty
c. frontalis suspension
d. levator muscle resection

Discussion   See Question O15.

Preferred Response   a. levator aponeurosis advancement

A 7-year-old boy is examined because of bilateral droopy eyelids since birth (see the figure). The visual acuity and ocular motility examinations are normal except for mild limitation of up gaze bilaterally. The eyelid measurements are as follows:

	Right Eye	Left Eye
Margin-reflex distance	0 mm	+0.5 mm
Levator function	3 mm	3 mm
Fissures	5 mm	6 mm
Eyelid crease	absent	absent

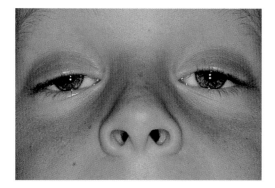

Congenital ptosis.

Which of the following is the *most* appropriate surgical management?

a. levator muscle resection
b. frontalis suspension
c. levator aponeurosis advancement
d. Fasanella-Servat procedure

Discussion

The procedures for ptosis correction are based on the amount of levator function and the amount of ptosis. A Fasanella-Servat procedure can be used for a small amount of ptosis (1 to 2 mm) and normal levator function.[9] This procedure consists of excision of the tarsus and Müller's muscle. The eyelid is everted and two hemostats are placed at the superior border of the tarsus, incorporating tarsus, conjunctiva, and Müller's muscle. A plicating suture is run across the eyelid at the eyelid crease superior to the hemostats. The tissue inferior to the hemostats is excised; the amount is based on the amount of ptosis. A levator aponeurosis advancement is used when levator function is good (10 to 15 mm, as in the patient in Question O14) and can be used for any degree of ptosis.[10] The procedure is done through an eyelid crease incision. The levator aponeurosis is identified beneath the preaponeurotic fat, an important surgical landmark of the eyelid that is identified after the orbital septum has been opened. The levator aponeurosis is separated from Müller's muscle, advanced, and attached to the tarsus. The amount of advancement is based on the desired eyelid height. If the levator function is poor to fair (3 to 7 mm) and the ptosis is moderate to severe or an eyelid crease is present, then a levator muscle resection is performed.[11] A frontalis suspension is used when levator function is very poor to absent and ptosis is severe. This procedure makes use of a "sling" from the eyelid to the frontalis muscle that lifts the ptotic eyelid with eyebrow elevation. Autogenous or donor fascia lata tissue is commonly used for this procedure. This procedure would be most appropriate for the patient in Question O15.[12]

Preferred Response

b. frontalis suspension

Severe involutional ptosis can be differentiated from severe congenital ptosis by all of the following *except*

a. amount of lid lag in down gaze
b. amount of levator muscle function
c. position of the upper eyelid crease
d. amount of ptosis

Discussion

Congenital ptosis has lid lag on down gaze and an increased amount of ptosis on up gaze, due in part to decreased elasticity of the dystrophic levator muscle complex. In involutional ptosis, the amount of ptosis is constant regardless of eyelid position. Levator muscle function is usually normal (10 to 15 mm) in involutional ptosis but typically fair (5 to 7 mm) or poor (4 mm or less) in congenital ptosis.[13] The amount of levator function in patients with congenital ptosis is critically important in deciding how much surgery to perform on the levator muscle. Patients with involutional ptosis are more likely to have an abnormally elevated eyelid crease due to elevation of the levator attachments to the skin and orbicularis muscle (see the figure, part A, page 166). Patients with congenital ptosis usually have a poorly defined or absent eyelid crease because the dystrophic levator muscle fails to develop these attachments (see the figure, part B). The amount of ptosis the patient may demonstrate can be identical in involutional and congenital cases.

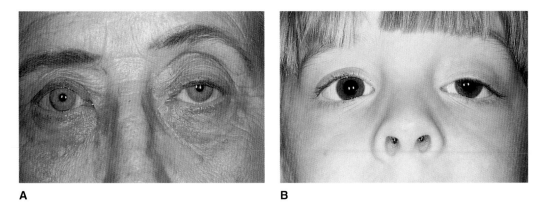

A   B

Comparison of involutional and congenital ptosis. **(A)** Involutional ptosis with elevated eyelid crease. **(B)** Congenital ptosis with faint eyelid crease. Notice that the amount of ptosis is about the same.

Preferred Response   d. amount of ptosis

A 32-year-old man has a painless mass located in the superior lateral aspect of the left upper eyelid, which has been present for 4 months. There is no history of trauma, surgery, or chronic conjunctivitis. The results of the ocular examination are normal except for the mobile, translucent mass shown on eversion of the upper eyelid (see the figure).

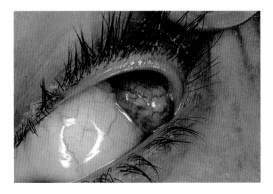

Lacrimal ductal cyst.

The *most* likely diagnosis is

a. lacrimal ductal cyst
b. lymphoma
c. lipodermoid
d. hematic cyst

Discussion   A lacrimal ductal cyst, or dacryops, is a cyst originating from the ductules of the palpebral lobe of the lacrimal gland. The cyst is translucent and may fluctuate in size with crying. Treatment consists of complete excision, with caution not to damage the lacrimal ductules in order to preserve tear secretion. The differential diagnosis includes a prolapsed lacrimal gland, lipodermoid, or a foreign-body granuloma. The pathogenesis is either trauma or inflammation of periductal structures with resultant ductule dilation that forms the cyst.[14,15] Lymphoid lesions are usually not cystic in appearance and do not fluctuate in size. A lipodermoid has connective tissue and fat composition and thus lacks cystic qualities. A hematic cyst is the result of persistent blood from a previous hemorrhage. The cyst is filled with blood breakdown products and thus is not translucent.

Preferred Response   a. lacrimal ductal cyst

A 55-year-old man reports an 8-month history of a lesion on the medial aspect of the right lower eyelid. The patient had an actinic keratosis removed elsewhere 3 years ago. The ocular examination is unremarkable except for the lesion seen in the figure.

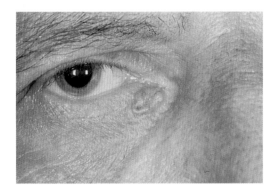

Basal cell carcinoma.

The *most* likely diagnosis is

a. sebaceous cell carcinoma
b. basal cell carcinoma
c. squamous cell carcinoma
d. seborrheic keratosis

Discussion   Sebaceous cell carcinoma is usually located in the upper eyelid and often masquerades as conjunctivitis or chalazion. This tumor has metastatic potential. Treatment consists of wide surgical excision with histopathologically controlled margins. Basal cell carcinoma is the most common eyelid tumor, representing 90% of malignant eyelid tumors. It is typically firm, with raised, pearly borders and a central crater.[16] It is commonly seen on sun-exposed skin. The diagnosis is suggested by the typical appearance, shown in figure. The medial lower eyelid is a frequent location. Treatment is surgical excision with controlled margins; controlled margins may be obtained with Mohs' surgery or frozen sections. A squamous cell carcinoma represents a more aggressive skin tumor and is less common than basal cell carcinoma. Clinically, it is a hyperkeratotic lesion with a poorly defined border. It is related to sun exposure, and actinic keratosis may be a precursor. Treatment consists of excision with histopathologically controlled margins. Seborrheic keratosis is an oily hyperkeratotic lesion that has a "stuck on" appearance. It is a benign lesion and may be treated with simple excision.

Preferred Response   b. basal cell carcinoma

An incisional biopsy is done on the patient in Question O18. The histopathology is shown in the figure.

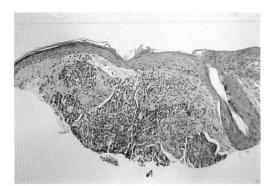

Histopathology of basal cell carcinoma. Note the tongues of basaloid cells in the superficial and deep dermis.

The *most* appropriate management is

a. observation
b. Mohs' surgery
c. radiation
d. liquid nitrogen

Discussion   It is important to obtain representative tissue when doing tissue biopsies. This tissue sample shows basal cell carcinoma. Note the nest and tongues of basaloid cells in the superficial and deep dermis. Complete excision with controlled tissue margins is the treatment of choice because of the destructive nature of these tumors. Mohs' micrographic surgery,[17] excision with frozen sections, or wide surgical resection with permanent section margins all would be satisfactory treatment options. Radiation therapy, although effective in certain cases, does not provide histologic evidence of tumor eradication and is usually not used as a primary treatment modality. Liquid nitrogen is used primarily to treat actinic keratosis.

Preferred Response   b. Mohs' surgery

A squamous cell carcinoma of the lower eyelid was excised with controlled margins. The figure shows the resultant defect.

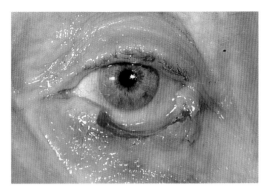

Left lower eyelid defect greater than 50%.

Which of the following is the *most* appropriate management?

a. observation
b. Hughes procedure
c. skin graft
d. Cutler-Beard procedure

Discussion

The defect shown in the figure above would require some surgical correction, since allowing the wound to granulate would likely result in a dysfunctional eyelid. Thus, observation would not be appropriate. A skin graft would provide an anterior lamella for the eyelid, but since the defect is over 50% of the eyelid, an adequate supportive base for the graft does not exist, and the graft would fail. A Cutler-Beard procedure is an eyelid-sharing procedure that uses the skin and muscle from the lower eyelid for reconstruction of upper eyelid defects.[18] A Hughes procedure (see the figure on page 170, part A) involves taking a tarsoconjunctival flap from the upper eyelid, leaving 3 to 4 mm of the upper tarsus intact, and advancing the remaining tarsus and conjunctiva into the lower eyelid defect.[19] This provides the posterior lamella of the eyelid. The anterior lamella is then formed by either a full-thickness skin graft or advancement of a skin–muscle flap from the lower eyelid or cheek. This would provide the most appropriate management for this defect. The postoperative appearance is shown in the figure, part B.

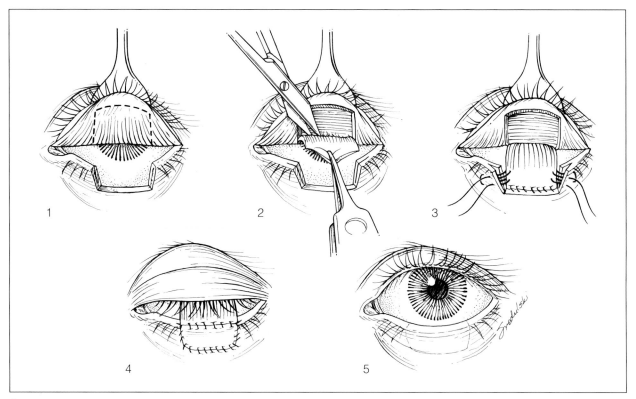

A

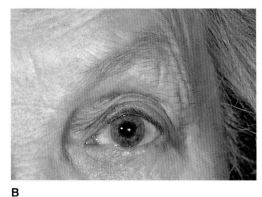

B

(A) Hughes procedure for lower eyelid defects.
(1) Tarsoconjunctival flap drawn 3–4 mm from eyelid margin to correspond to lower eyelid defect. (2) Flap made by dissecting tarsus from orbicularis and levator aponeurosis. (3) Flap positioned in the lower eyelid defect. (4) Anterior lamella made by using a skin graft or a myocutaneous advancement flap. (5) Flap separated in 4–6 weeks.
(B) Postoperative appearance of patient after Hughes procedure.

Preferred Response   b. Hughes procedure

A 68-year-old man complains of irritation and redness of the right eye that has been present for the past 2 months. He has recently been treated for recurrent chalazia and conjunctivitis without relief. The results of visual acuity and anterior and posterior segment examinations are normal. Examination of the regional lymph nodes yields negative results. The right upper eyelid is shown in the figure.

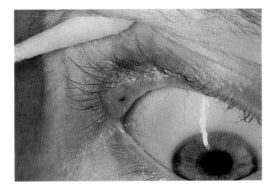

Sebaceous cell carcinoma.

The *most* likely diagnosis is

a. nevus
b. blepharitis
c. sebaceous cell carcinoma
d. viral conjunctivitis

Discussion

A conjunctival nevus is benign and similar to nevi located elsewhere on the body. The clinical appearance is often indicative of the type of nevus based on its epidermal location. Generally, flat nevi are junctional and elevated ones are compound, whereas dome-shaped or pedunculated nevi are intradermal. Sebaceous cell carcinoma often goes undiagnosed because it mimics other conditions, such as chalazion or blepharitis. Any loss of cilia or a unilateral blepharitis should alert the clinician to the possible diagnosis of sebaceous cell carcinoma. A full-thickness biopsy is required for examination of the meibomian glands located within the tarsal plate. Extension of this tumor by intraepithelial spread beyond the clinically involved area is common. Treatment consists of wide surgical excision with histopathologically controlled margins along with conjunctival mapping. Viral conjunctivitis can present with this history, but the results of the anterior segment and conjunctival examinations would be expected to be abnormal.

Preferred Response

c. sebaceous cell carcinoma

A 37-year-old woman is examined for irritation of the right eye. There is mild conjunctival injection and a follicular reaction. The external examination reveals the lesion shown in the figure.

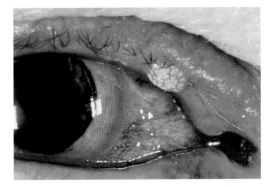

Molluscum contagiosum.

The *most* appropriate management for this patient is

a. excisional biopsy
b. incisional biopsy
c. observation
d. antiviral agents

Discussion   See Question O23.

Preferred Response   a. excisional biopsy

          The histopathology of the upper eyelid lesion depicted in Question O22 is shown in the figure.

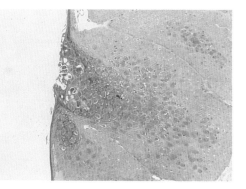

Histopathology of molluscum contagiosum showing large eosinophilic intracytoplasmic inclusion bodies.

The *most* likely diagnosis is

a. epithelial inclusion cyst
b. keratoacanthoma
c. nevus
d. molluscum contagiosum

Discussion   The diagnosis for the patient in Question O22 is molluscum contagiosum. This lesion is caused by a pox virus and is often found on the eyelid. The appearance is that of a dome-shaped nodule, often with central umbilication (see the figure below), or a flatter lesion with multiple small, whitish inclusions, as in this patient (see the figure in Question O22). The toxic reaction to the virus may cause a chronic follicular conjunctivitis to develop. The histopathology shows large eosinophilic intracytoplasmic inclusion bodies. Treatment consists of removal of the virus by complete excision or curettage of the lesion. An incisional biopsy would incompletely remove the lesion, allowing for continued viral shedding. Antiviral agents are not effective in the treatment of these lesions.

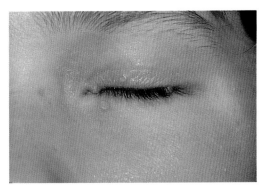

Multiple molluscum contagiosum lesions with more typical appearance of central umbilication.

Preferred Response   d. molluscum contagiosum

A 75-year-old man presents with the lesion shown in the figure. It has been present for 4 weeks, rapidly increasing in size, and it is painless.

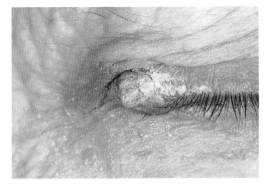

Keratoacanthoma.

All of the following are characteristics of this lesion *except*

a. malignant potential
b. keratin-filled crater
c. rapid growth
d. spontaneous resolution

Discussion   The clinical history of a rapidly growing lesion with a central crater is classic for a keratoacanthoma. Keratoacanthomas have a keratin-filled crater and occur on sun-exposed skin. These lesions do not have malignant potential and will frequently undergo spontaneous resolution. An important clinical note is that these lesions can be confused with squamous cell carcinoma if an incomplete biopsy is performed. If one suspects this diagnosis and elects to remove this lesion, an excisional biopsy should be performed for complete pathologic evaluation.

Preferred Response   a. malignant potential

A 47-year-old man with a 1-week history of eye discomfort is evaluated. The patient had an acoustic neuroma resected 3 months ago. The ocular examination shows 5 mm of lagophthalmos, exposure keratopathy, and inferior conjunctival injection. His lower eyelid is shown in the figure on page 174.

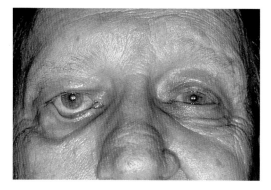

Paralytic ectropion.

The proper classification for the condition shown is

a. cicatricial ectropion
b. paralytic ectropion
c. involutional ectropion
d. mechanical ectropion

Discussion   This patient has suffered a facial nerve palsy after resection of an acoustic neuroma. The facial nerve is often unavoidably injured during this procedure, and recovery of function is unpredictable. The eyelid protractors (orbicularis oculi muscle) innervated by the facial nerve and responsible for eyelid closure are weakened, resulting in a paralytic ectropion. Shortening of the anterior lamella leads to a cicatricial ectropion. Involutional ectropion is the result of canthal tendon laxity and not orbicularis muscle weakness. Mechanical ectropion results from a mass effect on the lower eyelid that pulls it away from the globe.

Preferred Response   b. paralytic ectropion

The *least* appropriate management for the patient in Question O25 is

a. gold weight for the upper eyelid
b. lid tightening of the lower eyelid
c. complete tarsorrhaphy
d. eye lubricants

Discussion   Protection of the ocular surface is the primary goal in managing patients with facial nerve paralysis. The ocular surface lacks its normal protective mechanism of eyelid closure. Eye lubricants, such as artificial tears, viscous solutions, or ointments, become important for corneal protection. Tightening of the lower eyelid decreases the amount of inferior ocular surface exposed and may improve ocular surface lubrication through improved blinking. The placement of a gold weight in the upper eyelid allows complete closure of the upper eyelid with relaxation of the levator muscle.[20] The proper weight is determined by placing the gold weight on the upper eyelid and asking the patient to close the eyelids. The proper weight allows complete eyelid closure without resultant ptosis. The gold weights come in a set ranging from 0.6 g to 1.6 g. The gold weight is surgically secured to the tarsal plate. The figures (below) show the pre- and postoperative appearance of another patient with lagophthalmos but complete eyelid closure after gold-weight insertion to the right eyelid. A lateral tarsorrhaphy is often useful, but a complete tarsorrhaphy would be inappropriate. Today, most patients may be managed with reanimation techniques (gold weights, palpebral springs, and nerve grafting), reserving complete tarsorrhaphy for recalcitrant cases.

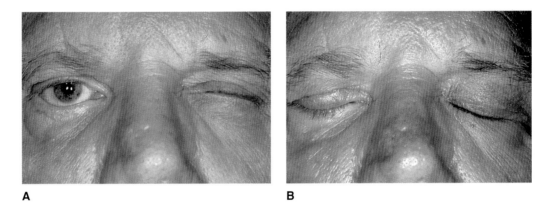

A   **B**

A patient with a facial nerve palsy before and after surgery. **(A)** Marked lagophthalmos with eyelid closure before surgery. **(B)** Complete eyelid closure after insertion of a 1.2 g gold weight in the right upper eyelid.

Preferred Response   c. complete tarsorrhaphy

O27

A patient suffered a facial burn 1 year ago, resulting in the eyelid position shown in the figure.

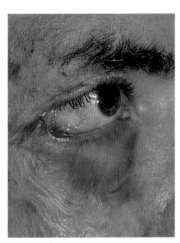

Cicatricial ectropion.

The *least* appropriate long-term management of this condition is

a. split-thickness skin graft
b. full-thickness skin graft
c. lid-tightening procedure
d. release of the cicatrix

Discussion

Management of a cicatricial process, such as a burn involving the eyelid, may be difficult. The cicatricial scar should first be allowed to mature for 6 to 12 months. The cicatrix should then be released to allow the eyelid to assume a normal position. Often the eyelid will require tightening because of the molding effect of the cicatrix. Once the eyelid is secured in a functional position, the resultant anterior lamella defect may be covered with a full-thickness skin graft. A full-thickness graft provides a better skin match and avoids the shrinkage associated with split-thickness grafts. Split-thickness skin grafts may occasionally be required in the acute management of patients sustaining severe periorbital burns.[21]

Preferred Response

a. split-thickness skin graft

A 22-year-old woman is examined for intermittent swelling of the medial canthal lesion shown in the figures. The visual acuity is normal. There is a past history of swelling of this lesion during upper respiratory tract infections.

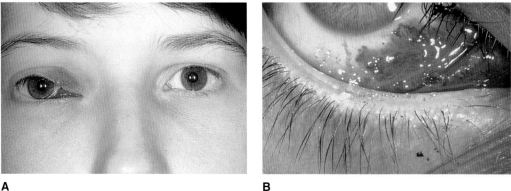

A   **B**

(A) Lymphangioma. **(B)** Elevated, reddish infiltrative lesion in a different patient with lymphangioma.

The *most* likely diagnosis is

a. lymphoma
b. neurofibroma
c. lymphangioma
d. leukemia

Discussion

Orbital lymphangiomas are benign, slowly growing tumors. The majority of cases are diagnosed in the first decade of life. These tumors can also involve the palatine and buccal mucosa, so examination of the oral cavity is suggested. A history of enlargement with upper respiratory infection (due to the lymphoid response within the tumor) is suggestive of this diagnosis. Often these tumors will enlarge with blood, either spontaneously or related to trauma ("chocolate cysts"). CT scanning or

MRI demonstrates an irregular, multiloculated cystic mass that appears to infiltrate the orbital tissues. Orbital lymphoma and leukemia are not cystic or infiltrative tumors. Neurofibromas may be infiltrative but are not cystic.

Preferred Response   c. lymphangioma

The patient in Question O28 later presents as shown in the figure. The visual acuity is 20/20 OU and the intraocular pressure is 18 mm Hg OU.

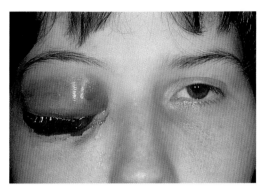

Lymphangioma after an acute bleeding episode.

The *most* appropriate management for this patient is

a. biopsy
b. observation
c. chemotherapy
d. radiation

Discussion   This patient has experienced an acute bleeding episode into the lymphangioma. There is now marked proptosis, decreased motility, and periocular swelling. The potential for visual loss is present during acute bleeding episodes. Attention should be directed toward reducing orbital and intraocular pressure and improving optic nerve function. Orbital decompression is indicated if optic nerve compromise occurs. Since the vision and intraocular pressure are normal in this patient, observation with reassurance of the patient is appropriate. If the diagnosis is unknown, a biopsy of the tumor is appropriate but it should be done after the acute event has resolved. Chemotherapy and radiation therapy are not indicated in the treatment of these tumors. Debulking of lymphangiomas may be useful in improving cosmesis or limiting complications.

Preferred Response   b. observation

O30

A 54-year-old woman is evaluated for painless bilateral proptosis. Her eyes were normal until 1 year ago. The CT scans are shown in the figures.

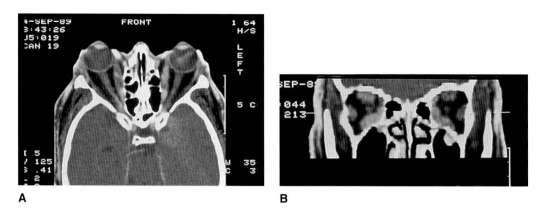

A   **B**

CT scans of thyroid-related orbitopathy. **(A)** Axial view showing fusiform shape to muscles. **(B)** Coronal view showing bilateral extraocular muscle enlargement.

Which of the eyelid findings listed below is *most* associated with this condition?

a. entropion
b. floppy eyelids
c. ectropion
d. eyelid retraction

Discussion

The axial and coronal CT scans (see the figures) show bilateral enlargement of the extraocular muscles. This CT finding is consistent with thyroid-related orbitopathy. Eyelid retraction is usually present when a patient presents with this diagnosis. Eyelid retraction is due to the combination of proptosis, adnexal fibrosis, and increased autonomic stimulation of the sympathetic-innervated muscles of the eyelids. Due to the proptosis and stretching of the eyelids, there is minimal laxity, ruling out floppy eyelids. Entropion and ectropion are not commonly associated with thyroid-related orbitopathy.

Preferred Response   d. eyelid retraction

O31

All of the following CT findings are commonly seen with thyroid-related orbitopathy *except*

a. bilateral extraocular muscle involvement
b. sparing of extraocular muscle tendons
c. involvement of extraocular muscle tendons
d. fusiform extraocular muscle involvement

Discussion

Thyroid-related orbitopathy is an immunologically related inflammatory condition that affects orbital tissues, particularly the extraocular muscles. The most common cause for unilateral or bilateral proptosis in an adult is thyroid-related orbitopathy. Even though the clinical findings may indicate a unilateral problem, a CT scan or MRI often shows bilateral disease. The CT findings consist of fusiform enlargement of the extraocular muscles, commonly the inferior and medial rectus muscles, with sparing of the tendons.

Preferred Response

c. involvement of extraocular muscle tendons

The patient in Question O30 returns 6 months later with decreased vision, worse in the left eye, and a relative afferent pupillary defect. The visual acuity is 20/50 OD and 20/200 OS. The Goldmann visual field of the left eye is shown in the figure.

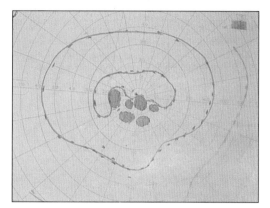

Goldmann visual field showing central and paracentral scotomas.

The *most* likely cause for the decreased vision is

a. corneal exposure
b. compressive optic neuropathy
c. refractive error
d. malingering

Discussion

Protecting the corneal surface may be challenging in patients with thyroid-related orbitopathy. The proptosis and eyelid retraction interfere with the normal ocular surface wetting that occurs with blinking. Frequent use of artificial lubricants, taping the eyelids closed at night, and moisture-chamber glasses all help keep the ocular surface lubricated. Corneal exposure, refractive error, or malingering will not give clinical findings of optic nerve dysfunction, such as a relative afferent pupillary defect. The most likely cause is compressive optic neuropathy that has produced central and paracentral scotomas and pupillary dysfunction.

Preferred Response

b. compressive optic neuropathy

The *least* appropriate management for the patient in Question O30 is

a. orbital decompression
b. corticosteroids
c. levothyroxine
d. radiation

Discussion

Compressive optic neuropathy is the most vision-threatening complication from thyroid-related orbitopathy. Treatment is directed toward decompressing the orbit either directly or by decreasing the inflammation. Surgical orbital decompression removes a portion of the orbital bones, allowing expansion of the orbital tissues into the surrounding paranasal sinuses. The inferior, medial, and lateral walls are usually removed.[22] Oral corticosteroids can decompress the orbit by decreasing orbital inflammation and edema. Orbital radiation also has a role in reversing compressive optic neuropathy.[23,24] It is used most frequently in the acute phase of the disease when there is marked orbital congestion. Radiation therapy is often combined with corticosteroid therapy in such cases. If the compressive optic neuropathy is severe, radiation treatment alone may not be a good option because of the time needed for it to take effect (usually several weeks). Medical thyroid replacement therapy is important in the systemic management of thyroid disease but has no role in reversing the orbital findings.

Preferred Response   c. levothyroxine

Which of the following procedures is *least* likely to improve the eyelid position and corneal exposure in the patient shown in the figure?

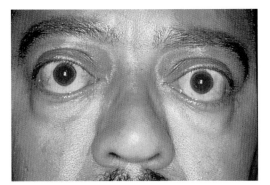

Marked lower eyelid retraction due to thyroid-related orbitopathy.

a. lid tightening (lateral tarsal strip)
b. levator recession/müllerectomy
c. lower lid retractor extirpation/spacer graft
d. lateral tarsorrhaphy

Discussion

Eyelid retraction predisposes thyroid patients to corneal exposure. The combination of an increased ocular surface exposure and an incomplete blink leads to this keratopathy. A lateral tarsorrhaphy would bring the lateral eyelids together and provide improved eye coverage. Levator recession and müllerectomy address upper eyelid retraction by allowing the eyelid to be lowered to a height that eliminates the superior scleral show. Lower eyelid retraction is treated by recession or extirpation of the lower eyelid retractors and sometimes placement of a "spacer" to elevate the eyelid and decrease inferior scleral show. Various materials are used as spacers, including sclera, ear cartilage, and hard-palate mucosa. Eliminating the eyelid retraction improves the ocular surface wetting. A lateral tarsal strip procedure would tighten the lower eyelid but might worsen the lower eyelid retraction unless the lower eyelid retractors are concurrently recessed or a spacer graft is inserted.

Preferred Response   a. lid tightening (lateral tarsal strip)

A patient is evaluated for ectropion of his left lower eyelid (see the figure, part A), which is causing epiphora. The ectropion has been present for 1 month. His ocular examination is otherwise normal. The patient's everted eyelid is shown in part B of the figure.

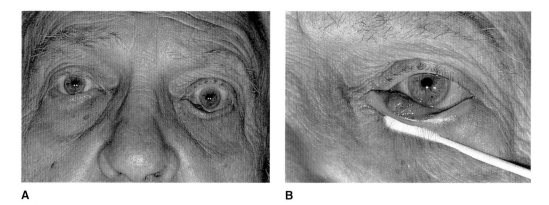

A   **B**

(A) Ectropion of the left lower eyelid. **(B)** Chalazion of the lower eyelid, causing the ectropion.

The *most* likely cause of the ectropion is

a. lymphoma
b. sarcoid
c. Kaposi's sarcoma
d. chalazion

Discussion   This lower eyelid ectropion is mechanical in nature and is caused by the chalazion shown in part B of the figure. A chalazion has its origin from the meibomian glands located within the tarsal plate. A lymphoma, sarcoid, and Kaposi's sarcoma originate elsewhere. A lymphoma would be subconjunctival and have a characteristic salmon color. Sarcoid lesions are usually conjunctival but are typically too small to cause ectropion. Kaposi's sarcoma of the conjunctiva was rare but now is seen more frequently in association with acquired immunodeficiency syndrome (AIDS).

Preferred Response   d. chalazion

During routine examination of a patient's inferior cul-de-sac, the lesion shown in the figure is observed. The patient is unaware of this lesion and is reportedly in good health. The results of the remainder of the ocular examination are normal.

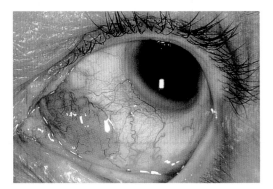

Subconjunctival lympho-proliferative lesion.

The *most* likely diagnosis is

a. chalazion
b. lymphoproliferative lesion
c. prolapsed orbital fat
d. Kaposi's sarcoma

Discussion

This lesion is suspicious because of its location and clinical features. The subconjunctival location and salmon color are characteristic of a lympho-proliferative lesion. Typically, lymphoproliferative lesions are located in the superior-anterior orbit. The type of lymphoproliferative lesion (benign reactive lymphoid hyperplasia, atypical lymphoid hyperplasia, malignant lymphoma) cannot be determined from the clinical appearance. Prolapsed orbital fat would be yellow, and one should see fat globules. Kaposi's sarcoma lesions are elevated and have a reddish color. Despite distinctive clinical features, tissue biopsy is the only way to make a definitive diagnosis in this patient.

Preferred Response

b. lymphoproliferative lesion

A biopsy is done on the patient in Question O36. The *least* useful test to perform on this biopsy would be

a. culture and sensitivity
b. cell-surface markers
c. permanent sections
d. electron microscopy

Discussion

Lesions suspected to be lymphomatous in nature should undergo biopsy. One should consult preoperatively with the pathologist to discuss the proper method of handling the tissue. The specimen should be divided into three sections. One section should go for permanent sections and be stored in formalin. The second section should be submitted on a saline wet gauze or sponge for immunopathologic studies to determine cell-surface markers. The third section can be stored in glutaraldehyde for electron microscopic studies if needed. Electron microscopic studies can aid in differentiating some of these tumors when there is confusion, but they are needed less commonly with current diagnostic testing. The clinical picture is not consistent with an infectious process, so cultures would be the least useful test in the management of this patient.

Preferred Response   a. culture and sensitivity

The 7-year-old girl shown in the figure is evaluated for left periorbital discomfort and tenderness that has been present for 24 hours. Her vision is 20/20 OD and 20/60 OS. The left globe is 3 mm proptotic and displaced inferiorly. Pain is present with eye movements. A mild left relative afferent pupillary defect is present. Fundus examination shows choroidal folds superiorly.

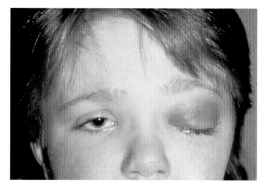

Left periorbital inflammation. Note demarcation of the erythema in left upper eyelid corresponding to the orbital septum.

The history and examination are *least* consistent with

a. preseptal cellulitis
b. rhabdomyosarcoma
c. orbital cellulitis
d. pseudotumor

Discussion   The development of periorbital swelling associated with painful eye movements and proptosis is consistent with the diagnosis of orbital cellulitis, pseudotumor, or rhabdomyosarcoma. Pain with eye movement, decreased visual acuity, and proptosis demonstrate extension of the process into the orbit. These findings are not consistent with the diagnosis of preseptal cellulitis. Imaging of the orbit is required to differentiate between orbital cellulitis, orbital abscess, and a neoplastic process.

Preferred Response   a. preseptal cellulitis

O39   The figures show the CT scans of the patient in Question O38.

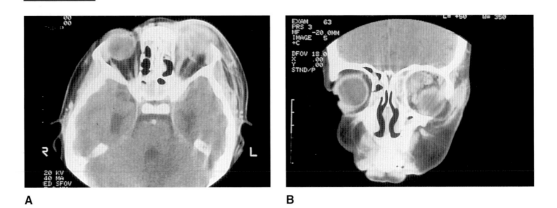

A   **B**

CT scans showing an orbital abscess. **(A)** Axial view demonstrating left proptosis. **(B)** Coronal view showing the abscess adjacent to the ethmoid sinus.

The appearance of these scans is *most* consistent with which of the following conditions?

a. orbital abscess
b. rhabdomyosarcoma
c. preseptal cellulitis
d. pseudotumor

Discussion   The CT scans demonstrate opacification of the ethmoid sinus with contiguous soft tissue swelling of the left orbit with lucent areas. The coronal view shows a well-defined opacity along the medial orbital wall adjacent to the ethmoid sinus. The diagnosis of an orbital abscess was made based on the presence of coexistent sinus disease combined with loculations within the orbit.[25] Pseudotumor is unlikely to cause this degree of sinus opacification. Rhabdomyosarcoma tends to have a more homogenous appearance on CT scan. Surgical exploration of the orbit combined with drainage of the affected paranasal sinuses is indicated, especially in the presence of pain and visual compromise.[26] Intravenous antibiotics should be started in the perioperative period. Initial treatment could be nafcillin 1 to 2 g every 4 hours with ceftazidime 1 to 2 g every 8 hours. In children, the dosages are nafcillin 150 mg/kg/day in 6 divided doses with ceftazidime 30 to 50 mg/kg every 8 hours. In children under 5 years old, *Haemophilus influenzae* should be considered, and amoxicillin and clavulanate potassium (Augmentin) is a good antibiotic choice. The antibiotics should be adjusted according to culture and sensitivity results.

Preferred Response   a. orbital abscess

You are asked to evaluate a 20-year-old man in the emergency room who has been hit over the left brow with a hockey stick. The visual acuity is 20/20 OD and 20/200 OS. A large hematoma is forming in the left upper eyelid, and the eyelid is tense. A left relative afferent pupillary defect is present. Anterior segment examination reveals a left subconjunctival hemorrhage with a microscopic hyphema. It is not possible to measure the intraocular pressure in the left eye; however, the left globe is tense to digital palpation. Dilated fundus examination of the left eye reveals peripheral retinal edema and pulsation of the central retinal artery.

The *most* appropriate emergent management is to

a. order an emergent CT scan
b. begin intravenous corticosteroids
c. perform a canthotomy and cantholysis
d. perform a paracentesis

Discussion

The clinical features of a tense upper eyelid, increased intraocular pressure, and pulsation of the central retinal artery are consistent with an acute orbital compartment syndrome. The orbital pressure needs to be lowered immediately. The most expeditious method is a canthotomy and cantholysis. Both the superior and inferior limbs of the lateral canthal tendon should be released for maximal decompression. Following this procedure, the fundus should be reexamined to make sure that arterial flow has been restored. The relative afferent pupillary defect may be due to a fracture of the optic canal; however, treatment should be directed toward lowering the intraorbital pressure before a CT scan is obtained. A paracentesis may lower the intraocular pressure transiently; however, this will not adequately address the compartment syndrome. Surgical or medical (corticosteroids) orbital decompression should be considered if the relative afferent pupillary defect does not resolve. This would indicate that a component of compressive optic neuropathy persists and should be treated.

Preferred Response   c. perform a canthotomy and cantholysis

O41

A previously healthy 6-year-old child presents with proptosis of the left eye. Family photographs reveal some prominence of the eye for the past year. One week prior to presentation, the child had a seizure of undetermined cause. Fundus examination reveals choroidal folds OS.

Which one of the following diagnostic tests is *least* useful in this case?

a. MRI
b. CT scan
c. echography
d. fluorescein angiography

Discussion   The findings of proptosis and choroidal folds suggest the presence of a mass behind the eye. A CT scan, MRI, or echographic examination of the orbit would all be reasonable imaging modalities to evaluate this patient. The occurrence of a seizure in this child raises the suspicion of intracranial involvement. MRI is often superior to CT scan in imaging lesions that involve both the orbit and intracranial structures, although CT scanning is usually preferred to MRI in lesions confined to the orbit. Fluorescein angiography is not likely to add any useful information regarding the cause of proptosis in this patient.

Preferred Response   d. fluorescein angiography

 The figures show the MRI results from the patient in Question O41.

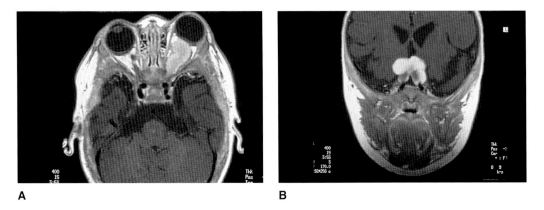

A   **B**

(A) MRI showing fusiform optic nerve enlargement that indents the back of the eye. **(B)** MRI showing intracranial extension of the optic nerve glioma.

The *most* likely diagnosis is

a. rhabdomyosarcoma
b. optic nerve meningioma
c. optic nerve glioma
d. leukemic infiltration of the optic nerve

Discussion   The transaxial MRI (T1-weighted with fat suppression) demonstrates an enhancing fusiform expansion of the left optic nerve (see the figure, part A). A noticeable kink is present in the midportion of the nerve. Both fusiform expansion of the optic nerve and a kink in its intraorbital course are typical features of an optic nerve glioma.[27] The coronal view (see the figure, part B) demonstrates intracranial spread of the glioma, which may account for the seizure in this child. Meningiomas tend to cause diffuse thickening of the optic nerve with either anterior or posterior expansion. One does not normally see kinking of the nerve with meningiomas. Rhabdomyosarcoma develops from mesenchymal tissue within the orbit and is not intrinsically confined to the optic nerve as demonstrated here.

Leukemic infiltration of the optic nerve generally results in irregular expansion of the nerve and not the fusiform expansion shown in this case.

Preferred Response   c. optic nerve glioma

A 55-year-old woman is examined for gradual visual loss in her left eye over 6 months. The visual acuity is 20/20 OD and 20/200 OS. She is found to have 3 mm proptosis and a left relative afferent pupillary defect. Part A of the figure shows the optic nerve head and part B shows the CT scan.

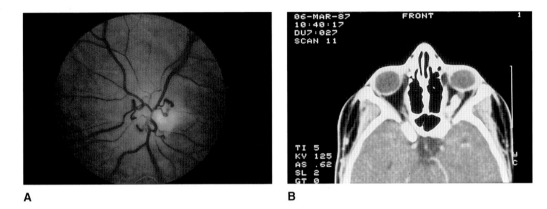

A   **B**

(A) Optic nerve with optociliary shunt vessels. **(B)** CT scan showing optic nerve enlargement with calcification.

The *least* appropriate management is

a. surgical debulking
b. complete surgical excision
c. radiation following incomplete surgical excision
d. chemotherapy

Discussion   The presence of optociliary shunt vessels (see the figure, part A) is highly suggestive of orbital meningioma, but is not pathognomonic. The CT scan (see the figure, part B) shows characteristics of an optic nerve meningioma. The visual acuity is reduced secondary to optic nerve compression from the meningioma. Treatment of optic nerve meningiomas is typically to follow the patient until either the vision is severely compromised or the tumor shows evidence of apical or intracranial extension. Well-defined meningiomas may be amenable to complete surgical excision. Meningiomas are traditionally considered to be radioresistant; however, the role of radiation for primary optic nerve meningiomas is being investigated. Kennerdell et al[28] have reported preservation of visual function in patients with primary optic nerve meningiomas treated with approximately 5500 rads. Chemotherapy does not have a role in the management of meningiomas.

Preferred Response   d. chemotherapy

Which of the following statements regarding meningiomas is *least* true?

a. Most optic nerve–sparing orbital meningiomas represent extensions of intracranial meningiomas.

b. Meningiomas in children are benign more frequently than meningiomas in adults.

c. Primary meningiomas of the optic nerve occur more frequently in females than in males.

d. Meningiomas occur more frequently in individuals with type 1 neurofibromatosis than in the general population.

Discussion

The majority (90%) of orbital meningiomas represent extensions of intracranial meningiomas from the sphenoid wing or olfactory groove. The remaining 10% of orbital meningiomas arise primarily from the optic nerve within the orbit.[29] Ectopic meningiomas arising elsewhere in the orbit have been reported; however, their pathogenesis remains controversial. The majority of studies on optic nerve meningiomas have found female preponderance, with approximately 60% occurring in females and 40% in males. Both meningiomas and gliomas occur more frequently in patients with type 1 neurofibromatosis. Primary optic nerve sheath meningiomas in individuals under 30 years of age often behave more aggressively, with intracranial spread occurring early in the course of the disease. This group of patients requires frequent imaging and consideration for earlier surgical intervention if apical extension of the tumor occurs or there is marked visual loss.[30]

Preferred Response

b. Meningiomas in children are benign more frequently than meningiomas in adults.

O45

The CT scan of a 61-year-old woman shows diffuse infiltration of the left inferior rectus muscle by metastatic breast carcinoma. All of the following statements about metastatic breast carcinoma to the orbit are true *except*

a. The breast is the most common primary site of metastatic orbital tumors in women.

b. The majority of women have diagnosed breast cancer at the time of orbital involvement.

c. Metastases to the choroid are more common than metastases to the orbit.

d. Enophthalmos is more common than proptosis in this condition.

Discussion

Tumors that metastasize to the orbit most commonly originate in the breast and lung.[31] Other sites of primary tumors seen with some frequency include the prostate and gastrointestinal tract. The majority of patients with metastatic breast carcinoma present with exophthalmos, although enophthalmos is associated with metastatic scirrhous adenocarcinoma of the breast.[32] Clinical series have demonstrated that approximately 90% of women have a history of breast cancer prior to developing orbital involvement.[33,34] Part A of the figure shows the patient's inability to depress the left eye; the CT scan (part B of the figure) shows diffuse involvement of the inferior rectus muscle. Choroidal metastasis is approximately 9 times more common than orbital disease in patients with breast cancer.[32]

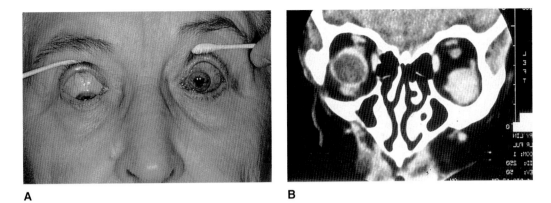

A **B**

Patient with metastatic breast carcinoma. **(A)** Inability to depress the left eye. **(B)** CT scan showing enlargement of inferior rectus muscle from breast carcinoma metastasis.

Preferred Response   d. Enophthalmos is more common than proptosis in this condition.

Potential advantages of MRI over CT scanning include all of the following *except*

a. MRI does not expose the patient to radiation.
b. MRI allows for better evaluation of lesions that extend from the orbit to the cranium.
c. MRI is unaffected by motion artifact.
d. MRI can generate high-quality axial, coronal, and sagittal images without repositioning the patient.

Discussion   Magnetic resonance imaging (MRI) is a valuable modality in the evaluation of orbital disease. Unlike computerized tomography (CT), MRI does not expose the patient to radiation. The image is generated by exposing the body tissue placed in a strong magnetic field to a radiofrequency pulse. MRI does require more time than a CT scan and is more sensitive to motion artifact. MRI may give superior detail of orbital soft tissue and is superior in evaluating processes that extend from the orbit into the cranium. It is not necessary to adjust the position of the patient to obtain axial, coronal, sagittal, parasagittal, or oblique images with a spatially coordinated MRI scanner. A CT scan image may be reconstructed in off-axis planes; however, the quality of the image is suboptimal.[35] Even with these advantages, MRI has not replaced CT scanning in the evaluation of orbital diseases. The majority of orbital processes can be adequately evaluated with a CT scan. CT scans provide bony imaging, important for orbital surgery, which is not present on MRI scans. CT scanning and MRI offer distinct advantages, and the appropriate selection should be based on the clinical situation.

Preferred Response   c. MRI is unaffected by motion artifact.

A 38-year-old woman presents with proptosis of her left eye. She complains of periodic headaches, especially in the brow area. On examination, her left eye is noted to be displaced inferiorly and laterally. The figures show the CT scans.

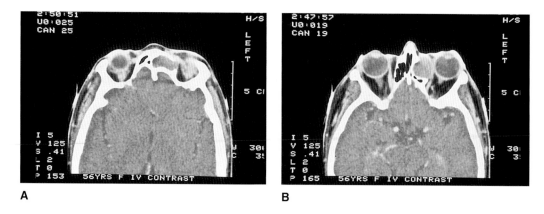

A   **B**

CT scans showing sinus mucocele. **(A)** Frontal sinus mucocele extending into orbit. **(B)** Ethmoid sinus component of mucocele displacing the eye.

The *most* likely diagnosis is

a. lymphangioma
b. lymphoma
c. orbital abscess
d. mucocele

Discussion

The most likely diagnosis is a left frontal sinus mucocele. Mucoceles are chronic cyst-like lesions filled with mucus and lined by respiratory epithelium. In order of decreasing frequency, mucoceles originate from the frontal, ethmoidal, sphenoid, and maxillary sinuses. Frontal and ethmoidal mucoceles account for approximately 95% of mucoceles. Obstruction of the natural ostia of the paranasal sinuses is the pathogenesis for mucocele formation. The obstruction may be secondary to trauma, inflammation, hyperviscous mucus (cystic fibrosis), polyps, or tumors.[36,37] The figures show CT scans with a soft tissue density expanding from the ethmoid and frontal sinuses through the medial wall of the orbit with secondary extension along the orbital roof.

Refer to Question O28 for a discussion of lymphangiomas. Orbital lymphomas tend to mold around structures within the orbit but usually do not cause bony erosion. In the absence of external signs of inflammation, the diagnosis of an orbital abscess is unlikely.

Preferred Response   d. mucocele

The *most* appropriate management of the patient in Question O47 is

a. observation
b. nasal decongestants and prophylactic oral antibiotics
c. drainage via percutaneous needle aspiration
d. surgical resection

Discussion

The management of mucoceles is surgical. Effective surgical management includes removal of the mucocele and its mucosal lining, combined with reestablishment of nasal sinus drainage. If drainage is not possible, then obliteration of the sinus is required to prevent recurrent mucocele formation. Mucoceles should be approached as a combined effort of the ophthalmologist and otolaryngologist. Observation increases the risk of developing infection (mucopyocele) and possible secondary orbital cellulitis. Needle aspiration is not an effective long-term management of this lesion, since the nasal sinus drainage obstruction remains. Nasal decongestants and antibiotics are ineffective in the management of established mucoceles.

Preferred Response

d. surgical resection

A 17-year-old boy is evaluated for a 2-day history of painful swelling of the right upper eyelid. The swelling began 24 hours after a wrestling tournament. The patient is healthy, with no history of past ocular problems. On examination the vision is 20/20 in each eye. Abduction of the right eye is limited and associated with pain. Moderate injection of the right temporal bulbar conjunctiva is present. The CT scans are shown in the figures.

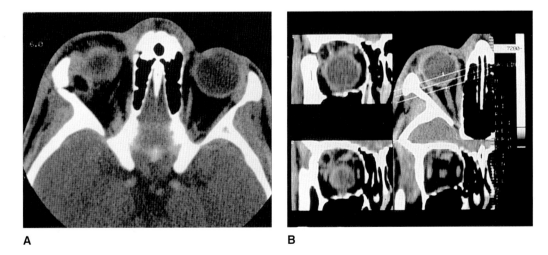

A   **B**

(A) Axial view CT scan showing a dermoid cyst. **(B)** Coronal view CT scan showing the cyst extending into the lateral orbital wall.

The *most* likely diagnosis is

a. fracture of the lateral wall of the orbit
b. orbital cellulitis
c. preseptal cellulitis
d. ruptured dermoid cyst

Discussion

The clinical presentation and CT scan appearance are consistent with a ruptured dermoid cyst in the area of the right frontozygomatic suture. It is probable that the patient sustained trauma to this area and ruptured the cyst while wrestling. However, this information was not volunteered. Dermoid cysts of the orbit tend to be associated with bony suture lines. The CT scans in this case depict a dermoid cyst extending from the lateral orbit through the frontozygomatic suture (see the figures). Orbital dermoid cysts, because of their location, are typically larger when diagnosed than anteriorly located dermoid cysts. The intense inflammatory reaction is secondary to the liberation of the dermoid cyst contents, which often include fat and hair. Fractures of the lateral orbital wall are often associated with fractures of the zygomatic complex, which is not shown in these CT scans. Fractures of the orbit may be associated with periorbital ecchymosis and hematoma formation, but not with inflammation. The presence of epibulbar injection suggests an inflammatory cause. There is no history of sinusitis, and the sinuses are clear on the CT scan, ruling out sinus infection as a cause. Pain with eye movement is not a feature of preseptal cellulitis.

Preferred Response

d. ruptured dermoid cyst

The *most* appropriate treatment for the patient in Question O49 is

a. intravenous antibiotics
b. oral prednisone
c. surgical excision
d. warm compresses

Discussion

The most appropriate therapy is surgical debridement of the dermoid combined with anti-inflammatory therapy. In this case the most direct exposure is through a lateral orbitotomy. Intravenous antibiotic therapy is not indicated because this is an inflammatory process rather than an infectious process. The inflammation is secondary to the dermoid contents within the orbit. Removal of the material will facilitate recovery and minimize the risk of excessive scar formation within the orbital tissues. Intravenous corticosteroids followed by oral prednisone should reverse the inflammatory signs and symptoms. Oral prednisone alone would help suppress the inflammatory response; however, the presence of ruptured dermoid contents may lead to chronic low-grade inflammation and possible fistula formation.[38]

Preferred Response

c. surgical excision

References

1. Nelson CC, Oestreicher J: Eyelid trauma. *Focal Points.* Vol IX, Module 10. San Francisco: American Academy of Ophthalmology; 1991.

2. Goldberg RA, Holds JB, Ebrahimpour J: Exposed hydroxyapatite orbital implants: report of six cases. *Ophthalmology* 1992;99:831–836.

3. Buettner H, Bartley GB: Tissue breakdown and exposure associated with orbital hydroxyapatite implants. *Am J Ophthalmol* 1992;113:669–673.

4. Fry CL, Leone CR Jr: Safe management of dermolipomas. *Arch Ophthalmol* 1994; 112:1114–1116.

5. Serdahl CL, Berris CE, Chole RA: Nasolacrimal duct obstruction after endoscopic sinus surgery. *Arch Ophthalmol* 1990;108:391–392.

6. Patipa M: Visual field loss in primary gaze and reading gaze due to acquired blepharoptosis and visual field improvement following ptosis surgery. *Arch Ophthalmol* 1992;110:63–67.

7. Wojno TH: Downgaze ptosis. *Ophthal Plast Reconstr Surg* 1993;9:83–88.

8. Dutton JJ: Evaluation of the ptosis patient. In: Dutton JJ: *A Color Atlas of Ptosis.* Singapore: PG Publishing; 1989.

9. Fasanella RM, Servat J: Levator resection for minimal ptosis: another simplified operation. *Arch Ophthalmol* 1961;65:493–496.

10. Anderson RL, Dixon RS: Aponeurotic ptosis surgery. *Arch Ophthalmol* 1979;97: 1123–1128.

11. Mauriello JA, Wagner RS, Caputo AR, et al: Treatment of congenital ptosis by maximum levator resection. *Ophthalmology* 1985;93:466–469.

12. Wagner RS, Mauriello JA, Nelson LB, et al: Treatment of congenital ptosis with frontalis suspension: a comparison of suspensory materials. *Ophthalmology* 1984; 91:245–247.

13. Callahan MA, Beard C: Examination and evaluation. In: Callahan M, Beard C, eds: *Beard's Ptosis.* 4th ed. Birmingham, AL: Aesculapius Publishing Co; 1990;88–95.

14. Nerad JA, Carter K, Folberg R: Simple dacryops. *Arch Ophthalmol* 1988;106:1129.

15. Bullock JD, Fleishman JA, Rosset JS: Lacrimal ductal cysts. *Ophthalmology* 1986;93:1355–1360.

16. Doxanos MT, Green WR, Iliff CE: Factors in the successful surgical management of basal cell carcinoma of the eyelids. *Am J Ophthalmol* 1981;91:726–736.

17. Mohs FE: Micrographic surgery for the microscopically controlled excision of eyelid cancers. *Arch Ophthalmol* 1986;104:901–909.

18. Cutler NL, Beard C: A method for partial and total upper lid reconstruction. *Am J Ophthalmol* 1955;39:1–7.

19. Hughes WL: Total lower lid reconstruction: technical details. *Trans Am Ophthalmol Soc* 1977;74:321–329.

20. Townsend DJ: Eyelid reanimation for the treatment of paralytic lagophthalmos: historical perspectives and current applications of the gold weight implant. *Ophthal Plast Reconstr Surg* 1992;8:196–201.

21. Kulwin DR, Kersten RC: Management of eyelid burns. *Focal Points.* Vol VIII, Module 2. San Francisco: American Academy of Ophthalmology; 1990.

22. Carter KD, Frueh BR, Hessburg TP, et al: Long-term efficacy of orbital decompression for compressive optic neuropathy of Graves' eye disease. *Ophthalmology* 1991;98:1435–1442.

23. Lloyd WC III, Leone CR Jr: Supervoltage orbital radiotherapy in 36 cases of Graves' disease. *Am J Ophthalmol* 1992;113:374–380.

24. Hurbli T, Char DH, Harris J, et al: Radiation therapy for thyroid eye diseases. *Am J Ophthalmol* 1985;99:633–637.

25. Krohel GB, Krauss HR, Winnick J: Orbital abscess: presentation, diagnosis, therapy, and sequelae. *Ophthalmology* 1982;89:492–498.

26. Harris GJ: Subperiosteal abscess of the orbit: age as a factor in the bacteriology and response to treatment. *Ophthalmology* 1994;101:585–595.

27. Jakobiec FA, Depot MJ, Kennerdell JS, et al: Combined clinical and computed tomographic diagnosis of orbital glioma and meningioma. *Ophthalmology* 1984;91:137–155.

28. Kennerdell JS, Maroon JC, Malton M, et al: The management of optic nerve sheath meningiomas. *Am J Ophthalmol* 1988;106:450–457.

29. Dutton JJ: Optic nerve sheath meningiomas. *Surv Ophthalmol* 1992;37:167–183.

30. Wright JE, McNab AA, McDonald WI: Primary optic nerve sheath meningioma. *Br J Ophthalmol* 1989;73:960–966.

31. Ferry AP: Carcinoma metastatic to the eye and orbit. I. A clinicopathologic study of 227 cases. *Arch Ophthalmol* 1974;92:276–286.

32. Shields CL, Shields JA, Peggs M: Tumors metastatic to the orbit. *Ophthal Plast Reconstr Surg* 1988;4:73–80.

33. Goldberg RA, Rootman J: Clinical characteristics of metastatic orbital tumors. *Ophthalmology* 1990;97:620–624.

34. Bullock JD, Yanes B: Ophthalmic manifestations of metastatic breast cancer. *Ophthalmology* 1980;87:961–973.

35. Wirtschafter JD, Berman EL, McDonald CS: *Magnetic Resonance Imaging and Computed Tomography.* Ophthalmology Monograph 6. San Francisco: American Academy of Ophthalmology; 1992.

36. Weaver DT, Bartley GB: Malignant neoplasia of the paranasal sinuses associated with mucocele. *Ophthalmology* 1991;98:342–346.

37. Rootman J, Allen L: Acquired lesions (mucocele). In: Rootman J, ed: *Diseases of the Orbit: A Multidisciplinary Approach.* Philadelphia: JB Lippincott; 1988:496–502.

38. Grove AS Jr: Giant dermoid cysts of the orbit. *Ophthalmology* 1979;86:1513–1520.

Additional Resources From the AAO

Basic and Clinical Science Course

Ophthalmic Pathology and Intraocular Tumors. Section 4. Updated annually.

Orbit, Eyelids, and Lacrimal System. Section 7. Updated annually.

Pediatric Ophthalmology and Strabismus. Section 6. Updated annually.

Focal Points

Boynton JR: *Management of Cicatricial Entropion, Trichiasis, and Distichiasis.* Vol XI, Module 12. 1993. (Item No. 029011)

Bullock JD, Goldberg SH, Felder DS: *Management of Malignant Eyelid Tumors.* Vol VII, Module 6. 1989. (Item No. 029007)

Cahill KV, Burns JA: *Management of Benign Eyelid Lesions.* Vol VII, Module 2. 1989. (Item No. 029007)

Dortzbach RK, McGetrick JJ: *Diagnosis and Treatment of Acquired Ptosis.* Vol II, Module 10. 1984. (Item No. 029002)

Dortzbach RK, Woog JJ: *Diagnosis and Management of Congenital Ptosis.* Vol V, Module 2. 1987. (Out of print)

Feldon SE: *Management of Thyroid Eye Disease.* Vol I, Module 14. 1983. (Item No. 029001)

Gavaris PT, Kaplan LJ: *Management of Entropion and Ectropion.* Vol I, Module 12. 1983. (Item No. 029001)

Kline LB: *Computed Tomography in Ophthalmology.* Vol III, Module 9. 1985. (Out of print)

Kulwin DR, Kersten RC: *Management of Eyelid Burns.* Vol VIII, Module 2. 1990. (Out of print)

Lauer SA: *Ectropion and Entropion.* Vol XII, Module 10. 1994. (Item No. 029012)

Lemke BN: *Management of Thyroid Eyelid Retraction.* Vol IX, Module 6. 1991. (Item No. 029009)

Nelson CC, Oestreicher J: *Eyelid Trauma.* Vol IX, Module 10. 1991. (Item No. 029009)

Nerad JA, Carter KD: *The Anophthalmic Socket.* Vol X, Module 9. 1992. (Item No. 029010)

Nunery WR: *Diagnosis and Management of Blunt Orbital Trauma.* Vol IV, Module 11. 1986. (Item No. 029004)

Stefanyszyn MA: *Orbital Tumors in Children.* Vol VIII, Module 9. 1990. (Out of print)

Steinkuller OG: *Orbital Cellulitis.* Vol IX, Module 11. 1991. (Item No. 029009)

Monographs

Stewart WB, ed: *Surgery of the Eyelid, Orbit, and Lacrimal System.* Vol 1. Ophthalmology Monograph 8. 1993. (Item No. 0210085)

Stewart WB, ed: *Surgery of the Eyelid, Orbit, and Lacrimal System.* Vol 2. Ophthalmology Monograph 8. 1994. (Item No. 0210086)

Wirtschafter JD, Berman EL, McDonald CS: *Magnetic Resonance Imaging and Computed Tomography: Clinical Neuro-Orbital Anatomy.* Ophthalmology Monograph 6. 1992. (Item No. 0210211)

Videotapes

Bergin DJ: *Management and Surgery of Congenital and Acquired Ptosis.* Clinical Skills Series. 1990. (Item No. 0250923)

Trauma to the Orbit, Eyelids, and Lacrimal System. Classic Series. 1982. (Item No. 0250513)

Wesley RE: *Ectropion and Entropion Repair of the Lower Lid.* Clinical Skills Series. 1989. (Item No. 0250773)

PEDIATRIC OPHTHALMOLOGY AND STRABISMUS

P1

A day-care worker has given birth to an infant with severe unilateral microphthalmia (see the figure) and a cataract. The mother reports possible exposure to chickenpox during her pregnancy.

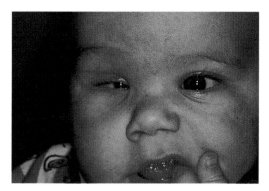

Unilateral microphthalmia secondary to congenital varicella.

Which of the following ocular abnormalities is least consistent with the diagnosis of an intrauterine varicella infection?

a. cataract
b. chorioretinitis
c. Horner's syndrome
d. aniridia

Discussion

A maternal infection with varicella can have devastating effects on the fetus. As many as one-fourth of cases result in intrauterine infection, with almost all of those cases occurring in the first and second trimesters of the pregnancy. Common nonocular manifestations include cicatricial skin lesions (see the figure on page 198), hypoplastic limbs, delayed development, and small size for gestational age. Chorioretinitis is probably the most common ocular finding. Other ocular manifestations include microphthalmia, cataract, Horner's syndrome, and optic nerve hypoplasia. Involvement may be unilateral or bilateral. Aniridia has not been reported as an ocular manifestation of congenital varicella syndrome.[1]

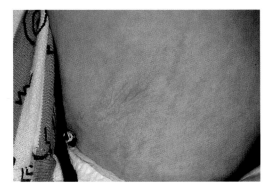

Cicatricial skin lesions secondary to congenital varicella.

Preferred Response   d. aniridia

You are asked to evaluate in the newborn nursery a low-birth-weight infant with possible eye anomalies. During your examination, you instruct the nursing personnel to dilate the child's eyes with a mixture of 0.5% cyclopentolate and 2.5% phenylephrine ophthalmic solution.

All of the following additional instructions should be given to the nursing personnel *except*

a. Delay the infant's feeding for at least 2 hours.
b. Temporarily occlude the nasolacrimal puncta after administering the drops.
c. Administer or increase supplemental oxygen.
d. Closely observe the vital signs.

Discussion   A 2.5% solution of phenylephrine has been reported to result in a significant elevation of systolic blood pressure in premature and low-birth-weight infants. Similarly, cyclopentolate has been associated with paralytic ileus and, at least in one instance, death. Based on this knowledge, it is reasonable to observe infants closely when these ocular drugs are being administered. Occlusion of the puncta will help decrease systemic absorption. Delaying feeding before administering the drops has been shown to reduce the incidence of gastrointestinal problems. Respiratory distress is not a common side effect of either of these drugs, and the administration of supplemental oxygen does not appear to be indicated unless the child demonstrates a decrease in PaO_2 during the examination. A commercially available solution of 0.2% cyclopentolate and 1.0% phenylephrine seems to provide adequate mydriasis in neonates with fewer side effects than the higher concentrations.[2]

Preferred Response   c. Administer or increase supplemental oxygen.

A 4-month-old infant girl is noted by her parents to have the unusual appearance of her right eye shown in the figure, part A. The otherwise healthy child was born 3 weeks prematurely with a birth weight of 5 pounds 6 ounces. Your examination reveals a normal left eye. The right eye demonstrates shallowing of the anterior chamber and a clear crystalline lens, as well as the retrolental and retinal abnormalities shown in the figures. Examinations of the parents and an older sibling are unremarkable.

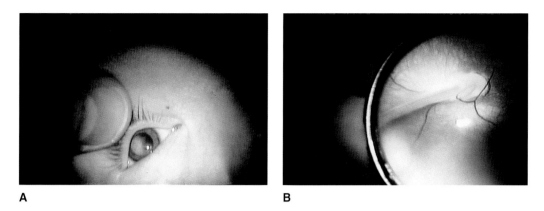

A   B

(A) Temporally located retrolental mass. **(B)** Retinal fold extending from the optic disc to the retinal periphery.

The *most* likely diagnosis is

a. persistent hyperplastic primary vitreous
b. Norrie's disease
c. incontinentia pigmenti
d. familial exudative vitreoretinopathy

Discussion   A funnel-shaped retinal detachment emanating from the optic nerve in an infant of normal birth weight is most consistent with a diagnosis of persistent hyperplastic primary vitreous (PHPV). PHPV is a predominantly unilateral congenital ocular anomaly characterized by incomplete atrophy of the fetal hyaloid vascular system. Commonly associated findings include microphthalmia, a retrolental fibrovascular mass, progressive lens swelling with cataract formation, and elongation of the ciliary processes. PHPV may present with involvement of the posterior segment of the eye only, characterized by tractional retinal folds and detachment. Other disorders to consider include familial exudative vitreoretinopathy (FEVR), Norrie's disease, incontinentia pigmenti, and retinopathy of prematurity. All of these conditions are usually bilateral. FEVR is an autosomal dominant condition with variable expressivity; examination of the parents or siblings will help in ruling it out. Most patients with FEVR are asymptomatic. Incontinentia pigmenti is inherited as an X-linked dominant disorder that is usually lethal in males. It has characteristic skin vesicles that cicatrize in infancy. Norrie's disease is a rare, X-linked, recessive condition characterized by progressive deafness and mental retardation after infancy. Female carriers are unaffected. Ocular manifestations include vitreous hemorrhages that lead to retinal detachment, rubeosis iridis, and phthisis bulbi. Norrie's disease can be confirmed in male patients by evaluation of the blood for the Norrie's gene.

Preferred Response   a. persistent hyperplastic primary vitreous

A 4-month-old infant boy presents with epiphora of the right eye that has been present since shortly after birth. Mucoid discharge can be expressed from the puncta with external pressure over the right nasolacrimal sac. The *most* reasonable treatment would be

a. observation
b. massage of the nasolacrimal sac
c. probing of the nasolacrimal duct
d. irrigation of the nasolacrimal duct

Discussion

Congenital obstruction of the nasolacrimal duct, or dacryostenosis, occurs in 1% to 6% of newborn infants. Most of the obstructions open spontaneously within the first 6 months of life. Thereafter, spontaneous resolution may still occur but is much less likely. Massage of the nasolacrimal sac appears to increase the rate of resolution of the obstruction, as compared with no massage. If massage is unsuccessful in clearing the obstruction, then probing of the nasolacrimal duct should be considered by 1 year of age.[3,4]

Preferred Response

b. massage of the nasolacrimal sac

P5

A 6-month-old infant boy demonstrates the ocular deviation shown in the figure. Each eye is able to abduct normally. The child was born after a normal, full-term pregnancy by a normal delivery.

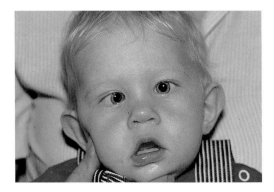

Congenital esotropia.

Considering the most likely diagnosis, all of the following statements about this condition are true *except*

a. Amblyopia is commonly associated.
b. Abduction and adduction movements are often asymmetric.
c. Vertical deviations are commonly associated.
d. Patients with this condition rarely require glasses during childhood.

Discussion

This infant shows an esotropia that is most consistent with a diagnosis of infantile, or congenital, esotropia. The relatively large size of the deviation and the patient's ability to abduct the eye tend to rule out causes such as sixth-nerve palsy and Duane's syndrome. Abduction can be difficult to test in an infant with this condition and may require stimulation of the oculovestibular reflex or a trial with monocular occlusion. Accommodative esotropia has been reported in children as young as 4 months of age and can usually be distinguished by a trial with glasses if a refractive error of more than 2 diopters of hyperopia is found. Amblyopia occurs in approximately 40% of children with infantile esotropia both before and after surgical correction.

Vertical deviations are commonly associated with congenital esotropia. Dissociated vertical deviations have been reported in up to 90% of cases, while inferior oblique overactions are nearly as common. Vertical deviations are usually not detected until after the first year of life. Both asymmetry of ocular smooth pursuit and monocular optokinetic nystagmus have been commonly associated with infantile esotropia. Children with this disorder demonstrate better temporal-to-nasal movements than nasal-to-temporal movements. Although surgery is the treatment of choice for infantile esotropia, a high percentage of patients develop a postsurgical accommodative component over time. In one study, 65% of surgically corrected patients with congenital esotropia required spectacle correction of their hyperopia to control the ocular alignment.[5]

Preferred Response

d. Patients with this condition rarely require glasses during childhood.

P6

A 2-week-old infant boy presents with the ocular findings shown in the figure. There is no history of ocular trauma or inflammation.

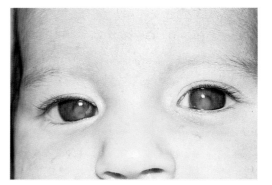

Peters' anomaly.

All of the following statements are true *except*

a. Glaucoma is commonly associated with this condition.
b. This condition is usually bilateral.
c. Systemic abnormalities are rare.
d. This condition may have been caused by neural crest dysgenesis.

Discussion

The ocular appearance shown in the figure is most consistent with a diagnosis of Peters' anomaly, which is characterized by a central corneal opacity without inflammation or vascularization. The lens or iris strands may be in contact with the corneal opacity. Peters' anomaly is thought to involve a dysgenesis of the neural crest cell layer (corneal stroma, Descemet's membrane, endothelium, and iris stroma) and surface ectoderm cell layer (lens) in the embryo. Most cases of Peters' anomaly are bilateral and more than 50% develop glaucoma. Other reported ocular anomalies are microcornea, microphthalmos, cornea plana, iris dysgenesis, and cataract. Systemic associations are well documented and include craniofacial, cardiovascular, and genitourinary anomalies. Peters' anomaly is usually sporadic, although both autosomal dominant and autosomal recessive inheritance have been described.[6,7]

Preferred Response

c. Systemic abnormalities are rare.

A 3-month-old infant presents with nystagmus and poor fixation responses. The undilated anterior segment findings, which are similar in both eyes, are shown in the figure. The posterior segment reveals small optic discs and indistinct foveae.

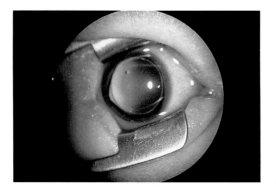

Aniridia.

What is the next *most* important step in managing this patient?

a. Obtain a family history.
b. Monitor for amblyopia.
c. Treat with tinted contact lenses.
d. Evaluate for Wilms' tumor.

Discussion

The ocular examination of this child is most consistent with a diagnosis of congenital aniridia. This is an uncommon ocular condition that affects primarily the iris but also often involves the cornea (pannus), the anterior chamber angle (glaucoma), the lens (cataract, subluxation), the retina (macular hypoplasia), and the optic nerve (hypoplasia). It is familial in approximately two-thirds of cases and is inherited as an autosomal dominant condition. One-third of cases are sporadic, with most of those cases considered to be new autosomal dominant mutations.

Although amblyopia can occur, the ocular pathology is the primary cause of reduced vision in patients with aniridia. Tinted glasses or contact lenses may improve the vision by reducing photophobia. The most important medical concern for patients with aniridia is the increased risk of developing Wilms' tumor. As many as one-third of sporadic cases of aniridia are associated with the development of Wilms' tumor in early childhood. Patients at risk for Wilms' tumor require frequent physical and abdominal ultrasound examinations. However, only one patient with familial aniridia has ever been reported to have developed Wilms' tumor.

Therefore, a positive family history significantly decreases the likelihood of developing Wilms' tumor and decreases the need for frequent repeated evaluations for this condition.[8]

Preferred Response a. Obtain a family history.

The 3-year-old child shown in the figure received surgery for esotropia at age 1 year. His parents are unhappy with his appearance of upturned eyes. In primary gaze, there is an 8-prism-diopter esotropia. A V pattern is present, with a difference in the deviation from down gaze to up gaze of 15 prism diopters. Under a cover, each eye has a very noticeable hyperdeviation but there is no corresponding hypodeviation on alternate-cover testing. On examination, you demonstrate elevation of each eye in adduction, a right hypertropia on left gaze, and a left hypertropia on right gaze.

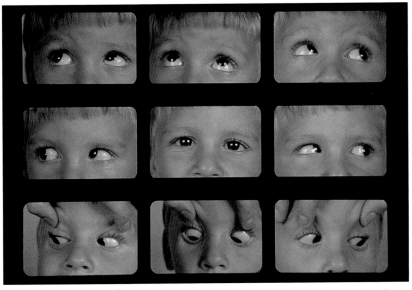

Bilateral elevation in adduction secondary to inferior oblique overaction and dissociated vertical deviations.

The *most* reasonable operation for this child would be

a. bilateral inferior oblique myectomy
b. bilateral superior rectus recession
c. bilateral inferior oblique recession with anterior displacement
d. bilateral inferior oblique and superior rectus recession

Discussion Elevation of either eye in adduction suggests the presence of one or more of the types of vertical deviations commonly associated with infantile esotropia and discussed in Question P5. The reversing hyperdeviations on side gaze and the V-pattern deviation indicate bilateral overaction of the inferior oblique muscles. The vertical deviations in primary gaze without a corresponding hypodeviation are suggestive of dissociated vertical deviation (DVD).

The treatment of choice for bilateral inferior oblique overaction is a weakening procedure (myectomy or recession) of the inferior oblique muscles. Treatment of DVD is more controversial. Some surgeons advocate superior rectus recession with or without posterior fixation sutures; others advocate inferior rectus resection. Inferior oblique weakening procedures alone will not correct DVD. Also, superior rectus recession alone will not help inferior oblique overaction. A combination of both procedures is possible; however, weakening both elevators may have a greater tendency than alternative procedures to result in problems with supraduction. Furthermore, quantifying the amount of surgery is difficult. A procedure currently advocated for treating inferior oblique overaction in combination with DVD is recession and anterior advancement of the inferior oblique muscle. The muscle is reattached adjacent to the lateral pole of the inferior rectus muscle. It is theorized that this procedure changes the action of the inferior oblique from an elevator to a depressor.[9]

Preferred Response   c. bilateral inferior oblique recession with anterior displacement

A 2-year-old child has been referred for wandering of one eye that has been evident for the past few months. Using binocular fixation-pattern techniques, you detect reduced vision in that eye. The anterior segment is normal, but the optic nerve is as shown in the figure. The posterior segment of the other eye is normal.

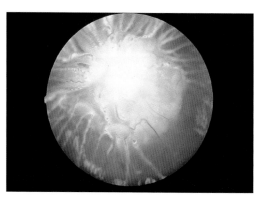

Morning glory disc anomaly.

Which of the following statements about the condition shown is true?

a. Visual acuity in the affected eye is usually better than 20/200.
b. The condition is associated with seizures and early death.
c. The condition is hereditary.
d. Retinal detachments are associated with this condition.

Discussion   The condition depicted in the photograph is most consistent with a diagnosis of morning glory anomaly of the optic disc, a nonhereditary congenital anomaly that is usually unilateral. It is characterized by an enlarged, excavated optic disc, a proliferation of glial tissue in the center of the optic nerve head, a peripapillary staphyloma, and an abnormal pattern of retinal vessels emanating from the optic nerve head. Visual acuity is usually poor. Retinal detachments have been reported in up to one-third of cases and are difficult to treat. Other associated ocular conditions include cataract, foveal hypoplasia, aniridia, and microphthalmos.

Systemic conditions reported with morning glory disc anomaly include basal encephalocele, absent corpus callosum, pituitary dysfunction, and renal abnormalities. Seizures and premature death are not characteristic. If nonocular conditions are suspected, a neurologic and endocrine workup may be warranted.[10, 11]

Preferred Response   d. Retinal detachments are associated with this condition.

P10   An otherwise healthy, 3-week-old newborn presents with bilateral conjunctivitis (see the figure).

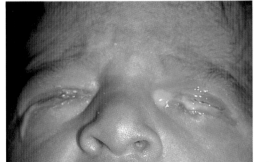

Neonatal conjunctivitis.

How would you initiate management?

a. Start broad-spectrum systemic antibiotics.
b. Start broad-spectrum topical antibiotics.
c. Obtain conjunctival specimens for microbiology.
d. Obtain blood cultures.

Discussion   Acute conjunctivitis of the newborn has a greater potential for ocular complications and systemic manifestations than conjunctivitis in older children or adults. Blindness, neurologic deficits, and death are known complications of neonatal conjunctivitis. Treatment should be based on laboratory results as well as clinical examination. Identification of the organism and appropriate treatment are critical for preventing permanent sequelae. Although the methods may differ depending on the laboratory facilities available, conjunctival scrapings should be obtained and fixed on a slide for Gram and Giemsa stains. Conjunctival specimens can be obtained with a moistened cotton applicator to inoculate blood agar, chocolate agar, Thayer-Martin agar, and viral transport medium. Only after these specimens are obtained should treatment be initiated.

Therapy should be based on the clinical impression, stains, and cultures. Gram-positive bacteria usually respond to topical erythromycin, while topical gentamicin or tobramycin is effective for most Gram-negative organisms. *Neisseria* requires systemic treatment, such as intramuscular ceftriaxone or intravenous cefotaxime or cefixime. Topical treatment consists of saline solution and erythromycin. Herpes simplex is treated with systemic acyclovir. Treatment of *Chlamydia* is discussed in Question P11. Unless the newborn has evidence of systemic involvement in the examination, blood cultures are not indicated.

Preferred Response   c. Obtain conjunctival specimens for microbiology.

All of the following statements about chlamydial conjunctivitis of the newborn are true *except*

a. It is the most common infectious cause of neonatal conjunctivitis.
b. It is commonly associated with pneumonitis.
c. Oral erythromycin should be prescribed.
d. Silver nitrate 1% solution provides prophylaxis.

Discussion

The most common infectious cause of neonatal conjunctivitis is *Chlamydia trachomatis*. Up to 10% of asymptomatic pregnant women have been shown to be culture positive for this organism. Approximately 30% to 40% of children born to untreated affected mothers will be infected. Approximately 15% of newborns with conjunctivitis develop chlamydial pneumonitis. Because of possible systemic involvement, oral erythromycin is the treatment of choice. Either erythromycin or tetracycline, given topically within 1 hour after birth, significantly decreases the likelihood of developing chlamydial conjunctivitis. Silver nitrate has little or no effect in preventing this infection.

Preferred Response   d. Silver nitrate 1% solution provides prophylaxis.

A mother complains that her 6-year-old daughter has had increased wandering of her left eye over the past year. Your examination notes an intermittent exotropia of 35 prism diopters with fixation at distance and 5 prism diopters of exophoria with fixation at near. Her uncorrected visual acuity is 20/20 OD and 20/20 OS. After a discussion with the mother, you decide on surgical treatment.

Which of the following tests would be *least* helpful in surgical management of this patient?

a. 30-minute occlusion test
b. +3.00 lens test
c. cycloplegic refraction
d. Worth four-dot test

Discussion

This case illustrates an exodeviation with a distance-to-near disparity. It is not clear from the information provided whether this is the patient's basic deviation, unaffected by fusional or accommodative convergence amplitudes. The occlusion test consists of occluding one eye for a specified period of time (usually at least 30 minutes) and reassessing the distance and near deviations without allowing the patient to regain fusion. Theoretically, this test will eliminate fusional convergence that is otherwise not detected with a traditional alternate prism-cover test. The +3.00 lens test measures the near deviation with and without the addition of a +3.00 sphere in front of both eyes. This test should eliminate accommodative convergence. Although each test may influence the other, in general both tests provide information on the mechanism of the distance-to-near disparity, which may suggest possible management options.

A refraction is mandatory in the evaluation of any strabismus case. For example, correction of an anisometropia may provide better control of the deviation. The Worth four-dot test provides the least useful information for the management of this patient. The fact that the patient has a phoria on near vision indicates the presence of fusion.

Preferred Response   d. Worth four-dot test

A 7-year-old boy complains of decreased vision in the right eye. The child also has lymphadenopathy, malaise, and a low-grade fever. On examination, the best-corrected visual acuity is counting fingers OD and 20/20 OS. The left fundus is normal; the right fundus is shown in the figure.

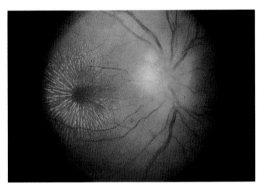

Optic disc edema and macular star secondary to cat-scratch disease.

All of the following diseases are consistent with the clinical picture *except*

a. multiple sclerosis
b. Lyme disease
c. syphilis
d. cat-scratch disease

Discussion   This condition is usually referred to as neuroretinitis. It differs from childhood optic neuritis in that it is almost always unilateral and associated with an exudative macular star. In the past, neuroretinitis was generally believed to be idiopathic, but recent studies suggest that cat-scratch disease is a common cause of this condition. The Gram-negative rod *Rochalimaea henselae* is suspected to be the causative agent of cat-scratch disease. Other known causes of neuroretinitis are Lyme disease and syphilis.

The child whose fundus is shown in the figure was scratched by a cat near his right eye 2 weeks before presenting with visual loss OD. Cat-scratch disease was suspected on the basis of the clinical history, lymphadenopathy, and low-grade fever. The diagnosis was later confirmed with an ELISA test. Trimethoprim with sulfamethoxazole may shorten the course of the disease. There is no increased risk of multiple sclerosis in a child with neuroretinitis.[12,13]

Preferred Response   a. multiple sclerosis

A 4-month-old boy is brought in for evaluation because of visual inattention and nystagmus. His pupils do not respond to light and he has a refractive error of +4.00 OU. Both fundi appear normal.

The *most* likely diagnosis is

a. Leber's optic neuropathy
b. cortical blindness
c. X-linked congenital stationary night blindness
d. Leber's congenital amaurosis

Discussion   Both Leber's congenital amaurosis and X-linked congenital stationary night blindness may be associated with nystagmus, decreased vision, and a normal-appearing fundus in infancy. X-linked congenital stationary night blindness is usually associated with a myopic refractive error, whereas 75% of children with Leber's congenital amaurosis have 3 diopters or more of hyperopia. The fundus may appear normal at a very early age, but arteriolar narrowing, pigmentary changes, and optic atrophy become evident with time. Nystagmus is usually not present in children with cortical blindness or Leber's optic neuropathy. In addition, pupillary responses should be normal with cortical blindness, and Leber's optic neuropathy is not seen in infants.[14]

Preferred Response   d. Leber's congenital amaurosis

A 6-month-old child is brought in for evaluation of nystagmus and decreased vision. His optic discs are shown in the figure.

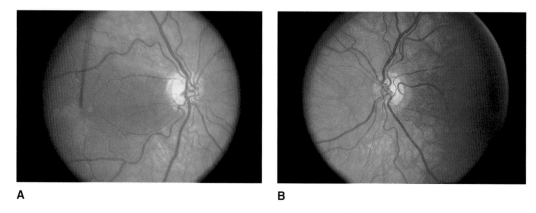

A   B

Optic nerve hypoplasia in a 6-month-old child. **(A)** Right eye. **(B)** Left eye.

Which of the following is the *least* important consideration in managing this patient?

a. inheritance pattern
b. pituitary hormonal dysfunction
c. association with brain anomalies
d. visual development

Discussion

This child has bilateral optic nerve hypoplasia. When combined with agenesis of the septum pellucidum or corpus callosum, optic nerve hypoplasia is called septo-optic dysplasia, or de Morsier's syndrome. Although rare cases have been reported of family members being affected by optic nerve hypoplasia, this disease is generally considered to be nonhereditary. Many children with this condition also have an endocrinopathy secondary to hypothalamic dysfunction. Recent neuroimaging studies have shown a variety of other brain anomalies that may be associated with optic nerve hypoplasia, including schizencephaly (focal absence of portions of the brain), neuronal migration abnormalities (ectopic gray matter in subcortical white matter), and posterior pituitary ectopia. Posterior pituitary ectopia in a child with optic nerve hypoplasia has been suggested to be a predictor of future endocrine problems. Visual acuity with complete optic nerve hypoplasia can vary but generally tends to be poor.[15]

Preferred Response

a. inheritance pattern

P16

A 5-year-old child with horizontal nystagmus sees 20/50 when her head is held straight but can see 20/25 by adopting a 45° left head turn. The nystagmus is unchanged when fixing on a near target.

Which surgical approach would be *most* likely to reduce her head turn?

a. Recess the right medial rectus and the left lateral rectus muscles. Resect the right lateral rectus and the left medial rectus muscles.
b. Recess both medial rectus muscles and resect both lateral rectus muscles.
c. Recess the left medial rectus and the right lateral rectus muscles. Resect the left lateral rectus and the right medial rectus muscles.
d. Recess the left medial rectus muscle and resect the left lateral rectus muscle.

Discussion

This child's excellent vision, combined with her large head turn, are most consistent with idiopathic or motor nystagmus. Presumably, the patient is adopting a head turn to fixate in null position. One surgical approach would be to create an exotropia that would stimulate a nystagmus-dampening convergence. In this case, the absence of a null position with convergence would make it unlikely that creating an exotropia would improve her head turn. Recession and resection of the horizontal extraocular muscles to move both eyes in the direction of the head turn is the treatment of choice. This procedure, originally described by Anderson and Kestenbaum, has undergone a number of variations to achieve the best head alignment while avoiding the development of strabismus. In this specific case, a recession of the left medial and right lateral rectus muscles with resection of the left lateral and right medial rectus muscles should achieve the desired goal.[16]

Preferred Response   c. Recess the left medial rectus and the right lateral rectus muscles. Resect the left lateral rectus and the right medial rectus muscles.

The child shown in the figure has had ptosis of the right upper eyelid since birth. When asked to fixate on a distant or near target, she demonstrates a chin-up head position. The alternate-cover test is normal. The induced prism test reveals a preference for the left eye, suggesting decreased vision in her right eye.

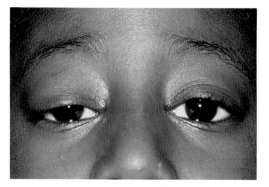

Congenital ptosis of the right upper eyelid.

The *most* likely cause of her reduced vision is

a. anisometropic amblyopia
b. deprivation amblyopia
c. strabismic amblyopia
d. chorioretinal coloboma

Discussion   About 20% of children with congenital ptosis have a significant refractive error, which frequently results in anisometropic amblyopia. The presence of a chin-up position does not rule out amblyopia. Since this child can clear the visual axis with a slight chin-up position, deprivation amblyopia is unlikely. The child is orthotropic, so strabismic amblyopia is also unlikely. Although chorioretinal coloboma can be present in a child with ptosis, it is not commonly associated with unilateral ptosis.[17,18]

Preferred Response   a. anisometropic amblyopia

A 2-year-old boy presents with a history of crossing of his left eye that has been noted by his parents over the past 3 months. Examination reveals a dense total cataract in the left eye. The anterior segment is otherwise normal. The right eye is normal. Both pupils react normally. The past medical history is unremarkable. The next step should be

a. ocular ultrasound
b. urinalysis for reducing substances
c. observation
d. cataract extraction

Discussion   The most common causes of unilateral cataracts in the pediatric population are trauma, posterior lenticonus, and persistent hyperplastic primary vitreous. Other less common but important causes include intraocular inflammation (ie, toxocariasis) and intraocular tumor (ie, retinoblastoma). Urinalysis for non–glucose-reducing substances after ingesting milk is a screening test for galactosemia; galactosemia would be highly unlikely. Most children with galactosemia present in infancy with feeding intolerance and hepatosplenomegaly. By 2 years of age, they usually manifest moderate to severe mental retardation. It would also be unusual for a galactosemic cataract to present unilaterally. Cataract extraction most likely would be indicated in this case; however, prior to cataract extraction, it would be important to assess the posterior segment of the affected eye. Ocular ultrasound provides the best method for assessing the status of the vitreous and retina.

Preferred Response   a. ocular ultrasound

You are asked to see a 6-month-old infant for suspected shaken baby syndrome. Assuming that the child was abused, what ocular abnormality are you *most* likely to find?

a. subconjunctival hemorrhage
b. retinal hemorrhage
c. iris sphincter tear
d. retinal fold

Discussion   Ocular findings occur in 30% to 40% of all child abuse cases and in more than 50% of the cases of shaken baby syndrome. Reported ocular manifestations include periorbital ecchymosis, subconjunctival hemorrhage, cataract, subluxated lens, iris tears, ocular motor palsies, optic atrophy, retinal folds, retinal detachment, and retinal hemorrhages. The most common ocular manifestation is retinal hemorrhage. The hemorrhages may affect any layer of the retina and may be of any size or shape (see the figure). They occur most frequently in the posterior pole. The pathophysiology of retinal hemorrhages in shaken baby syndrome is not completely known but appears to be due to acceleration and deceleration forces as well as to raised intraocular venous pressure at the time of the abuse.[19]

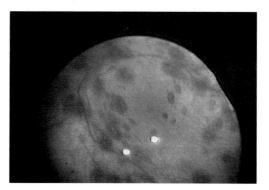

Retinal hemorrhages in suspected child abuse, as seen with a video indirect ophthalmoscope.

Preferred Response   b. retinal hemorrhage

P20

With regard to the patient in Question P19, which of the following statements is true?

a. Retinal hemorrhages associated with child abuse usually occur without intracranial hemorrhage.
b. Timing of the alleged abuse can be estimated by characteristics of the retinal hemorrhages.
c. Retinal hemorrhages in children can result from cardiopulmonary resuscitation.
d. Children diagnosed with shaken baby syndrome have a low incidence of permanent neurologic deficits.

Discussion

Retinal hemorrhages in children are highly suggestive, but not diagnostic, of child abuse. Although they can be an isolated finding, retinal hemorrhages are usually associated with coexisting intracranial hemorrhage. Neurologic evaluation is therefore appropriate. The clinical appearance of a retinal hemorrhage is not a good indicator of its age and should not be used to determine the timing of the trauma. Studies have suggested that permanent neurologic impairment occurs in one-third to three-fourths of children diagnosed with shaken baby syndrome. Although uncommon, retinal hemorrhages in children can be associated with cardiopulmonary resuscitation.

Preferred Response

c. Retinal hemorrhages in children can result from cardiopulmonary resuscitation.

A 3-year-old child was found by his pediatrician to have possible decreased acuity in one eye. Evaluation by an ophthalmologist using the illiterate E test demonstrated a visual acuity of 20/25 OD and 20/60 OS. Cycloplegic retinoscopy revealed mild hyperopia OD but an irregular streak OS that appears hyperopic in the lens periphery but myopic centrally. After a period of observation, the patient showed reduced acuity OS secondary to a lens opacity (see the figure).

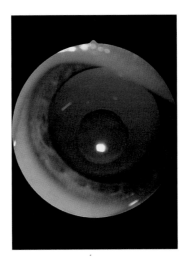

Posterior lenticonus.

This type of cataract is typically associated with

a. poor visual acuity outcome after surgery
b. progressive involvement of the fellow eye
c. an otherwise anatomically normal eye
d. galactosemia

Discussion

The history and findings are consistent with a cataract of the posterior lenticonus or lentiglobus type. Patients with this lenticular change typically undergo progressive visual loss and lens opacification. The lens changes involve a progressive bowing of the central 2 to 4 mm of the lens, perhaps because of intralenticular pressure that is being exerted as lens fibers are formed. The posterior bowing initially has an "oil droplet" appearance with a myopic change centrally and a normal peripheral lens. With time, the opacification increases and visual acuity loss becomes significant. With successful surgery and aggressive amblyopia therapy, visual acuity outcomes are often good, probably because the patient with posterior lenticonus often goes through the critical early period of visual development with a relatively clear lens. The remainder of the ocular anatomy and visual system in this condition is normal.

Almost all cases are unilateral and sporadic, although bilateral cases as well as familial cases have been described. Cataracts in infants with galactosemia are described as having an "oil droplet" appearance. However, such children would not be likely to reach age 3 years without ocular and medical detection of the systemic condition (see Question P18).[20]

Preferred Response

c. an otherwise anatomically normal eye

P22

A 3-year-old girl is referred by her pediatrician for ophthalmologic evaluation. She has had a recent episode of painful swelling of the right knee. Several months prior to that she had swelling of the left elbow. Which of the following statements is true?

a. Ocular involvement is unlikely because more than one joint is affected.
b. Initial ocular signs usually include conjunctival injection.
c. A positive antinuclear antibody (ANA) implies significant ocular risk.
d. If the patient has no ocular manifestations after 3 years, further ophthalmologic follow-up is usually unnecessary.

Discussion

Patients who have or are suspected of having juvenile rheumatoid arthritis (JRA) are at risk for developing eye problems, particularly, chronic anterior uveitis. Ocular involvement is an important cause of morbidity in these patients and may lead to significant visual loss. Young females with pauciarticular onset (involvement of one to four joints) who are ANA positive and rheumatoid-factor negative have an estimated risk of developing uveitis of as high as 91%. Patients with polyarticular onset are less likely to develop uveitis, although it can occur in this group. The iridocyclitis is typically quiet, without significant pain, discomfort, or conjunctival injection.

Patients with JRA of the pauciarticular, ANA-positive type require close follow-up (every 2 to 3 months) for many years, even in the absence of uveitis. It is unusual for the eyes to become involved after more than 7 years without ocular disease have passed since diagnosis. Of patients who will develop eye disease, 95% or more do so within 10 years after onset of the arthritis.[21,22]

Preferred Response

c. A positive antinuclear antibody (ANA) implies significant ocular risk.

The patient in Question P22 develops chronic anterior uveitis. In this case, all of the following statements are true *except*

a. The patient is also at risk for developing cataract, band keratopathy, and posterior synechiae.
b. If a cataract develops in this condition, visual acuity outcome is usually poor.
c. Visual prognosis is worse if the uveitis precedes the systemic condition.
d. Glaucoma is usually secondary to a pupillary-block mechanism.

Discussion

Patients with JRA and associated anterior uveitis are at high risk for developing complications such as cataract, band keratopathy, posterior synechiae, and secondary glaucoma. As many as 50% of such patients develop cataracts as a result of the chronic inflammation, chronic corticosteroid use, or both. However, with careful management, visual acuity outcomes may be good (20/40 or better) in as many as 75% of patients who develop cataracts. Secondary glaucoma typically has a pupillary-block component as a result of the inflammation-induced posterior synechiae. Visual loss and complications are strongly correlated with the degree of inflammation observed in the initial exam; those patients whose uveitis precedes the arthritis do worse than those whose arthritis antedates the uveitis.[23,24]

Preferred Response

b. If a cataract develops in this condition, visual acuity outcome is usually poor.

A child is referred for evaluation of an "abnormal pupil." The pupillary appearance is shown in the figure.

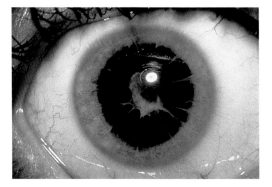

Persistent pupillary membrane.

This finding

a. is likely to lead to lens opacification
b. demonstrates a growth that should be surgically removed
c. represents failed regression of the primary vitreous
d. is compatible with good visual acuity

Discussion   Persistent pupillary membranes are usually seen in eyes that are otherwise anatomically normal. They result from incomplete involution of the tunica vasculosa lentis and can be unilateral or bilateral. They may range in size from nearly occluding the pupillary space—in which case surgical removal may be indicated—to relatively minor obstruction of the pupil. Significant regression of the pupillary membrane may occur during the first year of life. Secondary lens opacification may occur but is variable. Most cases of persistent pupillary membranes are sporadic, but autosomal dominant pedigrees have been reported. Despite the apparent severity of the membrane, visual impairment may not be significant enough to prompt surgical extraction. The patient should be followed closely, monitored for amblyopia, and treated with mydriatics in an attempt to improve acuity before surgery is performed.[25,26]

Preferred Response   d. is compatible with good visual acuity

An infant in the newborn nursery is found to have bilateral lens opacities of the type shown in the figure.

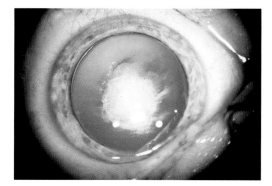

Congenital nuclear cataract.

All of the following are true about this condition *except*

a. Evaluation for systemic disease is not indicated.
b. Corneal diameter is usually small.
c. A family history of congenital cataracts is common.
d. The risk of glaucoma after cataract surgery is low.

Discussion   Bilateral, centrally located cataracts in a newborn child with the appearance shown in the figure are typical of congenital nuclear cataracts. The lens opacity initially involves the embryonic and fetal nucleus; however, there may be secondary involvement of surrounding cortex, often referred to as "riders." The presence of bilateral cataracts at birth warrants investigation to rule out systemic metabolic disease such as rubella, galactosemia, and Lowe syndrome. An exception is a healthy newborn with a family history of congenital cataracts. Most patients with nuclear cataracts have bilateral involvement and small corneas (<10 mm diameter at birth). An autosomal dominant inheritance pattern may be found in 50% or more of cases. These eyes are prone to development of glaucoma for many years after cataract surgery and should be watched carefully postoperatively.[27,28]

Preferred Response   d. The risk of glaucoma after cataract surgery is low.

A 16-year-old boy has a history of normal vision in both eyes. He presents complaining of a sudden decrease in vision in the right eye. His visual acuity is 20/200 OD and 20/15 OS. A relative afferent pupillary defect is present in the right eye, and confrontation visual fields reveal a dense central scotoma OD. Fundus examination reveals a normal macula with a hyperemic-appearing disc OD. The result of MRI of the head and optic nerves is normal.

If an abnormality in this patient's DNA related to visual loss were found, it would *most* likely reveal

a. a mutation in the rhodopsin gene on chromosome 3
b. a mutation on the X chromosome
c. a mutation of the mitochondrial DNA
d. chromosome 13 deletion

Discussion   This case is most consistent with a diagnosis of Leber's hereditary optic neuropathy. This condition is associated with mutations in the mitochondrial DNA in at least three loci: nucleotides 11778, 3460, and 14484. For reasons that are not well understood, males are affected more commonly than females. The disease is inherited from the maternal DNA, with a woman who harbors the mutation passing it to all of her offspring. Why only a fraction of the individuals who harbor the mutation will actually develop optic neuropathy is not currently understood. Molecular tests that reveal the presence of one of these three mutations are an extremely reliable way to make the diagnosis. The clinical presentation of Leber's hereditary optic neuropathy is not diagnostic of the condition. Neuroimaging should be considered in these patients at least once to rule out the possibility of a lesion of the optic nerve or brain. A mutation in the rhodopsin gene on chromosome 3 has been found in some types of retinitis pigmentosa. A mutation on the X chromosome has been associated with a number of ocular conditions, although not with Leber's hereditary optic neuropathy. Ocular manifestations of a chromosome 13 deletion include microphthalmia, colobomata, and retinoblastoma.

Preferred Response   c. a mutation of the mitochondrial DNA

A 6-year-old boy was noted to have abnormal vision on a school screening. The ophthalmologist finds his visual acuity to be 20/100 OD and 20/20 OS. When tested with a neutral-density filter, his acuity is 20/60 OD and 20/30 OS. He has a very small esotropia and a refractive error of +1.75 sphere OD and +1.00 sphere OS. He is treated with occlusion therapy of the left eye for 50% of his waking hours. After 3 months, his visual acuity is 20/80 OD and 20/20 OS.

What is the *most* likely reason for his poor response to treatment?

a. inadequate occlusion therapy
b. incomplete treatment of refractive error
c. irreversible functional amblyopia
d. subtle organic abnormality of the macula or optic nerve

Discussion

The most likely reason for the minimal improvement of vision in this case is inadequate occlusion therapy. To achieve an improvement in visual acuity with occlusion therapy, most experts recommend occlusion of the nonamblyopic eye for all or a majority of the hours the child is awake (high-percentage occlusion). Patching for 50% or less of waking hours is reserved for maintaining the existing level of acuity. Although reduced accommodation may be associated with amblyopia, it is unlikely that the uncorrected refractive error noted in this case would be severe enough to limit visual acuity improvement. Irreversible amblyopia could also be a factor, although it is unlikely. Most patients with strabismic or anisometropic amblyopia achieve ≥20/40 visual acuity following occlusion therapy. If an organic abnormality is the cause for decreased visual acuity, the acuity is usually worse when tested with a neutral-density filter.[29]

Preferred Response

a. inadequate occlusion therapy

Of the following case scenarios, which is the *least* likely to show visual improvement (≥20/40) with full-time occlusion therapy?

a. a 4-year-old child with esotropia of unknown duration whose visual acuity is 20/25 OD and 20/200 OS
b. an 8-year-old child with a refraction of +3.50 OD and +1.00 OS whose best-corrected visual acuity is 20/200 OD and 20/25 OS
c. a 2-year-old child following surgery and contact lens fitting for a unilateral traumatic cataract of 4 months' duration
d. a 2-year-old child found on routine examination to have an anomalous optic nerve head OD and who demonstrates poor fixation and following movements with that eye

Discussion

The patients in the cases presented may have permanent visual impairment as a result of irreversible functional amblyopia, organic amblyopia, or a combination of both. A 4-year-old child with strabismic amblyopia should be very responsive to amblyopia therapy; more than 90% of cases achieve 20/40 visual acuity or better. Most studies also suggest that more than 80% of the time an older child with anisometropic amblyopia will also respond to aggressive occlusion therapy. A young child with a unilateral acquired cataract has a worse prognosis than either of the first two choices but still may have a good result. In studies of acquired pediatric cataracts, between 54% and 79% of patients achieved ≥20/40 visual acuity. The worst prognosis appears to be a child with a unilateral optic nerve abnormality who presents with visual impairment. In one study of patients who presented with this clinical situation, the probability of obtaining a visual acuity of ≥20/40 was only 21%.[30]

Preferred Response   d. a 2-year-old child found on routine examination to have an anomalous optic nerve head OD and who demonstrates poor fixation and following movements with that eye

You are asked to examine a premature infant with bronchopulmonary dysplasia who is receiving supplemental oxygen by nasal cannula. You note the presence of 4 clock hours of stage 2, zone II retinopathy of prematurity (ROP) in the right eye and 2 clock hours of stage 1, zone II ROP in the left eye. The neonatologist would like your opinion on the level of oxygen to administer. Which one of the following approaches would you recommend?

a. Increase supplemental oxygen to maintain PaO_2 of 98%.
b. Decrease supplemental oxygen until ROP demonstrates regression.
c. Make no change in the supplemental oxygen.
d. Do not rely on the ocular condition in determining oxygen requirements.

Discussion   In the 1950s, ROP was associated with excessive supplemental oxygen. The presence of ROP suggested the need to reduce or eliminate supplemental oxygen when possible. Since that time, oxygen requirements have been more accurately measured and the amount of supplemental oxygen is carefully monitored. Recently, the rate of reduction of supplemental oxygen has been suggested as a contributing factor to the development of ROP. It is postulated that infants who have supplemental oxygen reduced too quickly may have a higher incidence and severity of ROP. A national collaborative study is currently under way to investigate this issue. At the present time, the best approach is probably to recommend that the neonatologist base the level of supplemental oxygen on the patient's systemic requirements rather than on the presence or absence of ROP.

Preferred Response   d. Do not rely on the ocular condition in determining oxygen requirements.

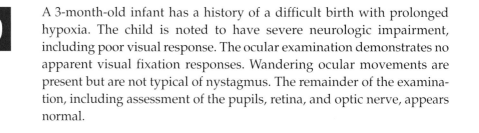

A 3-month-old infant has a history of a difficult birth with prolonged hypoxia. The child is noted to have severe neurologic impairment, including poor visual response. The ocular examination demonstrates no apparent visual fixation responses. Wandering ocular movements are present but are not typical of nystagmus. The remainder of the examination, including assessment of the pupils, retina, and optic nerve, appears normal.

Which of the following is the *best* method for predicting the visual outcome?

a. visual evoked responses
b. CT scan
c. electroretinogram
d. following the patient with sequential examinations

Discussion   An electroretinogram can aid in ruling out a retinal abnormality but is unlikely to be helpful in this case, since the damage is most likely at a higher level in the visual system. Many studies have attempted to use visual evoked response (VER) to help in determining visual prognosis in infants following cortical visual loss, but they have reported conflicting results. At the present time, it appears that the flash-evoked VER is not reliable enough to aid in predicting the visual outcome of infants who suffer a neurologic insult. CT scan or MRI of the brain may offer better clues than VERs in predicting visual outcome; however, the results are not conclusive. The best method for predicting a child's visual outcome appears to be sequential examinations during the first year or two of life.[31,32]

Preferred Response   d. following the patient with sequential examinations

A 38-year-old man was accidentally struck in the right eye with a bungee cord one day prior to your examination. The patient complains of double vision, especially when looking down. He has noticed no change in the vision in his right eye. There is a small laceration of the inferior conjunctiva. Ocular motility is shown in the figure. Forced-duction testing demonstrates slight restriction to elevation and depression. There is 1 mm of proptosis of the right eye. A CT scan of the orbit reveals soft-tissue swelling but no fracture.

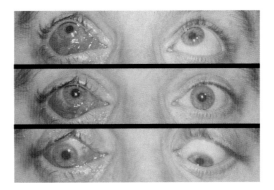

Right hypertropia following injury, with decreased infraduction.

What is the *most* likely cause for his ocular motility abnormality?

a. blowout fracture of the orbital floor
b. inferior rectus paresis
c. traumatic Brown's syndrome
d. laceration of the inferior rectus muscle

Discussion

This case demonstrates a traumatic motility disturbance characterized by a hyperdeviation and inability to depress the eye. The differential diagnosis should include a preexisting condition (ie, superior oblique palsy, old trauma), blowout fracture, and an acute injury to the inferior rectus muscle or its nerve. The history should help rule out a preexisting problem. A blowout fracture appears unlikely with a normal CT scan of good quality. Also, entrapment of orbital tissue would usually limit elevation as much or even more than depression in that eye. Forced-duction testing may be of help; however, it may be mildly abnormal (as in this case) because of orbital edema. The ocular motility abnormality with traumatic Brown's syndrome is a limitation to elevation, usually greater in adduction, and is often the result of injury to the superior nasal orbit.

Weakness of the inferior rectus muscle as a result of muscle or nerve trauma is the most likely explanation in this case. The lower eyelid lag in primary gaze shown in the figure, along with the conjunctival laceration, strongly suggests a laceration of the inferior rectus muscle with the muscle retracted from its insertion. Because a laceration of the inferior rectus is a likely cause, exploration of the muscle with repair and reattachment should be performed. Most strabismus surgeons advocate surgical exploration and repair during the acute phase with this type of injury, although others argue that repair at a later date is easier and equally successful.

Preferred Response

d. laceration of the inferior rectus muscle

A 27-year-old woman initially presents to you with a history of head injury 3 days previously in an automobile accident. The patient complains of constant double vision. The ocular versions are shown in the figure. The remainder of the examination is normal.

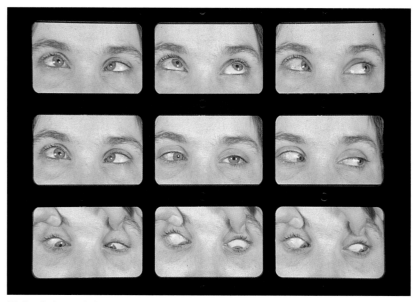

Right sixth cranial nerve palsy.

The *best* treatment option at this time would be

a. occlusion of the left eye and reevaluation in 1 to 2 weeks
b. botulinum toxin injection of the right medial rectus muscle
c. recession and resection procedure in the right eye
d. occlusion of the right eye and observation

Discussion

The best treatment option for this patient would be to occlude the paretic eye if desired to eliminate diplopia and then to follow the patient's progress. Occlusion of the unaffected eye in an attempt to decrease contracture of the medial rectus muscle has been proposed, but benefits of this approach have not been demonstrated, and most patients cannot tolerate seeing with only the affected eye. Because the patient is only 3 days postinjury, there is still a reasonable possibility of partial or complete recovery of lateral rectus function. Therefore, muscle surgery would not be appropriate at this time. To prevent contracture and to decrease symptoms, injection of botulinum toxin into the antagonist muscle is a reasonable option, although most experts would prefer to observe the patient for a few weeks to see if the palsy is resolving spontaneously. In some cases, prisms may offer relief from diplopia, although usually the deviation is too large and incomitant for the patient to benefit from this approach.

Preferred Response

d. occlusion of the right eye and observation

P33

Cytomegalovirus (CMV) is the most common intrauterine infection and has been isolated from the urine in up to 3% of newborns. A small percentage of these infants show clinical symptoms in the neonatal period and have widespread congenital anomalies. All of the following are typical congenital anomalies associated with intrauterine CMV infection *except*

a. hepatosplenomegaly
b. chorioretinitis
c. limb anomalies
d. microphthalmia

Discussion

The predominant abnormalities associated with CMV infection are related to damage to the central nervous system. Among the abnormalities noted are mental retardation, seizures, spasticity, and deafness. Other manifestations include premature birth, small size for gestational age, microcephaly, jaundice, hepatosplenomegaly, thrombocytopenia, and anemia. Reported ocular findings include chorioretinitis, microphthalmia, cataracts, and optic disc anomalies. Limb anomalies are not generally associated with intrauterine CMV infection.

Preferred Response

c. limb anomalies

A 30-year-old male accountant sustained a head injury as a result of an automobile accident 8 months previously. This patient's chief complaint is double vision when reading. There is no deviation in primary gaze, but a 15-prism-diopter esotropia is present in down gaze. There is a left hypertropia of 8 prism diopters in right gaze and a right hypertropia of 10 prism diopters in left gaze. Excyclotorsion of 6° is present in primary gaze, increasing to 15° in down gaze. Ocular versions demonstrate underaction of both superior oblique muscles.

What is the *best* treatment option for this patient?

a. reading glasses with prisms
b. bilateral superior oblique tucks
c. bilateral inferior oblique weakening procedures
d. advancement of the anterior fibers of both superior oblique muscles

Discussion

This patient demonstrates a common motility disturbance found with bilateral superior oblique palsies. These patients often fuse in primary gaze but have difficulty with reading as a result of the esotropia and torsion in down gaze. Some patients can compensate satisfactorily by holding their reading material in primary position. When presbyopia develops, however, bifocals do not work well and full-frame reading glasses are necessary. In a young patient whose occupation requires considerable near work, this approach would not seem reasonable. Prisms would not be helpful in this case because of the torsion. A surgical procedure would offer the most effective method for correcting this patient's problem. Inferior oblique weakening procedures will have minimal effect on the deviation in down gaze. Advancement of the anterior fibers of the superior oblique muscle (Harada-Ito procedure) will correct torsion and possibly some of the esodeviation in down gaze but will not significantly affect the vertical deviation on side gaze. Superior oblique tucks are the best procedure to improve the horizontal, vertical, and torsional misalignment problems.[33]

Preferred Response

b. bilateral superior oblique tucks

An 18-month-old child presents with a 6-month history of crossing of the left eye and a 6-week history of a white pupil in the same eye. The physical examination reveals a complete and diffuse haze in the vitreous. No retinal detail can be discerned. There is a suggestion of a mass lesion behind the haze. The CT scan is shown in the figure.

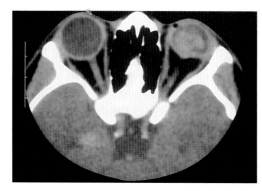

Orbital CT scan with intraocular mass lesion OS.

Appropriate management steps might include all of the following *except*

a. ultrasound
b. titer for toxocariasis
c. titer for toxoplasmosis
d. vitreous tap and histopathologic diagnosis

Discussion

This child's diagnosis is unilateral retinoblastoma. The presentation is atypical in that the mass lesion was not calcified on CT scan: the vast majority of retinoblastoma lesions of this size will demonstrate calcification on CT scan. (MRI will not demonstrate calcification.) Ultrasound may also detect calcification, but CT scan is likely to be more sensitive. Inflammatory mass lesions secondary to toxocariasis and toxoplasmosis should be considered in the differential diagnosis and titers obtained. A vitreous or aqueous tap in any eye that may harbor retinoblastoma is absolutely contraindicated. A tap may facilitate systemic spread and thus metastatic disease and death with this particular tumor. A blind eye harboring a mass in a child should be considered for enucleation if a neoplastic cause cannot be ruled out.

Preferred Response

d. vitreous tap and histopathologic diagnosis

All of the following are true about children with heritable retinoblastoma *except*

a. They may have a visible deletion at chromosome 13q14.
b. They may be unilaterally affected.
c. The majority have no family history.
d. Heritable and nonheritable retinoblastoma have an equal risk of secondary cancers.

Discussion

Approximately 40% of all cases of retinoblastoma are caused by a germinal mutation and are, therefore, heritable. Most of these cases are thought to be new mutations because a positive family history is present less than 10% of the time. It is important to note that 15% of sporadic, unilaterally affected patients have a heritable mutation and therefore must be followed closely. Between 1% and 3% of patients with retinoblastoma have a recognizable deletion at chromosome 13q14. These patients usually have a variety of systemic malformations. Secondary cancers are more common in patients with heritable retinoblastoma than in patients with nonheritable retinoblastoma.

Preferred Response

d. Heritable and nonheritable retinoblastoma have an equal risk of secondary cancers.

A 2-year-old boy presents with emesis, weight loss, and decreased appetite of 2 weeks' duration. The child has a history of retinoblastoma that required enucleation of the right eye and radiation of the left eye. He has been followed every 3 months by examination under anesthesia with no evidence of new or recurrent retinal tumors. A CT scan with contrast is obtained (see the figure).

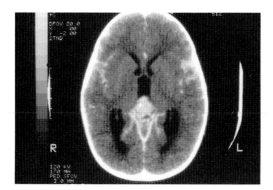

CT scan demonstrating a pineal mass with areas of calcification.

The findings on the scan are *most* likely

a. metastatic retinoblastoma
b. pineal blastoma
c. metastatic neuroblastoma
d. osteosarcoma

Discussion

Patients with heritable retinoblastoma are at significantly increased lifetime risk of developing secondary nonocular malignancies. The most common one is osteosarcoma. The role of radiation and chemotherapeutic agents in increasing this risk is not precisely known, but the overriding risk seems to be genetic. Another secondary cancer associated with bilateral retinoblastoma is a calcifying cancer of the pineal gland, or pineal blastoma. In patients with bilateral retinoblastoma, development of such a tumor is called "trilateral retinoblastoma." The CT scan demonstrates a mass with areas of calcification centered in the pineal gland and is consistent with this diagnosis. Prognosis for life with this particular triad is very poor. The differential diagnosis for the lesion seen on CT scan should include metastasis from retinoblastoma and other cancers, such as neuroblastoma, although the clinical presentation in this case is most consistent with a pineal blastoma.

Preferred Response

b. pineal blastoma

A 3-year-old girl presents to your office with wandering of the left eye that has been present for the past 3 months. Examination reveals 3 mm of proptosis of the left eye, a left relative afferent pupillary defect, and optic atrophy OS. Multiple skin lesions are noted on the child's body, as shown in the figure, part A. MRI is obtained, as shown in the figure, part B.

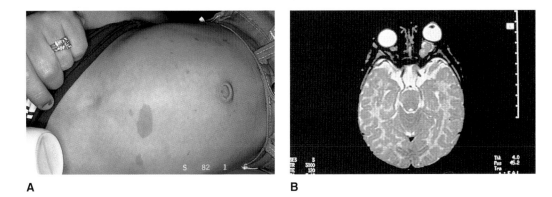

(A) Café-au-lait spot characteristic of neurofibromatosis type 1. **(B)** MRI showing glioma of the optic nerve and chiasm.

All of the following are true in this case *except*

a. In older patients, Lisch nodules are usually present.
b. The lesion present on the MRI is usually more aggressive in children than in adults.
c. Associated reactive meningeal hyperplasia may cause a biopsy to be misdiagnosed as meningioma.
d. Histologically, the lesion is a low-grade astrocytoma.

Discussion

The history, examination, and MRI findings are consistent with a diagnosis of optic nerve glioma, most likely associated with neurofibromatosis. Anterior visual pathway gliomas have been reported in 15% of patients with neurofibromatosis type 1. Bilaterality is especially associated with this condition. These tumors are often benign in children and may even undergo spontaneous regression. Their behavior in adults is much more aggressive and carries a poorer prognosis. Secondary reactive meningeal hyperplasia can be misdiagnosed on biopsy if a portion of the affected optic nerve is not included. Histologically, optic nerve gliomas are low-grade astrocytomas (grade 1–2) and most intraorbital lesions are of the pilocystic type. A rapid increase in proptosis can occur and is usually the result of mucoid degeneration.[34] Lisch nodules are present by age 6 years in more than 90% of patients with neurofibromatosis.[35]

Preferred Response

b. The lesion present on the MRI is usually more aggressive in children than in adults.

P39

A 20-year-old man has undergone a 4 mm right medial rectus recession for acquired esotropia. Shortly after surgery he developed exotropia and diplopia. The motility examination reveals a widened eyelid fissure with limited adduction of the operated eye. Cover testing shows exotropia in primary gaze that increases on left gaze (see the figure on page 226). The remainder of the ocular examination is normal.

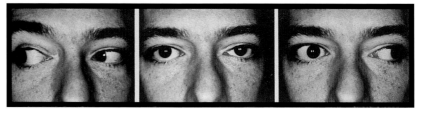

Secondary exotropia with limited adduction due to a slipped medial rectus muscle.

The *most* likely diagnosis is

a. partial third-nerve paresis
b. slipped medial rectus muscle
c. postoperative restriction
d. sensory exotropia

Discussion   Following recession surgery, the muscle can slip posteriorly within its sheath, resulting in unexpected underaction and incomitant strabismus. This occurs more commonly with surgery on the medial rectus when the muscle or tendon is not well secured to the suture. Signs of a slipped muscle include minimal to marked limitation of movement in the field of action of the muscle, proptosis, and eyelid fissure widening. Diplopia is often relieved by assuming a face turn opposite the muscle's field of action. In this case, the patient assumed a left face turn (placing eyes in right gaze). This clinical presentation can also be seen with partial third-nerve paresis, although the patient in this case has no history to support this diagnosis; in addition, vertical misalignment and pupil abnormalities are lacking. A postoperative restriction is unlikely when only medial rectus recessions have been performed. Palpebral fissure narrowing, rather than widening, would be more common in this situation. Forced ductions would also help to exclude this diagnosis. Since the patient has normal vision, sensory exotropia can be excluded. In this case, reoperation is necessary because the overweakened muscle is unlikely to recover full function over time. The medial rectus should be identified and advanced.

Preferred Response   b. slipped medial rectus muscle

A pediatrician calls to refer a 3-year-old Caucasian boy with a 1-week history of esotropia, abduction limitation, and face turn. There is no history of ocular disease or surgery. The patient is brought in for examination 3 days after the initial phone consultation. The parents have noted a slight improvement in the crossed eyes. The child has no history of trauma but did have a flu-like illness 1 week prior to onset of the esotropia. The ocular examination is normal.

Your workup at this time might include all of the following *except*

a. neurology referral
b. MRI
c. observation
d. erythrocyte sedimentation rate

Discussion

In childhood, almost 70% of abducens palsies can be accounted for by trauma, primary intracranial tumors (especially pontine gliomas and cerebellar astrocytomas), and congenital and postinfectious etiologies. Complete neurologic examination is appropriate to identify additional abnormalities that might suggest intracranial pathology. If other abnormalities are found, MRI should be considered to look for tumor. The most likely cause in this case is a sixth-nerve palsy secondary to viral infection. Since the patient is improving, continued observation is reasonable. An erythrocyte sedimentation rate (ESR) would not be helpful in this case. The ESR might be elevated as a result of the recent viral illness. More importantly, systemic conditions associated with an elevated ESR are not related to the development of sixth-nerve palsies in childhood.[36]

Preferred Response

d. erythrocyte sedimentation rate

P41

A 5-year-old boy who had allogenic bone marrow transplantation 1 year ago for acute lymphocytic leukemia presents for routine eye examination. All of the following are ocular complications of bone marrow transplantation *except*

a. cataract
b. superficial punctate keratopathy
c. iris heterochromia
d. retinal hemorrhage

Discussion

Ocular complications from bone marrow transplantation are related to the severity of graft-versus-host disease, the total dose and duration of corticosteroids, and the level of immunologic deficiency. Graft-versus-host disease can lead to significant problems with dry eyes and severe conjunctival scarring. Cataracts are thought to be related to the dose and duration of corticosteroids, although visually significant cataracts are uncommon. Cytomegalovirus (CMV) retinitis secondary to immunologic deficiency, especially with associated positive CMV cultures, may be seen in these children. Radiation retinopathy, which has been reported rarely, is characterized by retinal hemorrhages and cotton-wool spots and is thought to result from the combination of total body irradiation and chemotherapy. Iris heterochromia is not an ocular complication of the therapeutic management associated with bone marrow transplantation.[37]

Preferred Response

c. iris heterochromia

P42

A 13-year-old boy presents with a 6-month history of headaches, blurred vision, and intermittent crossed diplopia at near. His symptoms occur almost every day and are worse when he is tired. Your examination reveals an uncorrected acuity in each eye of 20/20. On a distant accommodative target, he is orthophoric. On a target at 1/3 m, he has a 15-prism-diopter exophoria. His near point of accommodation is 8 diopters in each eye. His fusional convergence amplitudes are 16 prism diopters to break and 12 to recover at 1/3 m, and 4 prism diopters to break and 2 to recover on a target at 6 m. Cycloplegic refraction reveals +0.75 sphere OD and +1.00 sphere OS.

The *best* treatment option is

a. correction of the cycloplegic refractive error
b. exercises for convergence insufficiency
c. glasses with base-in prisms
d. resection of both medial rectus muscles

Discussion

The best treatment option for this patient would be exercises for convergence insufficiency. Many motivated patients with symptomatic convergence insufficiency will improve with exercises if their symptoms are related to near work. A base-in prism may be helpful in selected patients, although the patient may compensate for the prism and increase the size of the deviation. Prisms are probably best reserved for elderly patients whose accommodation cannot be used to aid convergence and for patients unwilling to do exercises. Correction of the hyperopia is likely to decrease convergence and aggravate the symptoms. Surgery can benefit patients with moderate-to-large deviations who have failed to respond to exercises and prisms. A persistent esodeviation with diplopia is common following strabismus surgery for convergence insufficiency.

Preferred Response

b. exercises for convergence insufficiency

A 3-year-old girl has an esotropia that measures 18 prism diopters in primary position, 5 prism diopters in up gaze, and 35 prism diopters in down gaze. The ocular versions are shown in the figure. You plan to recess both medial rectus muscles for the esotropia.

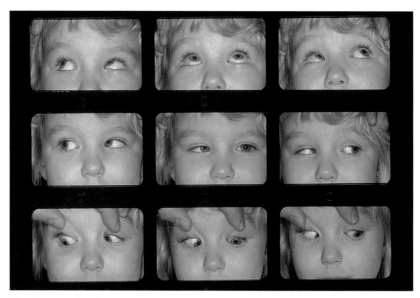

V-pattern esotropia.

How would you manage the V pattern?

a. Weaken both inferior oblique muscles.

b. Infraplace both medial rectus muscles.

c. Reassess the V pattern after correcting the horizontal deviation in primary gaze.

d. Perform bilateral superior oblique tenotomies.

Discussion

In general, the strabismus surgeon should attempt to correct all of the motility problems in one surgery, if possible, to spare the patient the risk and morbidity of additional procedures. Therefore, strabismus patterns should usually be managed at the same time as the horizontal strabismus surgery. Correction of A or V patterns depends on the amount of over- or underaction of the oblique muscles, which can be assessed in part by testing the ocular versions. Small to moderate A and V patterns are characterized by normal oblique muscle actions and are corrected by vertically displacing the horizontal rectus muscles. Large V patterns (20 prism diopter or more difference between up and down gaze) usually require oblique muscle surgery. In the case described above, the inferior oblique muscles demonstrate significant overaction consistent with a V pattern. In addition, measurements in side gaze are likely to reveal a right hypertropia in left gaze and a left hypertropia in right gaze that confirms the oblique muscle dysfunction. To correct the V pattern in this case, both inferior oblique muscles need to be weakened, which would be done at the same time as recession of the medial rectus muscles for the esodeviation. Bilateral superior oblique tenotomies are used to correct very large (>30 prism diopter) A patterns associated with superior oblique overaction.[38]

Preferred Response

a. Weaken both inferior oblique muscles.

A mother brings her 7-year-old son to you because he seems to be having trouble learning to spell and read. He is behind by at least one grade level in those areas. His math and art work are appropriate for his grade level. The patient's father had difficulty with school work as a child and currently wears glasses. The patient demonstrates 20/20 visual acuity in both eyes with a chart at 20 ft, but complains of difficulty with a near card and reads no better than 20/40. Your examination reveals +1.50 sphere OU and an exophoria of 2 prism diopters at near. Accommodative amplitudes and convergence fusional amplitudes are normal.

Which of the following statements is true?

a. The patient would benefit from orthoptic exercises.

b. The patient is probably going through a normal maturation process.

c. The patient should be evaluated for a possible learning disorder.

d. The patient should be treated with his hyperopic correction and a bifocal add.

Discussion

The history given for this child is more consistent with a learning disorder than an ocular problem. Inability to read and spell at grade level are rarely due to ocular abnormalities. Additional questioning about the child's ability to do near activities such as drawing or playing video games without difficulty may provide further evidence to rule out an ocular etiology. As in this case, children will occasionally demonstrate functional ocular complaints during the examination to explain poor academic performance. Accommodative insufficiency or convergence insufficiency can result in difficulty with near work and may require treatment with reading glasses or orthoptic exercises. In this case, however, accommodative amplitudes and convergence amplitudes are normal. Orthoptic exercises offer no help in the treatment of a learning disorder. This child should be referred to a well-established diagnostic and treatment program for evaluation of a possible learning disorder.

Preferred Response

c. The patient should be evaluated for a possible learning disorder.

Regarding developmental dyslexia, which of the following statements is true?

a. Dyslexia is not common in juvenile delinquents.
b. Dyslexics often present to ophthalmologists with visual symptoms.
c. Dyslexics rarely have a positive family history for dyslexia.
d. Dyslexics often have below-normal intelligence.

Discussion

Dyslexia is estimated to affect up to 8% of school-age children. As many as 75% of juvenile delinquents are thought to be dyslexic or to have learning disabilities. Recent evidence suggests that males and females may be affected nearly equally. A positive family history for learning disorders is not uncommon. If one parent is affected, a child has a five- to tenfold greater risk of have a reading disorder than a child of unaffected parents. Most dyslexics are of normal intelligence or even gifted. Since almost all dyslexics are visually normal, they frequently pass unsuspected through ophthalmology offices with vague complaints such as headaches with reading, blurry blackboards, words running together, or reading difficulties. Parental requests for routine checkups are often initiated by disappointing performance rather than by a desire for screening or preventive care, as is usually presumed. The value of a careful history and early recognition cannot be overestimated.[39]

Preferred Response

b. Dyslexics often present to ophthalmologists with visual symptoms.

A 7-year-old boy presents with a 9-month history of frequent episodes of blinking. The episodes are short in duration and occur randomly. Visual acuity is normal. The child's refractive error is +0.50 sphere in each eye. The remainder of the ocular examination is normal.

Which of the following statements is true?

a. A tear secretion test with and without anesthetic is likely to be diagnostic.
b. A conjunctival scraping to look for eosinophils and mast cells is indicated.
c. The blinking is most likely a habit.
d. The patient is likely to have a tic disorder.

Discussion

This patient most likely has a tic disorder. Tic disorders represent a clinical spectrum from the mild, transient form seen in up to 15% of children to the potentially devastating Tourette's syndrome, for which prevalence estimates vary from 1:200 to 1:2000. Tic disorders are characterized by involuntary, sudden, rapid, brief, repetitive, stereotyped, purposeless movements or vocalizations. There is often a positive family history, and males are more likely to be affected than females. Other behavioral problems are frequently associated with tic disorders; obsessive-compulsive disorder and attention-deficit hyperactivity disorder are the most common. Dry eye syndromes are very rare in children. It is unlikely with an otherwise normal examination that this child would have decreased tear secretion. Allergic or vernal conjunctivitis is more common; however, it is often seasonal and will usually demonstrate abnormalities on anterior segment examination.[40]

Preferred Response

d. The patient is likely to have a tic disorder.

A 29-year-old woman has a history of esotropia that was diagnosed at 4 years of age and treated with glasses and patching for a few months. She has had decreased vision in her right eye for as long as she can remember. She has noticed more crossing of her right eye in the past few years and would like it corrected. Her best-corrected visual acuity is 20/100 OD with a –0.50 sphere and 20/20 OS with a +0.50 sphere. Your examination reveals a 20-prism-diopter right esotropia in primary and side gaze. The esotropia decreases to 5 prism diopters in up gaze and increases to 30 prism diopters in down gaze. The remainder of her ocular examination is normal.

Which of the following would be the *best* procedure to correct this deviation?

a. resection of the right lateral rectus muscle and recession of the right medial rectus muscle (R and R OD)
b. bilateral recessions of the medial rectus muscles with infraplacement
c. R and R OD with infraplacement of the medial rectus muscle and supraplacement of the lateral rectus muscle
d. R and R OD and a weakening procedure on the right inferior oblique muscle

Discussion

This patient demonstrates a V-pattern esotropia and decreased visual acuity in the right eye, presumably resulting from amblyopia. The esotropia could be corrected with a recession and resection procedure of either eye or bilateral medial rectus recession. Because the patient has significant visual impairment, it is reasonable to restrict surgery to the poorer eye if possible. Correction of the V pattern can best be achieved by vertical displacement of the horizontal rectus muscles. In this case, the medial rectus should be infraplaced and the lateral rectus supraplaced. An inferior oblique muscle recession is indicated only if the inferior oblique muscle is overacting and there is an associated incomitant vertical deviation.[38]

Preferred Response

c. R and R OD with infraplacement of the medial rectus muscle and supraplacement of the lateral rectus muscle

A 4½-year-old girl presents with a 3-week history of a red eye. The slit-lamp findings are shown in the figure. The eye has light-perception vision, and there is no view of the posterior pole. The other eye is normal.

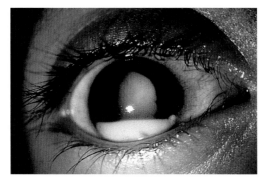

Pseudohypopyon secondary to retinoblastoma.

Appropriate investigation and management might include all of the following *except*

a. systemic evaluation for arthritis
b. angiotensin-converting enzyme (ACE) titer
c. an anterior chamber tap for cell identification and histopathology
d. CT scan of the head and orbits

Discussion

The pseudohypopyon in the figure is composed of retinoblastoma cells. The lack of view of the posterior pole is a contraindication to an anterior chamber tap without further investigations such as CT scan or ocular ultrasound to rule out the presence of a posterior-pole tumor. Surgical entry into an eye harboring a retinoblastoma can result in systemic spread of cancer and subsequent death. This child is slightly older than might be expected for a unilateral retinoblastoma; 90% present by age 3 years. There are cases of unilateral retinoblastoma, however, that initially present in late childhood. Retinoblastoma can present as a uveitis-like condition and even as a fulminant orbital cellulitis. A workup for juvenile rheumatoid arthritis and sarcoidosis is reasonable in the presence of childhood uveitis, but this particular child has a pseudohypopyon of large, white tumor cells that are atypical of bilateral granulomatous uveitis. Leukemia can also present as a hypopyon and must be included in the differential diagnosis for this patient. However, in this case, a CT scan of the child's orbits demonstrated a large calcified intraocular mass consistent with retinoblastoma.[41]

Preferred Response

c. an anterior chamber tap for cell identification and histopathology

A 6-week-old infant presents to the ophthalmologist with a history of a bluish mass in the medial canthal area that has been present since birth (see the figure). A pediatric otorhinolaryngologist evaluated the patient and noted a mass lesion in the nose.

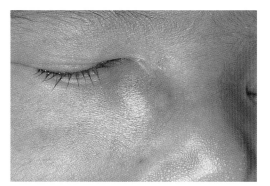

Blue-colored medial canthal mass secondary to amniotocele.

Which of the following is the *most* likely diagnosis?

a. nasal encephalocele
b. amniotocele
c. metastatic neuroblastoma
d. dermoid

Discussion

The location and appearance of this bluish mass in the area of the lacrimal sac is classic for an amniotocele. This condition represents a congenital proximal and distal obstruction of the lacrimal system that can become infected and abscessed, leading to systemic sepsis. An amniotocele can appear as a mass in the nose and can lead to respiratory symptoms. Nasal encephaloceles are rare but should be included in the differential diagnosis. However, the lacrimal sac location is quite distinctive for amniotocele. The location and appearance also make dermoid or neuroblastoma very unlikely; clinical examination should help distinguish these entities. Gentle massage of an amniotocele may express material from the nasolacrimal duct and decompress it. In some cases, a CT scan or MRI may be indicated. Although some cases have resolved with only massage, the presence of an amniotocele is usually an indication for nasolacrimal duct probing.[42]

Preferred Response

b. amniotocele

A 6-week-old infant was discharged from the hospital at 3 days of age with essentially the same appearance as shown in the figure. No further evaluation or treatment was recommended.

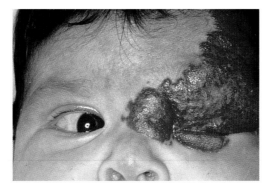

Periorbital infantile capillary hemangioma.

The *most* serious consequence of further lack of intervention in this child would be

a. metastatic disease and death
b. dense and irreversible amblyopia OS
c. permanent levator damage in the left upper eyelid
d. glaucoma OS

Discussion

The figure shows an infantile capillary hemangioma that is causing complete obscuration of the visual axis of the left eye. The lesion is benign. The distribution of the lesion approximates that of a port-wine stain, which could be associated with Sturge-Weber syndrome (encephalotrigeminal angiomatosis) and glaucoma. The appearance, however, is most consistent with an infantile capillary hemangioma. If left untreated, a capillary hemangioma will almost always regress over several years. In this case, however, the lesion obscures the visual axis and is likely to result in dense and irreversible amblyopia if not treated within the first few months of life. Systemic or intralesional corticosteroids have proven effective in "shrinking" capillary hemangiomas in these situations, although there are potentially serious side effects from this form of therapy. Systemic or intralesional corticosteroids in combination with occlusion therapy of the right eye would be the most reasonable treatment for this patient.[43]

Preferred Response

b. dense and irreversible amblyopia OS

References

1. Lambert SR, Taylor D, Kriss A, et al: Ocular manifestations of the congenital varicella syndrome. *Arch Ophthalmol* 1989;107:52–56.
2. Hermansen MC, Hasan S: Abolition of feeding intolerance following ophthalmologic examination of neonates. *J Pediatr Ophthalmol Strab* 1985;22:256–257.
3. Kushner BJ: Congenital nasolacrimal system obstruction. *Arch Ophthalmol* 1982;100: 597–600.
4. Katowitz JA, Welsh MG: Timing of initial probing and irrigation in congenital nasolacrimal duct obstruction. *Ophthalmology* 1987;94:698–705.
5. Nelson LB, Wagner RS, Simon JW, et al: Congenital esotropia. *Surv Ophthalmol* 1987;31:363–383.
6. Kivlin JD, Fineman RM, Crandall AS, et al: Peters' anomaly as a consequence of genetic and nongenetic syndromes. *Arch Ophthalmol* 1986;104:61–64.
7. Traboulsi EI, Maumenee IH: Peters' anomaly and associated congenital malformations. *Arch Ophthalmol* 1992;110:1739–1742.
8. Nelson LB, Spaeth GL, Nowinski TS, et al: Aniridia: a review. *Surv Ophthalmol* 1984;28:621–642.
9. Burke JP, Scott WE, Kutschke PJ: Anterior transposition of the inferior oblique muscle for dissociated vertical deviation. *Ophthalmology* 1993;100:245–250.
10. Traboulsi EI, O'Neill JF: The spectrum in the morphology of the so-called morning glory disc anomaly. *J Pediatr Ophthalmol Strab* 1988;25:93–98.
11. Eustis HS, Sanders MR, Zimmerman T: Morning glory syndrome in children: association with endocrine and central nervous system anomalies. *Arch Ophthalmol* 1994;112:204–207.
12. Margo CE, Hamed LM: Neuroretinitis. *Ophthalmol Clin North Am* 1993;6:273–280.
13. Margileth AM, Hayden GF: Cat scratch disease: from feline affection to human infection. *N Engl J Med* 1993;329:53–54.
14. Lambert SR, Taylor D, Kriss A: The infant with nystagmus, normal appearing fundi, but an abnormal ERG. *Surv Ophthalmol* 1989;34:173–186.
15. Brodsky MC, Glasier CM: Optic nerve hypoplasia: clinical significance of associated central nervous system abnormalities on magnetic resonance imaging. *Arch Ophthalmol* 1993;111:66–74.
16. Zubcov AA, Stark N, Weber A, et al: Improvement of visual acuity after surgery for nystagmus. *Ophthalmology* 1993;100:1488–1497.
17. Merriam WW, Ellis FD, Helveston EM: Congenital blepharoptosis, anisometropia, and amblyopia. *Am J Ophthalmol* 1980;89:401–407.
18. McCulloch DL, Wright KW: Unilateral congenital ptosis: compensatory head posturing and amblyopia. *Ophthal Plast Reconstr Surg* 1993;9:196–200.
19. Karr B, Taylor D: Fundus hemorrhages in infancy. *Surv Ophthalmol* 1992;37:1–17.
20. Cheng KP, Hiles DA, Biglan AW, et al: Management of posterior lenticonus. *J Pediatr Ophthalmol Strab* 1991;28:143–149.
21. Kanski JJ: Uveitis in juvenile chronic arthritis. *Clin Exp Rheumatol* 1990;8:499–503.
22. Malagon C, Van Kerckhove C, Giannini EH, et al: The iridocyclitis of early onset pauciarticular juvenile rheumatoid arthritis: outcome in immunogenetically characterized patients. *J Rheumatol* 1992;19:160–163.
23. Foster CS, Barrett F: Cataract development and cataract surgery in patients with juvenile rheumatoid arthritis-associated iridocyclitis. *Ophthalmology* 1993;100: 809–817.
24. Wolf MD, Lichter PR, Ragsdale CG: Prognostic factors in the uveitis of juvenile rheumatoid arthritis. *Ophthalmology* 1987;94:1242–1248.
25. Mader TH, Wergeland FL Jr, Chismire KJ, et al: Enlarged pupillary membranes. *J Pediatr Ophthalmol Strab* 1988;25:73–74.

26. Miller SD, Judisch GF: Persistent pupillary membrane: successful medical management. *Arch Ophthalmol* 1979;97:1911–1913.

27. Del Monte MA: Diagnosis and management of congenital and developmental cataracts. *Ophthalmol Clin North Am* 1990;3:205–219.

28. Parks MM, Johnson DA, Reed GW: Long-term visual results and complications in children with aphakia: a function of cataract type. *Ophthalmology* 1993;100:826–841.

29. *Amblyopia*. Preferred Practice Pattern. San Francisco: American Academy of Ophthalmology; 1992.

30. Bradford GM, Kutschke PJ, Scott WE: Results of amblyopia therapy in eyes with unilateral structural abnormalities. *Ophthalmology* 1992;99:1616–1621.

31. Lambert SR, Hoyt CS, Jan JE, et al: Visual recovery from hypoxic cortical blindness during childhood: computed tomographic and magnetic resonance imaging predictors. *Arch Ophthalmol* 1987;105:1371–1377.

32. Granet DB, Hertele RW, Quinn GE, et al: The visual-evoked response in infants with central visual impairment. *Am J Ophthalmol* 1993;116:437–443.

33. Morris RJ, Scott WE, Keech RV: Superior oblique tuck surgery in the management of superior oblique palsies. *J Pediatr Ophthalmol Strab* 1992;29:337–346.

34. Imes RK, Hoyt WF: Childhood chiasmal gliomas: update on the fate of patients in the 1969 San Francisco Study. *Br J Ophthalmol* 1986;70:179–182.

35. Lewis RA, Riccardi VM: Von Recklinghausen neurofibromatosis: incidence of iris hamartomata. *Ophthalmology* 1981;88:348–354.

36. Kodsi SR, Younge BR: Acquired oculomotor, trochlear, and abducens cranial nerve palsies in pediatric patients. *Am J Ophthalmol* 1992;114:568–574.

37. Dunn JP, Jabs DA, Wingard J, et al: Bone marrow transplantation and cataract development. *Arch Ophthalmol* 1993;111:1367–1373.

38. Scott WE, Drummond GT, Keech RV: Vertical offsets of horizontal recti muscles in the management of A and V pattern strabismus. *Aust NZ J Ophthalmol* 1989;17:281–288.

39. Rumsey JM: The biology of developmental dyslexia. *JAMA* 1992;268:912–915.

40. Singer HS, Walkup JT: Tourette syndrome and other tic disorders: diagnosis, pathophysiology, and treatment. *Medicine* 1991;70:15–32.

41. Murphree L, Munier FL: Retinoblastoma. In: Ryan SJ, ed-in-chief: *Retina, Basic Science and Inherited Retinal Disease and Tumors*. 2nd ed. St Louis: CV Mosby Co; 1994:1:571–626.

42. Weinstein GS, Biglan AW, Patterson JH: Congenital lacrimal sac mucoceles. *Am J Ophthalmol* 1982;94:106–110.

43. Haik BG, Karcioglu ZA, Gordon RA, et al: Capillary hemangioma (infantile periocular hemangioma). *Surv Ophthalmol* 1994;38:399–426.

Additional Resources From the AAO

Academy Statements

BB and Pellet Guns Are a Major Cause of Devastating Ocular Injuries in Children. Public Health Note. 1992.

Infant and Children's Vision Screening. Policy Statement. 1991.

Learning Disabilities, Dyslexia, and Vision. Policy Statement. 1992.

Basic and Clinical Science Course

Pediatric Ophthalmology and Strabismus. Section 6. Updated annually.

Focal Points

Archer SM: *Esotropia*. Vol XII, Module 12. 1994. (Item No. 029012)

Borchert MS: *Nystagmus in Childhood*. Vol IX, Module 8. 1991. (Item No. 029009)

Dinning WJ: *Uveitis and Juvenile Chronic Arthritis (Juvenile Rheumatoid Arthritis).* Vol VIII, Module 5. 1990. (Out of print)

Helveston EM: *Management of Dyslexia and Related Learning Disabilities.* Vol III, Module 1. 1985. (Out of print)

Hiatt RL: *Diagnostic and Therapeutic Applications of Prisms.* Vol IV, Module 5. 1986. (Out of print)

Hoyt CS: *Management of Congenital Cataracts.* Vol I, Module 6. 1983. (Item No. 029001)

Lambert SR, Boothe RG: *Amblyopia: Basic and Clinical Science Perspectives.* Vol XII, Module 8. 1994. (Item No. 029012)

Palmer EA: *Current Management of Retinopathy of Prematurity.* Vol XI, Module 3. 1993. (Item No. 029011)

Scott AB: *Botulinum Toxin Treatment of Strabismus.* Vol VII, Module 12. 1989. (Item No. 029007)

Scott WE, Arthur BW: *Current Approaches to Superior Oblique Muscle Surgery.* Vol VI, Module 3. 1988. (Item No. 029006)

Stefanyszyn MA: *Orbital Tumors in Children.* Vol VIII, Module 9. 1990. (Out of print)

Stevens JCL: *Retinoblastoma.* Vol VIII, Module 1. 1990. (Out of print)

Wright KW: *Current Approaches to Inferior Oblique Muscle Surgery.* Vol IV, Module 6. 1986. (Item No. 029004)

Monograph   Fishman GA, Sokol S: *Electrophysiologic Testing in Disorders of the Retina, Optic Nerve, and Visual Pathway.* Ophthalmology Monograph 2. 1990. (Item No. 0210020)

Preferred Practice Patterns   *Amblyopia.* 1992. (Item No. 110014)

Comprehensive Pediatric Eye Evaluation. 1992. (Item No. 110016)

Esotropia. 1992. (Item No. 110015)

Publication   Edelman PM, ed: *Orthoptics: A Syllabus of Ocular Motility.* 2nd ed. 1992. (Item No. 0230108)

Slide-Script   Day SH: *Understanding and Preventing Amblyopia.* Eye Care Skills for the Primary Care Physician Series. 1987. (Item No. 0240277)

Videotapes   Palmer EA: *Clinical Management of Retinopathy of Prematurity.* Clinical Short Subjects Series. 1988. (Item No. 0251063)

Price RL, Beauchamp GR: *Strabismus Surgery: Oblique Procedures.* Clinical Skills Series. 1989. (Item No. 0250743)

Price RL, Beauchamp GR: *Strabismus Surgery: Rectus Recession and Resection.* Clinical Skills Series. 1989. (Item No. 0250753)

Smelser G, Ozanics V: *Embryology of the Eye.* Classic Series. 1977. (Item No. 0250233)

Wilson EM Jr: *Ocular Motility Evaluation of Strabismus and Myasthenia Gravis.* Clinical Skills Series. 1993. (Item No. 0250943)

RETINA AND VITREOUS

R1

A healthy 28-year-old man presents with a 1-week history of pain, redness, and floaters in his left eye. Examination reveals visual acuity of 20/20 OD and 20/25 OS. The right eye is normal on examination. Significant findings on examination of the left eye are mild ciliary injection, fine keratic precipitates, mild anterior chamber cell, clear lens, and moderate anterior vitreous cell. The posterior pole appears normal except for a slightly hazy view secondary to vitreous debris. The lesion shown in the figure is present in the peripheral retina.

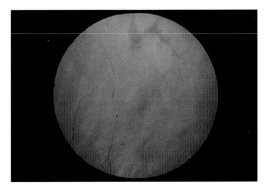

Peripheral retinal necrosis with associated retinal hemorrhage.

Given the patient's clinical presentation, what is the *most* likely diagnosis?

a. toxoplasmosis
b. cytomegalovirus retinitis
c. acute retinal necrosis syndrome
d. peripheral uveitis

Discussion

While toxoplasmosis, cytomegalovirus (CMV) retinitis, and peripheral uveitis all can produce anterior chamber reaction and vitritis, these conditions rarely cause a red, painful eye. CMV retinitis may produce areas of retinal necrosis similar to that seen in this patient but is rare in a nonimmunosuppressed patient. Acute retinal necrosis (ARN) syndrome has been reported in a wide age range of patients, but it is more common in patients in their twenties. ARN syndrome typically is manifested by pain, redness, floaters, mild or no decrease in visual acuity, mild anterior chamber reaction, obliterative retinal and choroidal vasculitis, peripheral retinal necrosis, and vitritis. ARN syndrome occurs bilaterally in one-third of patients, but the second eye typically may not become involved for weeks to months.[1] Visual loss in ARN syndrome is most often either from optic neuritis, which may occur early in the disease, or from retinal detachment and proliferative vitreoretinopathy, which is a frequent late complication. Diagnosis of ARN syndrome is made based on the clinical appearance and retinal examination. There are no noninvasive laboratory studies to diagnose ARN syndrome. Serologic titers for toxoplasmosis or cytomegalovirus, if positive, do not indicate that these entities are the cause of the retinal findings. Treatment for ARN syndrome should be instituted if clinical suspicion is high. If the disease is unresponsive to therapy, retinal biopsy submitted for light and electron microscopy and/or ELISA analysis may be necessary to obtain a diagnosis.

Preferred Response   c. acute retinal necrosis syndrome

Following completion of the diagnostic workup, the *most* appropriate initial treatment for the patient in Question R1 is

a. intravenous acyclovir for a minimum of 5 to 10 days, followed by oral acyclovir
b. intravenous ganciclovir induction for 2 weeks, followed by daily maintenance ganciclovir
c. oral prednisone 60 mg to 80 mg per day
d. laser demarcation of peripheral retinal lesions

Discussion   Herpes viruses, particularly herpes simplex and varicella zoster, have been implicated in the pathogenesis of ARN syndrome.[1] Consequently, the antiviral agent acyclovir has been used in its treatment. Acyclovir has been shown to hasten the regression of retinal lesions and to reduce the likelihood of involvement of the fellow eye, but not to prevent the development of retinal detachment and other complications.[2] Although it has activity against both herpes simplex and varicella zoster, ganciclovir is not recommended for treatment of ARN syndrome because of its greater potential systemic complications, such as neutropenia, and the need for intravenous administration. Systemic prednisone may be beneficial for treatment of the associated ocular inflammation and vitritis, but it has no beneficial effect on the retinal lesions. Prophylactic laser demarcation of the areas of peripheral retinal necrosis may help prevent extensive retinal detachment but does not stop the progression of retinitis. Systemic prednisone or laser demarcation should be administered only with concurrent antiviral therapy.

Preferred Response   a. intravenous acyclovir for a minimum of 5 to 10 days, followed by oral acyclovir

On routine ophthalmoscopic examination, a healthy 45-year-old woman is noted to have the retinal lesion depicted in the figure.

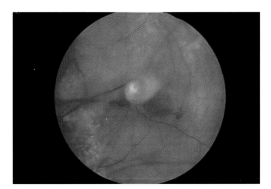

Retinal capillary hemangioma, partially fibrosed. Note large feeder vessels and adjacent hemorrhage and intraretinal exudate.

Which of the following courses of management is *most* appropriate?

a. Observe the lesion for change; no additional evaluation is necessary.
b. Ablate the lesion by laser photocoagulation or cryotherapy. If a detailed family history is negative, no additional evaluation is necessary.
c. Observe the lesion. Order a CT scan or MRI of the head, abdomen, and upper cervical spinal cord and obtain a detailed family history.
d. Ablate the lesion by laser photocoagulation or cryotherapy. Regardless of the findings of a detailed family history, order a CT scan or MRI of the head, abdomen, and upper cervical spinal cord.

Discussion

The lesion in the figure is a retinal capillary hemangioma, which is characteristic of von Hippel-Lindau (VHL) disease. VHL disease has an autosomal dominant inheritance pattern with variable expression. It is one of the phakomatoses and is characterized by capillary hemangiomas of the retina, cerebellum, spinal cord, and viscera as well as by visceral cysts and tumors, which are often silent initially but may prove lethal. Retinal capillary hemangiomas often are the first manifestation of VHL disease to be diagnosed and frequently are asymptomatic. A characteristic feature of retinal capillary hemangiomas is the prominent feeding and draining vessels. Given the potential lethality of VHL disease and the frequently asymptomatic lesions, a careful family history and radiologic imaging of the head, abdomen, and spinal cord should be performed on all patients without an obvious ophthalmologic reason for retinal capillary hemangioma. The retinal capillary hemangiomas associated with VHL disease progress variably but may lead to significant visual loss; therefore, treatment with either laser photocoagulation or cryotherapy should be performed, preferably when the tumor is small.

Preferred Response

d. Ablate the lesion by laser photocoagulation or cryotherapy. Regardless of the findings of a detailed family history, order a CT scan or MRI of the head, abdomen, and upper cervical spinal cord.

R4

All of the following are risk factors for the development of neovascular age-related macular degeneration *except*

a. increased serum cholesterol level
b. cigarette smoking
c. exogenous estrogen use in postmenopausal women
d. soft drusen

Discussion

The Eye Disease Case-Control Study Group studied patients with neovascular age-related macular degeneration and control patients without macular degeneration. Cigarette smoking and elevated serum cholesterol levels were characteristics found significantly more often in patients with neovascular age-related macular degeneration than in control patients.[3] Cigarette smoking had been linked previously by the Macular Photocoagulation Study Group as a risk factor for recurrent choroidal neovascularization. Clinical characteristics such as large, bilateral, soft drusen and pigment irregularities in the macula have also been linked to an increased risk of choroidal neovascularization. Exogenous estrogen use in postmenopausal women and increased serum carotenoid levels were factors found to be associated with a decreased risk of neovascular age-related macular degeneration.[3]

Preferred Response   c. exogenous estrogen use in postmenopausal women

R5

A 72-year-old woman presents with metamorphopsia and blurred vision OD of 1 month's duration. On examination, her visual acuity is 20/30 OD and 20/20 OS. Mild cataract is present symmetrically in both eyes. In the posterior pole OD, a large, smooth, dome-shaped elevation is noted without associated hemorrhage, lipid, or serous retinal detachment. Soft drusen are scattered in the posterior pole of both eyes. The early view (see the figure, part A) and late view (see the figure, part B) of the fluorescein angiogram are shown.

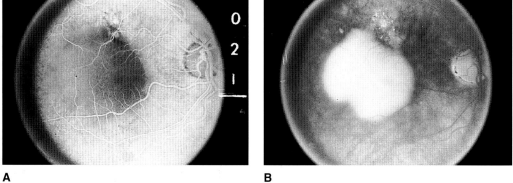

A   **B**

Early venous-phase fluorescein angiogram **(A)** demonstrating early filling of large central retinal pigment epithelial (RPE) detachment, which fills completely and uniformly in later phases **(B).** A small hyperfluorescent area superior to the RPE detachment could represent an area of poorly defined choroidal neovascularization, but there is no angiographic confirmation of this extending beneath the fovea.

All of the following statements regarding the patient's condition are correct *except*

a. Indocyanine green angiography may be helpful in further assessing this patient.
b. This patient's risk of developing exudative age-related macular degeneration in her fellow eye is between 4% and 12% annually.
c. A retinal pigment epithelial tear may complicate treatment of this lesion.
d. There is angiographic evidence of choroidal neovascularization beneath the fovea.

Discussion

This patient has exudative age-related macular degeneration (ARMD) and presents with a serous retinal pigment epithelial (RPE) detachment OD. It has been estimated that patients with exudative ARMD in one eye have a 4% to 12% annual risk of developing exudative ARMD in the fellow eye. RPE detachments may have associated choroidal neovascular membranes, the presence of which may be suggested by an overlying serous retinal detachment, subretinal lipid, subretinal or sub-RPE hemorrhage, choroidal folds, or irregularity or notching of the RPE detachment on fluorescein angiography. The fluorescein angiogram in this patient shows no angiographic signs that definitively indicate choroidal neovascularization. Indocyanine green (ICG) angiography is an imaging technique that uses indocyanine green dye, the absorption and emission of which are in the near-infrared range, allowing visualization through overlying hemorrhage, melanin, lipid, and xanthophyll. Because of these properties, ICG angiography may be particularly useful in identifying occult or poorly defined choroidal neovascular membranes. Laser photocoagulation may be attempted if choroidal neovascularization can be identified within an RPE detachment; however, RPE tears may either develop spontaneously or complicate laser photocoagulation.

Preferred Response

d. There is angiographic evidence of choroidal neovascularization beneath the fovea.

R6

A 78-year-old man presents with the fundus and angiographic findings shown in the figures.

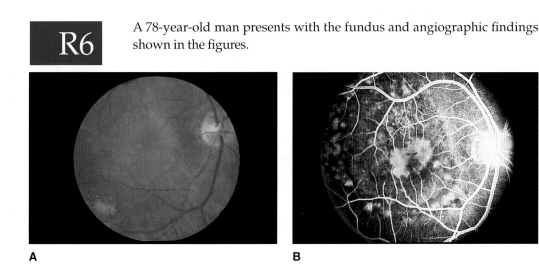

A   **B**

Subfoveal choroidal neovascular membrane in a clinical photograph (**A**) and a fluorescein angiogram (**B**) in a patient with age-related macular degeneration.

Which of the following is *most* important in determining if treatment with laser photocoagulation should be recommended?

a. lesion size and initial visual acuity
b. a lesion with well-defined borders
c. a lesion with features of classic choroidal neovascularization
d. a disciform scar in the fellow eye

Discussion

The Macular Photocoagulation Study Group originally reported beneficial effects of laser photocoagulation on visual acuity in eyes with subfoveal choroidal neovascular membranes (CNVM) when well-demarcated lesions beneath the foveal center with features of classic choroidal neovascularization were present. All eyes, whether treated or untreated, experienced a decrease in visual acuity over time. Those eyes that received laser photocoagulation to ablate the entire CNVM had less of a decline in visual acuity at 12 to 42 months' followup compared to untreated eyes. However, eyes that received treatment experienced a greater initial decline in visual acuity compared to untreated eyes. A subsequent investigation (New Choroidal Neovascularization Study) evaluated the outcome of laser photocoagulation vs observation in patients who were categorized by initial visual acuity and size of subfoveal CNVM.[4] This study grouped patients into four groups (A–D). Eyes in group A (a small lesion with moderate or poor initial visual acuity or a medium-sized lesion with poor visual acuity) had the best visual outcome with treatment. Eyes in group D (a large lesion with moderate or good visual acuity) had the worst visual outcome with treatment. Therefore, patients being considered for treatment must be evaluated based on lesion size and initial visual acuity and must be counseled carefully regarding the immediate effects and expectations of laser treatment. The presence or absence of a well-defined or classic CNVM vs either an occult or poorly defined lesion in the affected eye or a disciform scar in the fellow eye was not used to determine which eyes would benefit from treatment in the New Choroidal Neovascularization Study.

Preferred Response   a. lesion size and initial visual acuity

In the emergency room you are asked to examine the fundi of an obtunded 2-year-old girl who has no visible signs of external injury. She has no known prior medical problems. Examination reveals large, dome-shaped hemorrhages beneath the internal limiting membrane (ILM) in the posterior pole in both eyes (left eye shown in the figure). A few scattered retinal hemorrhages are visible in the retinal periphery of both eyes. A small, circumferential retinal fold extends around the margin of the sub-ILM hemorrhage in each eye.

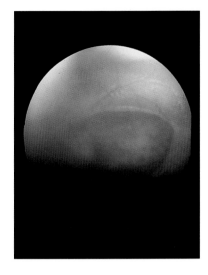

Fundus of left eye shows large, central, sub–internal limiting membrane hemorrhage with the optic disc hazily visible on the left and the superotemporal vascular arcade at the top.

Which of the following is the *most* likely cause of the retinal abnormalities?

a. juvenile retinoschisis
b. acute myelogenous leukemia
c. child abuse
d. retinal macroaneurysm

Discussion

Child abuse must be strongly considered in an obtunded child when the fundus contains a large central hemorrhage beneath the internal limiting membrane. The sub-ILM hemorrhage may be surrounded by a circumferential retinal fold that is usually at or near the posterior vascular arcades.[5,6] With time, the sub-ILM hemorrhage resolves and only schisis of the ILM may remain visible. The retinal folds also resolve over time, with arcuate white lines at the level of the RPE sometimes remaining visible in the area of the previous retinal folds.[5] These fundus findings may be present in the absence of other external findings of injury in cases of child abuse, particularly in the shaken baby syndrome. Other conditions that may lead to retinal or vitreous hemorrhages include juvenile retinoschisis, blood dyscrasias, or retinal macroaneurysms. Retinal macroaneurysms are unusual in children; they occur most often in adult patients with hypertension. Vitreous hemorrhage or hemorrhage within a schisis cavity may occur in juvenile retinoschisis, but a single posterior schisis cavity would be unusual. Also, X-linked juvenile retinoschisis is not seen in females. Blood dyscrasias, such as acute myelogenous leukemia, may produce anemia, thrombocytopenia, or hyperviscosity and may lead to retinal hemorrhages or vitreous hemorrhage. However, these conditions are rare and they typically cause blot or nerve-fiber hemorrhages rather than sub-ILM hemorrhages.

Preferred Response   c. child abuse

A 70-year-old woman presents for followup examination 2 months after trabeculectomy in her left eye. She is without complaints; her best-corrected visual acuity is 20/25 OU with $-1.00 + 0.50 \times 120$ OD and $-0.50 + 0.25 \times 30$ OS; IOP is 19 mm Hg OD and 13 mm Hg OS. External and ocular motility examinations are normal. A good filtering bleb is visible superonasally OS; the conjunctiva is white OU; the anterior chamber is quiet and deep OU; and mild nuclear sclerosis and cortical lens opacities are present OU. Fundus examination in the right eye is normal. The left fundus and corresponding fluorescein angiogram are shown in the figures.

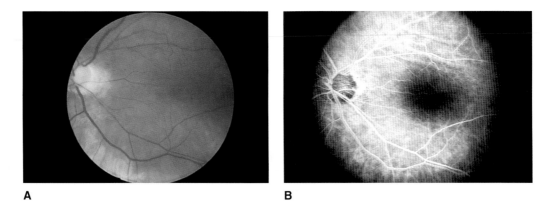

A   **B**

Choroidal folds are not well visualized in the clinical photograph **(A)** but are seen in the fluorescein angiogram **(B)** as alternating hypofluorescent and hyperfluorescent lines.

The choroidal abnormality is *most* likely the result of

a. choroidal neovascularization
b. retrobulbar tumor
c. previous hypotony
d. epiretinal membrane

Discussion   The fundus photograph of the left eye shows subtle, parallel, hypopigmented lines in the choroid superior to the macula. These lines are better distinguished in the fluorescein angiogram as alternating hypofluorescent and hyperfluorescent lines, which are characteristic of choroidal folds. Choroidal folds typically occur in the posterior pole and may be bilateral or unilateral. There is no age or sex predilection. Frequently they produce no symptoms, blurred vision, or metamorphopsia. The differential diagnosis of choroidal folds is extensive and includes idiopathic origin as well as orbital tumors, hyperopia, scleritis, hypotony, thyroid ophthalmopathy, choroidal neovascularization, intraocular neoplasm, optic nerve abnormalities, and previous scleral surgery.[7] Choroidal folds may be parallel, concentric, radiating, or in an irregular pattern depending on the cause. They are best visualized by fluorescein angiography as alternating hyperfluorescent and hypofluorescent lines in the choroid that are visible in the earliest phases of the angiogram and slowly fade. Retinal folds caused by epiretinal membranes do not produce such angiographic findings; therefore, the fluorescein angiogram may be useful in distinguishing between choroidal and retinal folds as well as in ruling out choroidal neovascularization, as in this case. Ultrasonography and computerized tomography may be used to rule out a retrobulbar tumor. Treatment of the underlying condition that produces choroidal folds usually results in resolution, although this change may occur gradually. Therefore, choroidal folds that occur with hypotony following glaucoma filtering surgery may still be visible for some time following normalization of the intraocular pressure.

Preferred Response   c. previous hypotony

A 28-year-old man with acquired immunodeficiency syndrome (AIDS) presents with the right fundus shown in the figure.

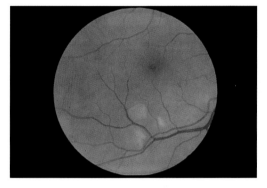

White intraretinal lesions above the inferotemporal arcade consistent with cotton-wool spots or early CMV retinitis.

Which of the following statements regarding the patient's condition is *most* accurate?

a. The lesions most likely represent early CMV retinitis, if the patient's CD4 lymphocyte count is less than 50 cells/mm^3.
b. The lesions most likely are cotton-wool spots, which are a manifestation of human immunodeficiency virus (HIV)-related noninfectious retinal vasculopathy and do not require close followup.
c. The lesions may represent either cotton-wool spots or early CMV retinitis. Close observation of the patient for change in these lesions, with documentation of the fundus by photographs, is indicated.
d. If the patient is without symptoms and no retinal hemorrhage is associated with these lesions, they do not represent CMV retinitis.

Discussion   These white retinal lesions may represent either cotton-wool spots, a manifestation of HIV-related noninfectious retinal vasculopathy, or the earliest manifestation of CMV retinitis. Both the retinal vasculopathy associated with HIV infections and CMV retinitis are typically late manifestations of AIDS. CMV retinitis, in particular, is more common when CD4 lymphocyte counts are reduced to 50 cells/mm^3 or less.[8] CMV retinitis often may present without symptoms, and although the retinal lesions are characteristically areas of hemorrhagic retinal necrosis, atypical presentations of CMV retinitis may occur. Therefore, the safest course in this case is to document the fundus appearance with photographs and observe closely for any enlargement or change in these lesions, which would indicate CMV retinitis.

Preferred Response

c. The lesions may represent either cotton-wool spots or early CMV retinitis. Close observation of the patient for change in these lesions, with documentation of the fundus by photographs, is indicated.

R10

A 32-year-old man with a history of AIDS and CMV retinitis OU initially received ganciclovir but was switched to foscarnet 6 months later when recurrence of the CMV retinitis indicated resistance to ganciclovir. Following foscarnet therapy, all CMV activity in the retina resolved. The patient now presents with the fundus appearance shown in the figure. His creatinine clearance is currently reduced and his white blood cell count is critically low.

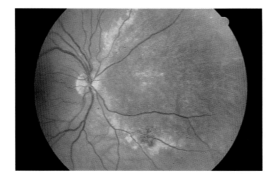

Recurrent CMV retinitis in the nasal retina of the right eye.

Which treatment plan would be the *most* desirable in this patient?

a. Stop intravenous foscarnet and either give intravitreal ganciclovir or foscarnet by injection, or use a sustained-release ganciclovir device intravitreally.
b. Repeat induction doses of foscarnet intravenously.
c. Continue foscarnet and start induction doses of ganciclovir intravenously.
d. Add zidovudine (AZT) to the current foscarnet therapy.

Discussion

The patient's fundus examination indicates another recurrence of CMV retinitis, which requires additional anti-CMV therapy. The reduced creatinine clearance indicates nephrotoxicity from foscarnet, and further systemic treatment with foscarnet, particularly high induction doses, must be avoided to prevent further renal impairment. Frequently, early renal impairment may reverse if the foscarnet is stopped. In this patient, foscarnet must be discontinued to prevent further nephrotoxicity. Systemic ganciclovir can worsen the neutropenia and therefore should be avoided in this patient. Intravitreal therapy with ganciclovir or foscarnet may be used when systemic complications prevent systemic administration of effective doses of these drugs. Viral resistance to both ganciclovir and foscarnet has been noted.[9] Although this patient previously developed resistance to ganciclovir, the drug once withdrawn may again be effective when reinstituted. Therefore, either intravitreal ganciclovir by injection or sustained-release device or intravitreal foscarnet would be the therapy of choice.[10,11] AZT has anti-HIV activity, which may improve the patient's immune status, but it has no specific activity against CMV.

Preferred Response

a. Stop intravenous foscarnet and either give intravitreal ganciclovir or foscarnet by injection, or use a sustained-release ganciclovir device intravitreally.

R11

All of the following statements about central retinal artery occlusion are true *except*

a. Electroretinography shows a diminished A-wave.
b. Long-term survival is decreased in patients who have had retinal artery occlusions.
c. Iris neovascularization may occur in 5% of patients.
d. Emboli more commonly cause retinal arterial occlusions than thrombosis or vascular narrowing from atherosclerosis.

Discussion

Retinal arterial occlusions may occur from many causes, including embolism, thrombosis, or narrowing from atherosclerosis; vasculitis; arterial spasm as in migraine; and extravascular compression. Of the many potential causes, emboli originating from the carotid arteries are the most common cause of retinal artery occlusion. Multiple reports have noted decreased life expectancy for patients with retinal artery obstructions. Since the central retinal artery supplies the inner retina, the B-wave is diminished on the electroretinogram. Iris neovascularization and neovascular glaucoma occur infrequently (approximately 5%) following central retinal artery occlusion. The development of iris neovascularization may not always be the direct result of the retinal artery occlusion, since significant carotid artery narrowing has frequently been noted on the ipsilateral side.[12]

Preferred Response

a. Electroretinography shows a diminished A-wave.

An 84-year-old woman with a history of bilateral pseudophakia presents with a 7-day history of sudden, decreased vision in her right eye without associated pain, redness, or photophobia. Examination reveals best-corrected visual acuity of counting fingers at 2 feet OD and 20/25 OS. Examination of the right eye shows an afferent pupillary defect, inferior keratic precipitates, and mild flare and cell. The vitreous in the right eye contains clumps of white, cellular debris. The right fundus is shown in the figure (see page 250). Posterior chamber IOLs are in position with central posterior capsular openings OU. The left eye is normal. The patient was diagnosed 4 years ago with tuberculosis and was treated medically for it for 1 year.

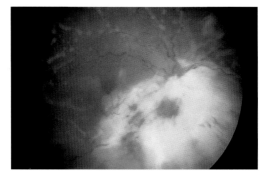

Cryptococcal chorioretinitis/ endophthalmitis with vitreous, retinal, and perivascular inflammatory infiltrates.

Which of the following is *least* likely to be helpful in establishing a diagnosis in this patient?

a. fluorescein angiography
b. vitreous biopsy for cytology and microbiology
c. magnetic resonance imaging (MRI) of the head and orbits
d. referral to an internist for evaluation of possible systemic malignancy, immunosuppression, or reactivation of tuberculosis

Discussion

This patient presents with panuveitis, including vitritis, retinal vasculitis, and retinitis, with involvement of the optic nerve head. Given the patient's age, clinical presentation, ocular findings, and previous history of tuberculosis, an infectious or neoplastic cause is most likely. Tuberculosis would be high in the differential diagnosis. Other organisms, particularly fungal, should also be strongly considered. The patient is not known to be immunosuppressed, but a thorough evaluation, including complete blood count with differential and HIV testing, should be performed. Evidence of extraocular malignancy or active tuberculosis should also be evaluated. MRI may provide information about involvement of the optic nerve or central nervous system. Vitrectomy for vitreous biopsy should be performed in this patient and the specimen sent for both microbiologic and cytologic examination. Although there is clinical evidence of retinal vascular inflammation, fluorescein angiography is unlikely to provide any useful information in establishing a diagnosis.

Preferred Response   a. fluorescein angiography

A vitreous biopsy of the patient in Question R12 demonstrates cryptococcal organisms on fungal stain and culture. All of the following statements about endogenous ocular cryptococcal infections are true *except*

a. Cryptococcal meningitis is frequently associated with ocular cryptococcal infections.
b. Cryptococcal infections occur only in immunosuppressed patients.
c. Ocular involvement frequently is the result of direct extension along the optic nerve or by hematogenous spread.
d. Chorioretinitis is the most common intraocular presentation of *Cryptococcus*.

Discussion   Cryptococcal infections are caused by *Cryptococcus neoformans*, a ubiquitous fungus found in bird droppings. Cryptococcal infections are more common in, but not limited to, immunocompromised patients. Chorioretinitis with or without vitritis is the most common intraocular presentation of cryptococcosis; cryptococcal endophthalmitis is rare.[13] Many disorders must be considered in the differential diagnosis of chorioretinal lesions with vitritis, such as those seen in cryptococcosis. Similar lesions may be found in tuberculosis, sarcoidosis, CMV retinitis, candidiasis, and toxoplasmosis. Acute retinal necrosis syndrome also presents with retinal inflammation and vitritis but, given this patient's age, would be unlikely. Large-cell lymphoma should also be considered in the differential diagnosis. Ocular cryptococcal organisms may gain access to the eye by hematogenous spread, by direct inoculation as in trauma, or by direct extension along the optic nerve from the often accompanying cryptococcal meningitis, which is often fatal.

Preferred Response   b. Cryptococcal infections occur only in immunosuppressed patients.

A 24-year-old man with a 10-year history of insulin-dependent diabetes mellitus presents with a visual acuity of 20/25 OD and 20/200 OS. Examination of the macula in the right eye demonstrates hard exudate and retinal thickening to within 500 microns of the foveal center. A small area of flat retinal neovascularization is present in the right eye off the superotemporal arcade. The vitreous in the right eye is clear. Examination of the left eye demonstrates diffuse retinal thickening throughout the macula, scattered hard exudates, and blot hemorrhages. Marked neovascularization of the disc is present in the left eye, as well as nasal retinal neovascularization with mild vitreous hemorrhage.

The *best* sequence of photocoagulation treatment for this patient is

a. initial focal photocoagulation OU, followed by panretinal photocoagulation OU
b. initial panretinal photocoagulation OU, followed by focal photocoagulation OS
c. initial panretinal photocoagulation OS, followed by focal photocoagulation OU
d. initial panretinal and focal photocoagulation OS, followed by focal photocoagulation OD

Discussion   According to the criteria of the Diabetic Retinopathy Study[14] and the Early Treatment Diabetic Retinopathy Study (ETDRS),[15] this patient has both high-risk proliferative diabetic retinopathy (PDR) in the left eye and clinically significant diabetic macular edema in both eyes. Therefore, panretinal photocoagulation in the left eye and focal photocoagulation in both eyes are needed. However, panretinal photocoagulation has been shown to exacerbate coexisting diabetic macular edema.[16] The ETDRS found that to reduce the effects of panretinal photocoagulation on diabetic macular edema, the procedure is best delayed until focal photocoagulation is completed. However, in cases in which high-risk PDR characteristics and diabetic macular edema coexist, the ETDRS does not recommend delaying panretinal photocoagulation in lieu of focal photocoagulation.[16] Therefore, in this patient concurrent focal and panretinal photocoagulation would be the best choice to initiate treatment for the high-risk PDR in the left eye while reducing the effects of panretinal photocoagulation on the diabetic macular edema.

Preferred Response

d. initial panretinal and focal photocoagulation OS, followed by focal photocoagulation OD

The Diabetes Control and Complications Trial was a multicenter, randomized clinical trial in which insulin-dependent diabetic patients with either no retinopathy or mild to moderate nonproliferative retinopathy were treated either with conventional insulin therapy or intensive insulin therapy that consisted of either three or more insulin injections daily or an insulin pump.

All of the following statements about the findings of this trial are true *except*

a. In patients initially without retinopathy, intensive insulin therapy reduced the risk of onset of retinopathy by 76% compared to patients in the conventional therapy group.
b. In patients initially with mild to moderate nonproliferative retinopathy, intensive insulin therapy slowed the progression of retinopathy by 54% compared to patients in the conventional therapy group.
c. In patients with mild to moderate nonproliferative retinopathy, intensive therapy reduced the development of proliferative or severe nonproliferative retinopathy by 47% compared to conventional insulin therapy.
d. No transient early worsening of retinopathy with intensive insulin therapy was noted in patients with mild to moderate retinopathy, as reported in previous trials.

Discussion

The Diabetes Control and Complications Trial demonstrated that intensive insulin therapy that maintained serum glucose at much tighter, lower levels than conventional therapy (1) reduced the risk of development of retinopathy in patients without retinopathy by 76%; (2) reduced the risk of development of proliferative or severe nonproliferative retinopathy in patients with mild to moderate nonproliferative retinopathy by 47%; and (3) slowed the progression of retinopathy by 54% in patients with mild to moderate nonproliferative retinopathy. With intensive therapy, however, patients with mild to moderate retinopathy often experienced a transient worsening of their retinopathy over the first year of treatment. Ultimately, these patients demonstrated a significant reduction in the risk of progression of their retinopathy, the development of proliferative or severe nonproliferative retinopathy, or the need for photocoagulation, as compared to patients treated with conventional therapy.[17]

Preferred Response

d. No transient early worsening of retinopathy with intensive insulin therapy was noted in patients with mild to moderate retinopathy, as reported in previous trials.

A 60-year-old hypertensive woman with insulin-dependent diabetes mellitus of 27 years' duration presents with complaints of gradual decrease in visual acuity in her right eye. On examination, her visual acuity is 20/60 OD and 20/30 OS. Previously, she had laser photocoagulation for clinically significant diabetic macular edema OU. The fundus photograph (see the figure, part A) and fluorescein angiogram (see the figure, part B) for the right eye are shown.

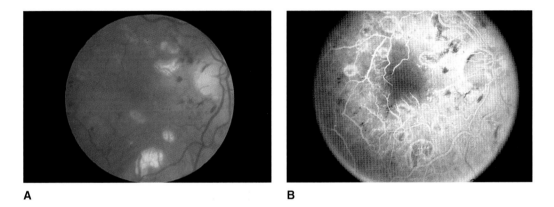

A   **B**

Fundus photograph **(A)** and mid-venous phase fluorescein angiogram **(B)** of right eye demonstrating background diabetic retinopathy with macular ischemia.

Which of the following statements about this patient is *most* accurate?

a. Focal laser photocoagulation OD is the treatment of choice.

b. There is no visible abnormality on either the fundus photograph or fluorescein angiogram OD to explain the patient's decrease in visual acuity. Therefore, optic nerve dysfunction should be considered.

c. Macular ischemia most likely accounts for the patient's decrease in visual acuity in the right eye.

d. Modified grid photocoagulation OD is the treatment of choice.

Discussion

The fluorescein angiogram demonstrates an enlarged foveal avascular zone, previous photocoagulation scars, and a few microaneurysms near the foveal region. Therefore, this patient's decrease in visual acuity is most likely secondary to macular ischemia from closure of perifoveal capillaries. Laser photocoagulation provides no benefit in treating visual loss from macular ischemia. Macular ischemia may coexist with clinically significant macular edema, in which case laser photocoagulation may be used to treat the macular edema component; however, visual improvement is uncertain following laser photocoagulation in such cases.

Preferred Response   c. Macular ischemia most likely accounts for the patient's decrease in visual acuity in the right eye.

All of the following statements about *Propionibacterium acnes* endophthalmitis are correct *except*

a. *Propionibacterium* may cause a recurrent granulomatous iridocyclitis that may not develop until months after cataract surgery.
b. Nd:YAG laser capsulotomy may cause a flare-up of the intraocular inflammation in *Propionibacterium* endophthalmitis.
c. *Propionibacterium acnes* is frequently found in the normal flora of the conjunctiva.
d. Inflammation associated with *Propionibacterium* endophthalmitis typically increases with topical corticosteroid use.

Discussion   *Propionibacterium acnes* is a Gram-positive, anaerobic, pleomorphic bacillus that is commonly present in the normal conjunctival flora. It has been recognized as a cause of chronic, recurrent, often granulomatous inflammation following cataract extraction (see the figure, part A). The inflammation typically associated with *Propionibacterium acnes* may not develop for weeks to months after uncomplicated cataract surgery. The organism may be sequestered in the capsular bag and a characteristic capsular plaque may be visible (see the figure, part B). Flare-up of intraocular inflammation has been reported following Nd:YAG laser capsulotomy, which may expose or release more organisms.[18] Inflammation from *Propionibacterium acnes* typically shows a transient response to corticosteroids, but intraocular administration of antibiotic with or without vitrectomy, capsulectomy, and/or IOL removal or exchange are the preferred treatments for *Propionibacterium acnes* endophthalmitis.

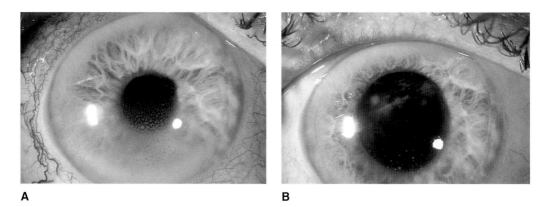

A   **B**

Keratic precipitates **(A)** and capsular plaque **(B)** in *Propionibacterium acnes* endophthalmitis.

Preferred Response   d. Inflammation associated with *Propionibacterium* endophthalmitis typically increases with topical corticosteroid use.

R18

A 74-year-old woman who underwent trabeculectomy in her left eye 2 years ago for primary open-angle glaucoma presents with a 2-day history of decreased vision and redness OS. On examination, her visual acuity is 20/25 OD and 20/200 OS. Intraocular pressure is 15 mm Hg OD and 22 mm Hg OS. The slit-lamp appearance OS is shown in the figure. A 1 mm hypopyon and moderate vitreous cell are also present.

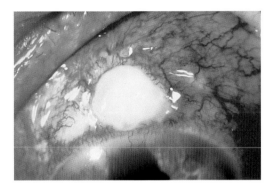

Opacified filtering bleb in a patient with endophthalmitis.

Which of the following statements regarding the patient's condition is *least* correct?

a. It is unusual to see this complication after filtration surgery unless the filtration bleb is Seidel-positive.
b. *Streptococcus* or *Haemophilus* organisms are most commonly associated with this condition.
c. Closed vitrectomy with injection of broad-spectrum intravitreal antibiotics such as an aminoglycoside and vancomycin would be an appropriate course of management in this patient.
d. Filtering procedures using antimetabolites such as 5-fluorouracil have a higher risk of this complication.

Discussion

Late endophthalmitis following filtration surgery has been estimated to occur in up to 3% of patients.[19] The organisms causing late endophthalmitis gain entry to the eye through the filtering bleb, possibly penetrating intact conjunctiva or entering through microscopic breaks. Therefore, patients with bleb-associated infections may often present as Seidel-negative. Studies have shown that the thin-walled blebs associated with the use of antimetabolites such as 5-fluorouracil have a higher incidence of bleb-associated endophthalmitis. *Streptococcus* and *Haemophilus* organisms are most commonly associated with this condition. Given the frequency of more aggressive organisms associated with bleb-related endophthalmitis, an initial treatment involving closed vitrectomy with injection of broad-spectrum intravitreal antibiotics such as an aminoglycoside (amikacin 400 µg in 0.1 cc balanced salt solution [BSS]) and vancomycin (1 mg in 0.1 cc BSS) would be appropriate. Cases of isolated bleb infection without vitreous involvement may be successfully treated with intensive topical antibiotics and intravenous antibiotics alone.[20]

Preferred Response

a. It is unusual to see this complication after filtration surgery unless the filtration bleb is Seidel-positive.

R19

In the evaluation and treatment of diabetic retinopathy, fluorescein angiography is *least* useful

a. to determine areas of capillary closure
b. to determine the presence of clinically significant diabetic macular edema prior to recommending photocoagulation
c. to determine the location of diffuse retinal leakage from incompetent retinal capillaries or intraretinal microvascular abnormalities prior to photocoagulation
d. to determine the location of retinal microaneurysms prior to photocoagulation

Discussion

The Early Treatment Diabetic Retinopathy Study defined clinically significant diabetic macular edema by biomicroscopic examination of the macula and not by fluorescein angiography.[15] Therefore, recommendations for photocoagulation should be based on biomicroscopic determination of: (1) retinal thickening at or within 500 microns of the center of the fovea; (2) hard exudate at or within 500 microns of the center of the fovea if associated with thickening of adjacent retina; or (3) a zone or zones of retinal thickening 1 disc area or larger, any part of which is within 1 disc diameter of the center of the fovea.[21] Fluorescein angiography may be useful in evaluating the presence and location of capillary closure, particularly when there is clinically unexplainable visual loss. Fluorescein angiography is also useful prior to photocoagulation to determine the location of leaking retinal microaneurysms or areas of diffuse retinal leakage that require treatment.

Preferred Response

b. to determine the presence of clinically significant diabetic macular edema prior to recommending photocoagulation

R20

A 26-year-old myopic man presents with a 5-day history of photopsias, small scotomas, and blurred vision in both eyes. He is recovering from a recent flu-like illness. Examination reveals best-corrected visual acuity of 20/50 OD and 20/40 OS. Slit-lamp examination shows mild flare and cell in both anterior chambers and mild vitreous cell in both eyes. The fundus findings are similar in both eyes; the right fundus is shown in the figure.

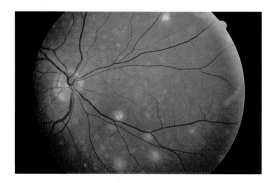

Multifocal choroiditis demonstrating chorioretinal scars in the nasal retina.

Which of the following diagnoses is *most* likely in this patient?

a. presumed ocular histoplasmosis syndrome
b. multifocal choroiditis
c. birdshot retinochoroidopathy
d. acute posterior multifocal placoid pigment epitheliopathy

Discussion

The clinical picture in this patient represents an inflammatory process of the choroid and retina. Inflammatory retinal and choroidal diseases are classified based on ophthalmoscopic findings and clinical course of the disease, with overlap between many of the diagnoses. Of the choices given, multifocal choroiditis best fits the clinical history and appearance in this patient. The patient's young age is consistent with any of the listed diagnoses except birdshot retinochoroidopathy, which is more common in patients between ages 40 and 60. Bilateral ocular involvement is seen in all of the diagnoses. A preceding viral illness is a frequent history given by patients with either multifocal choroiditis or acute posterior multifocal placoid pigment epitheliopathy. Vitritis is a finding in multifocal choroiditis, birdshot retinochoroidopathy, and acute posterior multifocal placoid pigment epitheliopathy. Acute posterior multifocal placoid pigment epitheliopathy causes multiple yellow-white, flat, round or irregular lesions at the level of the pigment epithelium and choroid, typically larger than the lesions present in this patient. Presumed ocular histoplasmosis syndrome commonly produces peripapillary scarring (not present in this patient) in addition to typical punched-out, peripheral chorioretinal scars and lack of vitreous cells.

Preferred Response

b. multifocal choroiditis

A 32-year-old man presents without complaints for routine examination. On indirect ophthalmoscopy, multiple patches of peripheral lattice degeneration containing multiple atrophic retinal holes are noted in the superior retina OD. Lattice degeneration without retinal breaks is noted inferiorly OS. Which of the following statements regarding prophylactic treatment is *most* correct?

a. Only the patient's right eye should be prophylactically treated with laser photocoagulation or cryoretinopexy.
b. Both of the patient's eyes should be prophylactically treated with laser photocoagulation or cryoretinopexy.
c. If there is a prior history of retinal detachment in the left eye, prophylactic laser photocoagulation or cryoretinopexy should be considered in the right eye.
d. The patient's right eye should receive prophylactic treatment with laser photocoagulation or cryoretinopexy prior to cataract surgery.

Discussion

Lattice degeneration occurs in 6% to 8% of the population, with 20% to 30% of patients with lattice degeneration also having coexisting retinal holes. The decision to treat prophylactically is based on the risk of developing a retinal detachment without treatment, how much the treatment will reduce the risk of retinal detachment, and the risks of treatment. The rate of retinal detachment in eyes with lattice degeneration has been estimated to be less than 1%.[22] Retinal breaks following cataract surgery are less likely to be associated with lattice degeneration than with the development of new flap tears. There are no studies documenting the value of prophylactic treatment in eyes with lattice degeneration except in the fellow phakic eyes with lattice degeneration of previous retinal detachment patients. In untreated eyes, a 2.5 times greater risk (1.8% vs 5%) of a new tear or detachment was found than in treated eyes.[23]

Preferred Response

c. If there is a prior history of retinal detachment in the left eye, prophylactic laser photocoagulation or cryoretinopexy should be considered in the right eye.

R22

A 12-year-old boy presents with a nonpenetrating BB gun injury in the right eye. His visual acuity is 20/400 OD and 20/20 OS. Slit-lamp examination reveals a focal conjunctival hemorrhage temporally OD with no evidence of scleral laceration. The anterior segment appears normal except for moderate cell and flare OD. Mild diffuse vitreous hemorrhage is present with dense hemorrhage inferiorly OD. Retinal examination OD reveals an area of hemorrhagic and necrotic retina temporally with accompanying RPE and choroidal disruption and bare sclera visible, as shown in the figure. Commotio retinae surrounds the area of retinal and choroidal loss and extends into the macula. Cystoid edema is present in the macula. No other retinal breaks are visible, although vitreous hemorrhage prevents complete examination of the peripheral retina.

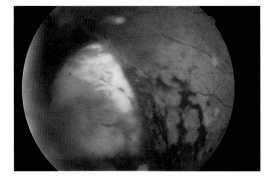

Chorioretinitis sclopetaria in the temporal peripheral retina of the right eye.

Which of the following is *least* likely to result in later decreased visual acuity in this patient?

a. retinal detachment resulting from the necrotic retinal break
b. retinal detachment resulting from a peripheral retinal break, if present
c. granular pigmentation in the macula following resolution of the commotio retinae
d. macular hole

Discussion   This patient presents with chorioretinitis sclopetaria, which is seen frequently in severe blunt injuries such as BB gun injuries. Ragged retinal breaks extending posteriorly are often visible. However, these retinal breaks, although large, rarely result in retinal detachment.[24] Blunt injuries commonly result in retinal dialyses or breaks at the posterior vitreous base. Retinal detachments from such retinal breaks rarely develop acutely following blunt trauma because of the solid vitreous present in the young patients who often sustain these injuries.[24] Frequently, commotio retinae and macular edema may also complicate severe blunt injuries. Commotio retinae may result in a decrease in visual acuity, if the macula is involved. It resolves rapidly, often resulting in a granular pigmentation. Macular holes may also develop following blunt injury, resulting in a decrease in central vision. Patients who sustain severe nonpenetrating blunt ocular injury should undergo a complete ophthalmic examination, including gonioscopy and dilated retinal examination. Initial therapy should include topical corticosteroids and cycloplegics. Follow-up retinal examination is necessary, once vitreous hemorrhage has cleared, to rule out peripheral retinal breaks that can produce late retinal detachments.

Preferred Response   a. retinal detachment resulting from the necrotic retinal break

Indications for immediate or early pars plana vitrectomy in a penetrating injury include all of the following *except*

a. intraocular foreign body
b. early endophthalmitis
c. retinal detachment with vitreous hemorrhage
d. vitreous incarceration in a posterior scleral wound that cannot be closed by an external approach

Discussion   Immediate or early pars plana vitrectomy is indicated when an intraocular foreign body is present to decrease the risk of endophthalmitis or to reduce the inflammatory effects that the intraocular foreign body may have on ocular tissues. Traumatic endophthalmitis, particularly that following an intraocular foreign body, may be associated with aggressive organisms such as *Bacillus cereus*. Although the benefit of pars plana vitrectomy in endophthalmitis is a matter of debate, the procedure is advisable when potentially aggressive organisms are likely to be present. Early (not necessarily immediate) pars plana vitrectomy should be performed to repair retinal detachment when vitreous hemorrhage prevents adequate visualization to allow scleral buckling. Vitreous incarceration in a posterior scleral wound also requires pars plana vitrectomy; however, when an unclosed posterior wound is present, pars plana vitrectomy should be delayed 7 days to allow possible spontaneous closure of the wound prior to proceeding with vitrectomy.

Preferred Response   d. vitreous incarceration in a posterior scleral wound that cannot be closed by an external approach

All of the following statements about peripheral uveitis are true *except*

a. The most common causes of reduction in visual acuity in peripheral uveitis are cystoid macular edema and vitreous debris.
b. Fluorescein angiography may demonstrate staining of peripheral retinal vessels.
c. An indication for initiating treatment for peripheral uveitis is a reduction in visual acuity to less than 20/25.
d. Lyme disease, Fuchs' heterochromic cyclitis, *Toxocara canis*, toxoplasmosis, and retinoblastoma are included in the differential diagnosis of peripheral uveitis.

Discussion

Peripheral uveitis (formerly called pars planitis) is a panuveitis that most commonly occurs bilaterally in patients under age 30. Symptoms most frequently include floaters and painless decrease in vision. Characteristic ocular findings include pars plana–ora serrata exudate (snowbank), vitreous debris, posterior subcapsular cataract, cystoid macular edema, optic disc edema, and retinal vasculitis. Less commonly, retinal neovascularization, peripheral angiomalike lesions, and tractional/rhegmatogenous retinal detachment may develop. Decrease in visual acuity most commonly occurs as the result of either vitreous debris or cystoid macular edema. Fluorescein angiography may demonstrate cystoid macular edema, optic nerve papillitis, and retinal vascular staining. There are no diagnostic tests specific for peripheral uveitis; diagnosis is based on the clinical appearance and the exclusion of other diagnoses. Other ocular inflammatory conditions involving the anterior and posterior segments that present without pain or injection should be considered, including Lyme disease, Fuchs' heterochromic cyclitis, *Toxocara canis*, juvenile rheumatoid arthritis, and toxoplasmosis. In younger children, retinoblastoma must also be considered in the differential diagnosis. Initial therapeutic intervention with corticosteroids is started if visual acuity decreases below 20/40[25] but earlier therapy may be considered in certain clinical situations.

Preferred Response

c. An indication for initiating treatment for peripheral uveitis is a reduction in visual acuity to less than 20/25.

A healthy 22-year-old man presents with a 6-month history of floaters OU and a 1-month history of painless decrease in visual acuity OS. Examination reveals a visual acuity of 20/25 OD and 20/50 OS, no injection, quiet anterior chamber, clear lens, mild to moderate anterior vitreous cell, and a thick white deposit of debris over the inferior ora serrata/pars plana in both eyes. The figures show the patient's fundus appearance (part A) and fluorescein angiogram (part B) of the left eye. Systemic evaluation, including chest x-ray, PPD, FTA-ABS, and titers for *Toxoplasma*, Lyme disease, and *Toxocara canis*, is normal.

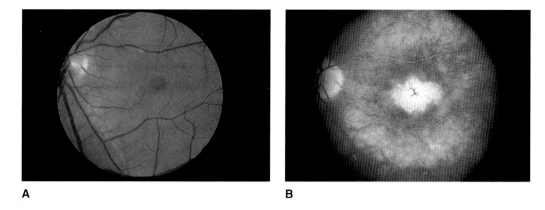

A   **B**

Cystoid macular edema in peripheral uveitis, shown clinically **(A)** and on fluorescein angiography **(B).**

Initial treatment should consist of

a. systemic prednisone beginning at 60 mg po qd for 2 weeks
b. topical prednisolone acetate OS
c. posterior subtenon's or transseptal injection of corticosteroid OS
d. cryotherapy to the area of pars plana debris OS

Discussion   With a negative diagnostic workup, the clinical description is most consistent with a diagnosis of peripheral uveitis. Treatment OS is indicated, since visual acuity is reduced to 20/50 and cystoid macular edema is present. The use of topical corticosteroids is indicated in peripheral uveitis for treatment of anterior chamber inflammation but is not effective in the treatment of posterior segment involvement. Subtenon's or transseptal injection of corticosteroid is an effective initial treatment for cystoid macular edema or vitreous debris from peripheral uveitis and has fewer systemic side effects than systemically administered corticosteroids. Cryotherapy, using a freeze-refreeze technique to the area of pars plana exudate, can also be an effective treatment for peripheral uveitis but its use is limited to patients with neovascularization of the vitreous base, poor response to corticosteroids, or intolerance of corticosteroids.[26]

Preferred Response   c. posterior subtenon's or transseptal injection of corticosteroid OS

All of the following statements about retinal detachment patient selection for pneumatic retinopexy are true *except*

a. Retinal break(s) should be located within the superior two-thirds of the fundus.
b. Retinal break(s) should be located within 1 clock hour of each other.
c. Patients with proliferative vitreoretinopathy (PVR) grade C or higher or severe glaucoma should not be considered candidates for pneumatic retinopexy.
d. Aphakic or pseudophakic patients have the same rate of success with pneumatic retinopexy as phakic patients.

Discussion   Published studies demonstrate that pneumatic retinopexy for retinal detachment may have a degree of success comparable to scleral buckling in selected cases. Most studies limited patient selection to those retinal detachments that had retinal breaks within the superior two-thirds of the fundus and all were located within 1 clock hour of each other. Patients with PVR grade C or higher, in which the retina may be stiff or the retinal breaks may be under traction, are considered poor candidates for pneumatic retinopexy. Patients with a history of severe glaucoma may also be poor candidates because of the significant rise in intraocular pressure that can occur immediately following gas injection. Although failure rates are reportedly higher in pseudophakic or aphakic patients (compared to phakic patients) following either pneumatic retinopexy or scleral buckling,[27] pseudophakia or aphakia is generally not considered an absolute contraindication to pneumatic retinopexy.

Preferred Response   d. Aphakic or pseudophakic patients have the same rate of success with pneumatic retinopexy as phakic patients.

A 60-year-old man presents with a 3-day history of photopsias and new floaters in his left eye. His visual acuity is 20/20 OU. Slit-lamp examination shows mild nuclear sclerosis and clear anterior vitreous bilaterally. On fundus examination, a posterior vitreous detachment (PVD) is seen only in the left eye.

All of the following statements are true *except*

a. If hemorrhage or pigment granules are not present in the vitreous, depressed examination of the peripheral retina is not necessary.

b. Approximately 15% of patients who present with acute, symptomatic PVD will have a retinal tear.

c. In the majority of cases, when the fellow eye develops a PVD it will likely respond in the same way (ie, symptoms, complications) as the first eye did upon developing PVD.

d. Myopia, diabetic retinopathy, vitreous hemorrhage, and surgical aphakia all predispose the patient to vitreous detachment at an earlier age.

Discussion   Symptomatic PVD is characterized by photopsias and/or floaters, symptoms that may also occur with the development of a retinal tear. Since approximately 15% of patients presenting with an acute, symptomatic PVD will have a retinal tear, all such patients should have a dilated examination of the peripheral retina with indirect ophthalmoscopy and scleral depression to look for peripheral retinal breaks.[22] The presence of hemorrhage or pigment (Shafer's sign) in the vitreous correlates highly with the presence of a retinal break.[28] However, absence of Shafer's sign does not negate the need for careful examination of the peripheral retina. Posterior vitreous detachment is more common with increasing age, but myopia, vitreous hemorrhage, surgical aphakia, and diabetic retinopathy, particularly following panretinal photocoagulation, all have been associated with the development of posterior vitreous detachment at an earlier age. Fellow eyes of patients who have developed a PVD in one eye most often follow a similar course (symptoms, complications) when a PVD develops.[29]

Preferred Response

a. If hemorrhage or pigment granules are not present in the vitreous, depressed examination of the peripheral retina is not necessary.

An increased rate of proliferative vitreoretinopathy (PVR) has been associated with all of the following *except*

a. vitreous hemorrhage
b. scleral buckling surgery rather than closed vitrectomy for the repair of retinal detachment
c. large and/or multiple retinal breaks
d. cryoretinopexy

Discussion

Vitreous hemorrhage, cryoretinopexy, large or multiple retinal breaks, and vitrectomy surgery have all been associated with an increased risk of developing PVR. Cryoretinopexy has been associated with both the dispersion of retinal pigment epithelial cells into the vitreous and the breakdown of the blood-retinal barrier (releasing serum components), both of which may participate in the pathogenesis of PVR. Scleral buckling surgery, unlike vitreous surgery, has not been linked to an increased risk of PVR, perhaps because it produces less breakdown of the blood-retinal barrier.[30]

Preferred Response

b. scleral buckling surgery rather than closed vitrectomy for the repair of retinal detachment

All of the following statements about the use of indirect ophthalmoscopy to screen for retinopathy of prematurity are true *except*

a. Screening should be performed prior to hospital discharge or by 4 to 6 weeks of age.
b. Screening should be performed on all premature neonates of less than 30 weeks' gestation.
c. Screening should be performed on all premature neonates with a birth weight of less than 1300 g.
d. Screening should be repeated biweekly on neonates who demonstrate retinopathy of prematurity on the initial examination.

Discussion

Multiple risk factors have been associated with the development of retinopathy of prematurity in premature neonates, including low birth weight, low gestational age, oxygen therapy,[31] apnea, sepsis, and others. Premature infants with a birth weight of 1300 g or less, of gestational age of 30 weeks or less, or who require supplemental oxygen are particularly at greater risk of developing retinopathy of prematurity. Initial examination of the peripheral retina by indirect ophthalmoscopy in these neonates is recommended prior to hospital discharge or by 4 to 6 weeks of age. Repeat retinal examinations are performed every 2 weeks until the retina becomes fully vascularized or retinopathy of prematurity is noted. If retinopathy of prematurity develops, weekly examinations should be performed to watch for possible progression to threshold disease.[32]

Preferred Response

d. Screening should be repeated biweekly on neonates who demonstrate retinopathy of prematurity on the initial examination.

On routine ophthalmoscopic examination, a 62-year-old woman is noted to have asymptomatic, bilateral, smooth peripheral elevations in the inferotemporal retina that extend slightly posterior to the equator. Visual acuity is 20/20 OU. Which of the following statements is true?

a. Laser demarcation along the posterior border of these lesions will prevent extension into the macula.
b. Retinal detachment frequently occurs in such a case if an inner-layer retinal break is present.
c. Retinal detachment will not occur unless a retinal break is present in the outer layer or full-thickness retina.
d. Retinal detachments associated with outer-layer breaks typically progress rapidly.

Discussion

Senile or acquired retinoschisis is present in up to 4% of normal patients over age 40. This frequently bilateral condition typically develops from a splitting of the outer plexiform layer in the peripheral retina. Smooth, tense, peripheral retinal elevations develop, most commonly in the inferotemporal quadrant, although less frequently other quadrants may be involved.[7] Retinal breaks may develop in either or both the inner or outer retinal layers or the adjacent full-thickness retina. Retinal detachments associated with retinoschisis occur infrequently but may develop when either an outer-layer retinal break alone or both inner- and outer-layer retinal breaks are present.[33] Retinal detachments associated with senile retinoschisis are rare and typically progress slowly; therefore, outer-layer breaks may not routinely require prophylactic treatment.[22] Retinal cryotherapy or scatter photocoagulation may be used over the area of retinoschisis and outer-layer retinal hole formation if the detachment progresses. Typically, senile retinoschisis does not progress posteriorly. Attempts to demarcate the area of retinoschisis by laser photocoagulation will not prevent posterior extension. Unlike in juvenile retinoschisis, macular function remains normal.

Preferred Response

c. Retinal detachment will not occur unless a retinal break is present in the outer layer or full-thickness retina.

The results of an ultrasound test are shown in the figure.

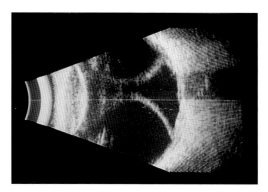

Ultrasound test demonstrating serous choroidal detachment.

All of the following statements about this nonmobile ultrasound finding are true *except*

a. Surgical drainage is indicated in most cases.
b. Excessive panretinal photocoagulation may produce this lesion.
c. A shallow anterior chamber may be associated with this lesion.
d. A double-peaked spike is a characteristic finding observed on A-scan.

Discussion

The smooth, relatively nonmobile, dome-shaped lesions depicted in the periphery on B-scan are consistent with serous choroidal detachment. Typically, serous choroidal detachments are peripheral and are tethered at the vortex vein ampullae. In massive choroidal detachments, the elevations may insert near the edge of the optic disc rather than from its center as in retinal detachments. A-scan shows a characteristic thick, double-peaked, high spike. Serous choroidal detachments may develop in association with inflammation, hypotony, or compromise of vortex vein outflow such as may occur postoperatively, following trauma, following panretinal photocoagulation, or with many other conditions. With large choroidal detachments, an anterior displacement of the lens–iris diaphragm may occur, causing a shallowing of the anterior chamber. In most cases, the serous choroidal detachment will spontaneously resolve and requires no specific treatment. In other situations, such as coexisting wound leak or cyclodialysis cleft, the underlying cause for hypotony must be treated to hasten resolution of the choroidal detachment. Treatment of underlying inflammation with topical or systemic corticosteroids may be helpful. Most serous choroidal detachments resolve so that surgical drainage of choroidal fluid need only be considered for "kissing" choroidal detachments that cause retinal apposition. In such circumstances, drainage should probably be performed within 5 days of apposition.

Preferred Response

a. Surgical drainage is indicated in most cases.

A 54-year-old woman complains that 1 month ago she developed metamorphopsia, followed by a sudden decrease in central vision in her left eye. Her visual acuity is 20/20 OD and 20/100 OS. Anterior segment examination demonstrates trace nuclear sclerosis OU. Her fundi are shown in the figures.

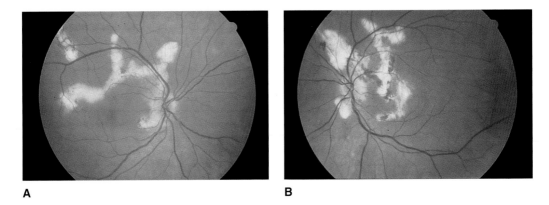

A   **B**

Serpiginous choroidopathy showing inactive chorioretinal scars, right eye **(A)** and left eye **(B)**.
A disciform scar from previous choroidal neovascularization is visible in the fovea of the left eye.

All of the following statements about this patient's ocular condition are true *except*

a. Visual loss may occur from progression of this condition into the fovea.
b. Visual loss may occur from a secondary subretinal neovascular membrane involving the fovea.
c. Visual loss may occur secondary to optic nerve involvement.
d. Recurrences are common and typically progress outward from the optic disc from the edge of old lesions.

Discussion

Serpiginous choroidopathy, or geographic helicoid peripapillary choroidopathy, is a bilateral but frequently asymmetric disease that occurs most commonly in patients in their thirties to fifties. The active lesions appear as yellow-gray, opaque, linear or serpentine lesions within the choroid/RPE and emanate from the peripapillary region. As these lesions heal, chorioretinal atrophy remains in the areas of previous inflammation, as seen in the figure. Recurrences are common, with new areas of activity developing at the margins of old lesions.[7] Visual loss may develop if recurrent disease spreads into the fovea or if choroidal neovascularization develops from the edge of chorioretinal atrophy and involves the fovea. This condition does not affect the optic nerve even though it typically progresses centripetally from the peripapillary region.

Preferred Response

c. Visual loss may occur secondary to optic nerve involvement.

A 67-year-old woman presents with a history of uncomplicated extracapsular cataract extraction with a posterior chamber IOL in her left eye 3 years ago and bilateral iritis beginning 2 years ago. Visual acuity is 20/40 OD and 20/25 OS. Slit-lamp examination shows quiet anterior chambers OU, mild nuclear sclerosis OD, and a posterior chamber IOL in good position with a central posterior capsular opening OS. Mild anterior vitreous cell is present OU. The patient's fundi are shown in the figures. Fluorescein angiography confirms cystoid macular edema OU and scattered postequatorial hypofluorescent lesions corresponding to the hypopigmented lesions in the fundus photographs.

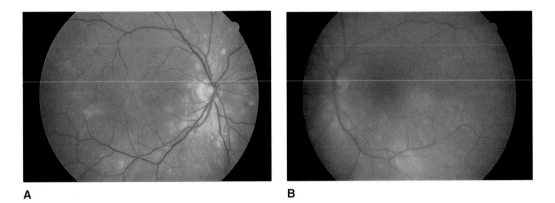

A   **B**

Fundus photographs of the right eye **(A)** and the left eye **(B)** show the hypopigmented lesions near the posterior vascular arcades which are characteristic of vitiliginous chorioretinitis.

All of the following statements about this patient's condition are true *except*

a. HLA-A29 antigen is frequently present.
b. Serous retinal detachments may be seen.
c. Most such patients respond poorly to corticosteroid therapy.
d. Although visual acuity may be affected, most such patients retain useful central vision in at least one eye for many years.

Discussion

This clinical picture describes vitiliginous chorioretinitis (birdshot retinochoroidopathy). This condition typically occurs in women in their forties to sixties and is characterized by multiple depigmented patches in the postequatorial choroid and RPE, cystoid macular edema, vitreous inflammation, and papilledema.[34] HLA-A29 antigen is found in approximately 80% of patients. Central vision may be affected by cystoid macular edema, secondary changes in the RPE, or rarely by choroidal neovascularization. Vitiliginous chorioretinitis has periodic exacerbations but progresses slowly; useful central vision may be maintained for many years in at least one eye. No therapy, including corticosteroids, has been shown to be effective. The differential diagnosis may include conditions with similar-appearing choroidal lesions or vitreous inflammation such as Vogt-Koyanagi-Harada syndrome, serpiginous choroiditis, acute posterior multifocal placoid pigment epitheliopathy, sarcoidosis, sympathetic ophthalmia, presumed ocular histoplasmosis syndrome, multifocal choroiditis, and large-cell lymphoma. Serous retinal detachments, which are typically associated with Vogt-Koyanagi-Harada syndrome, are not seen in vitiliginous chorioretinitis.

Preferred Response   b. Serous retinal detachments may be seen.

A 67-year-old woman presents with a 1-week history of sudden, painless loss of vision in her right eye. She notes no preceding or associated symptoms. She has hypertension that is controlled by medication but no history of diabetes mellitus. On examination, her visual acuity is counting fingers at 1 foot OD and 20/20 OS. Anterior segment examination is normal. Fundus examination reveals a dense vitreous hemorrhage OD. The left fundus exam demonstrates a few drusen in the macula but no other abnormalities. Ultrasonography of the right eye is shown in the figure.

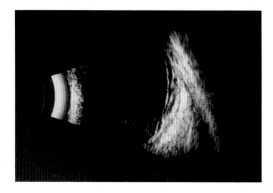

Ultrasonograph of extra-macular disciform lesion.

The *least* likely cause for her vitreous hemorrhage is

a. retinal tear
b. retinal vein occlusion
c. melanoma
d. extramacular disciform lesion

Discussion   All of the above diagnoses can be associated with vitreous hemorrhage. Among these diagnoses, melanoma most rarely causes a dense vitreous hemorrhage.[35] Retinal tear formation may cause dense vitreous hemorrhage and may have preceding symptoms of photopsias. Retinal vein occlusion may also cause vitreous hemorrhage and frequently may be related to a history of systemic hypertension. Choroidal neovascularization, including that which produces extramacular disciform lesions, can cause vitreous hemorrhage and may have no preceding symptoms. Ultrasonography would be particularly helpful in this patient to look for evidence of retinal tear or detachment, choroidal mass with low internal reflectivity suggestive of choroidal melanoma, or a flatter high internal reflective lesion suggestive of an extramacular disciform lesion. Sequential ultrasound may show reduction in the size of the lesion when an extramacular disciform lesion is present. The ultrasound in this patient showed the typical flat choroidal lesion associated with an extramacular disciform lesion (see the figure above), which appeared smaller 3 months later (see the figure on the following page).

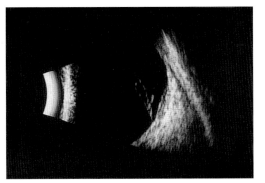

The same lesion as in the figure above, reduced in size on ultrasonography performed 3 months later.

Preferred Response   c. melanoma

A subfoveal yellow lesion in the macula of a 62-year-old woman is shown in the fundus photograph (see the figure, part A) and fluorescein angiogram (see the figure, part B).

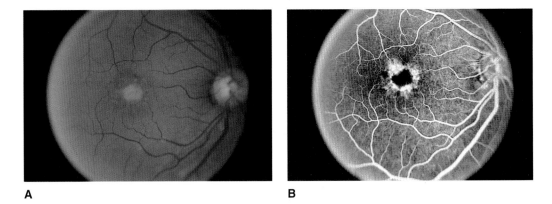

A   **B**

Adult vitelliform dystrophy. **(A)** Typical yellow subfoveal lesion. **(B)** Lesion is hypofluorescent with surrounding hyperfluorescence on corresponding fluorescein angiogram.

Which of the following is true?

a. The lesion is typically associated with severely decreased visual acuity.
b. The lesion has a high risk of developing choroidal neovascularization.
c. The lesion is typically hypofluorescent on fluorescein angiography and is surrounded by an incomplete ring of hyperfluorescence that fades in the late angiogram.
d. The lesion is likely to undergo rapid changes with time.

Discussion   Adult vitelliform dystrophy, also known as adult-onset foveomacular dystrophy or adult Best's disease, is a common uniocular or bilateral maculopathy that occurs in middle-aged or older adults.[36] The typical lesion is a small (one-half to one-third disc diameter) subretinal yellow lesion (see the figure, part A), which can be either subfoveal or parafoveal. Within the center of the lesion, there may be an area of black hyperpigmentation. On fluorescein angiography, the yellow lesion is typically hypofluorescent and is surrounded by an incomplete ring of hyperfluorescence that fades in the late angiogram (see the figure, part B). Some reports have described an autosomal dominant inheritance pattern but other reports have failed to identify a genetic pattern. The visual prognosis tends to remain relatively good (in the range of 20/25 to 20/40), with concurrent mild metamorphopsia. In some patients in their sixties, yellow material disappears and is replaced by atrophy of the RPE. In these eyes, there is a marked decrease in visual acuity. Patients with adult-onset foveomacular dystrophy do not have a high risk of developing choroidal neovascularization; however, choroidal neovascularization can occur when any process disrupts the RPE.

Preferred Response   c. The lesion is typically hypofluorescent on fluorescein angiography and is surrounded by an incomplete ring of hyperfluorescence that fades in the late angiogram.

Following an uneventful cataract extraction, a 66-year-old woman is referred to you because of an elevated gray choroidal mass in her left eye. Her left eye has a visual acuity of 20/25 and shows no evidence of inflammation. In the superior periphery, there is a large, dome-shaped, gray choroidal mass as shown in the figure, part A. A minimal amount of subretinal fluid is present around the margins of the lesion. Echographic examination (see the figure, parts B and C) shows that the lesion has a regular internal acoustic pattern and is of very low reflectivity.

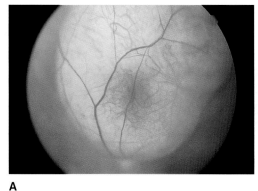

A

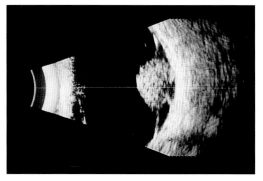

B

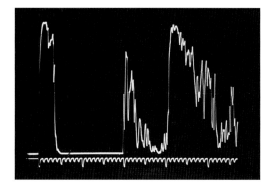

C

Amelanotic choroidal melanoma. **(A)** Superior amelanotic choroidal mass. **(B)** The mass appears mushroom-shaped on B-scan. **(C)** The mass is of low internal reflectivity on the A-scan.

The choroidal mass is *most* consistent with

a. scleritis
b. choroidal detachment
c. choroidal metastasis
d. amelanotic choroidal melanoma

Discussion

Eyes with scleritis typically show inflammatory signs. Choroidal detachments do not present as a single dome-shaped lesion posteriorly but typically involve the peripheral choroid and extend to the ora serrata (see the figure at Question R31). A choroidal metastasis typically presents as a white choroidal lesion, but the internal acoustic pattern is very irregular with medium to high frequencies. Choroidal melanomas are usually dome-shaped or mushroom-shaped lesions, and the degree of pigmentation varies considerably from amelanotic to markedly pigmented. The internal acoustic pattern described above is classic for malignant choroidal melanoma.

Preferred Response

d. amelanotic choroidal melanoma

A 64-year-old man is referred to you because of an elevated, brown choroidal mass involving the inferior quadrant of his left eye. On echographic examination, the lesion shows a pattern highly consistent with malignant melanoma. A subsequent metastatic workup is completely negative.

Factors predictive of subsequent metastatic disease include all of the following *except*

a. cell type
b. extrascleral extension
c. extension through Bruch's membrane
d. location of the anterior tumor margin

Discussion

A variety of factors have been shown to increase the risk of subsequent tumor-related death following enucleation or radiation therapy for malignant melanoma. Tumors composed primarily of epithelioid cells (versus spindle A, spindle B, or mixed-cell type) have a poor prognosis. Extrascleral extension of the tumor is also a grave prognostic sign. Kaplan-Meier survival curves show a steadily worsening prognosis with every 2 mm increase in the largest tumor dimension. Tumors that involve the anterior choroid, particularly the ciliary body, have also been shown to have a poor prognosis. Extension through Bruch's membrane is not predictive of later metastatic disease.

Preferred Response

c. extension through Bruch's membrane

A 60-year-old man has bilateral graying of the retina temporal to the fovea (see the figure, part A), subtle angiographic evidence of staining in this area (see the figure, part B), and visual acuity of 20/25 OU.

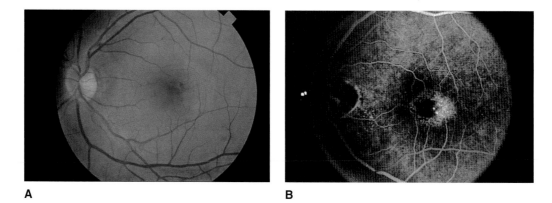

A　　　　　　　　　　　　　　　　**B**

Idiopathic juxtafoveolar retinal telangiectasis seen as retinal graying temporal to left fovea **(A),** which stains late on the fluorescein angiogram **(B).**

The *most* likely diagnosis is

a. cone dystrophy
b. age-related macular degeneration
c. idiopathic juxtafoveolar retinal telangiectasis
d. chloroquine toxicity

Discussion

Cone dystrophy and chloroquine toxicity characteristically produce a perifoveal ring of retinal pigment epithelial depigmentation, causing a bull's-eye pattern on fluorescein angiography. In age-related macular degeneration, one would expect to see drusen with or without the atrophic or exudative changes of advanced disease. Idiopathic juxtafoveolar retinal telangiectasis (of the acquired type) produces a gray zone in the parafoveolar retina with late staining on the angiogram. Patients initially have minimal or no symptoms and mild visual loss.[37] Although background diabetic retinopathy could also present with this appearance, microaneurysms outside of this region would most likely be noted as well and the patient would have a history of diabetes mellitus.

Preferred Response　　　c. idiopathic juxtafoveolar retinal telangiectasis

The *early* manifestations of the condition diagnosed in Question R38 include all of the following *except*

a. pigmentary migration into the retina
b. temporal graying of the macula
c. a diffuse pattern of late staining surrounding the fovea on fluorescein angiography
d. asymmetric presentation

Discussion   Many patients with idiopathic juxtafoveolar retinal telangiectasis present with symptoms in one eye only. The early angiographic findings reveal late staining of the retina, often in an oval configuration. The earliest clinical feature is graying of the retina temporal to the fovea. Only in the later stages of the disease does pigmentary migration occur.[37] This acquired form of idiopathic juxtafoveolar retinal telangiectasis usually presents in the middle-aged to elderly population. Most patients retain good vision in at least one eye. The most common cause of visual loss is atrophy of the retinal pigment epithelium. Choroidal neovascular membranes may also occur.

Preferred Response   a. pigmentary migration into the retina

A patient with diabetes presents with an optic disc appearance as shown in the figure.

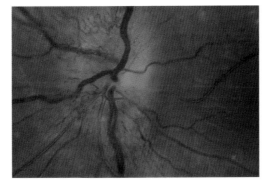

Diabetic papillopathy.

Which of the following statements about the condition illustrated is true?

a. It only afflicts patients in diabetic ketoacidosis.
b. It usually causes severe and permanent visual acuity loss.
c. It is characterized by disc edema in one or both eyes.
d. It is treated with panretinal photocoagulation.

Discussion   Diabetic papillopathy is an uncommon condition of unknown etiology characterized by true optic nerve head swelling.[38] Patients may have unilateral or bilateral disc edema. In patients with bilateral disc swelling, conditions that cause increased intracranial pressure must be ruled out. Diabetic papillopathy may occur in younger or older patients or may be accompanied by background or proliferative diabetic retinopathy. The majority of patients suffer only minimal deficits in visual acuity with a mild afferent pupillary defect or visual field loss. Most patients with diabetic papillopathy are not ill on presentation or in poor glycemic control. Laser treatment is not indicated.

Preferred Response   c. It is characterized by disc edema in one or both eyes.

R41

The parents of a 2-year-old girl report that she has had "bobbing eyes" and light sensitivity since birth. In your office, the girl shows good visual attention but has bilateral pendular nystagmus and squints in bright light. The retina appears normal, but the foveal reflex is blunted. Dark-adapted scotopic electroretinogram (ERG) responses are normal, but light-adapted photopic signals are greatly diminished. No relatives are similarly affected.

This patient *most* likely has

a. congenital stationary night blindness (CSNB)
b. Leber's congenital amaurosis
c. achromatopsia
d. Stargardt's disease

Discussion

The early onset of photophobia and nystagmus point to a congenital cone dysfunction. The loss of photopic ERG response, including photopic flicker response, and the patient's essentially normal rod function confirm the generalized cone abnormality. While CSNB can reduce acuity and cause nystagmus, the congenital loss of night vision from rod system abnormalities would cause an abnormal scotopic ERG. CSNB is frequently an X-linked recessive trait that affects males. In Leber's congenital amaurosis, overall vision is very limited because of generalized retinal dysfunction that causes loss of both rod and cone ERG responses. Stargardt's disease becomes evident during the grade school and teenage years and typically shows a nearly normal rod and cone ERG. Achromatopsia causes total color blindness from a congenital absence of cone photoreceptors. It is autosomal recessive and rarely affects more than the current generation. Ultimate acuity ranges from 20/100 to 20/200 and is best in dimmer light or with sunglasses.

Preferred Response   c. achromatopsia

R42

A 12-year-old boy fails his school vision screening test. His medical history is benign. Middle-aged relatives of both sexes for three generations reportedly have had central visual loss. His best-corrected visual acuities are 20/80 OD and 20/20 OS. The disc, vessels, and retinal periphery of both eyes appear normal but the macula of the right eye has a fibrotic scar and the left eye shows a yellow, round, circumscribed lesion of one disc diameter (see the figure) that blocks fluorescence on fluorescein angiogram. The ERG is normal, but the electrooculogram ratio (light peak/dark trough) is reduced.

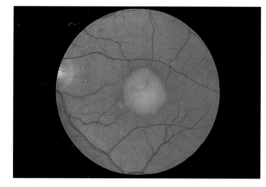

Best's vitelliform macular dystrophy with typical macular "egg yolk" lesion.

The *most* likely diagnosis is

a. neuronal ceroid lipofuscinosis
b. Bardet-Biedl syndrome
c. Best's vitelliform macular dystrophy
d. Stargardt's disease

Discussion

Neuronal ceroid lipofuscinosis causes a hyperfluorescent bull's-eye maculopathy from generalized cone dystrophy, with seizures and progressive dementia in school-age years. In Stargardt's disease, the macular RPE atrophy causes hyperfluorescence against the abnormally dark background of the "silent choroid" sign. Bardet-Biedl syndrome frequently has atrophic maculopathy, but the diffuse photoreceptor loss causes reduced ERG amplitudes by a young age. Bardet-Biedl syndrome is autosomal recessive, and patients frequently have extra digits on their hands or feet. In Best's vitelliform macular dystrophy, visual acuity typically is excellent until the "egg yolk" ruptures or involutes. The yellow lesion is hypofluorescent in the early phases of the fluorescein angiogram but can stain and become hyperfluorescent in the later stages.[7] The condition is transmitted from an affected parent as an autosomal dominant trait. The electrooculogram is characteristically subnormal despite a normal ERG.

Preferred Response

c. Best's vitelliform macular dystrophy

A 47-year-old woman in good health with a history of autosomal dominant retinitis pigmentosa presents with complaints of further decline in visual acuity in both eyes. On examination, her visual acuity is 20/100 OD and 20/70 OS. Mild posterior subcapsular cataract is present in both lenses. Moderate fine cell is seen on biomicroscopy of the vitreous of both eyes. The fundi are shown in the figures on page 276 (right eye: parts A and B; left eye: parts C and D). The patient's sister has retinitis pigmentosa that required retinal laser treatment 2 years earlier.

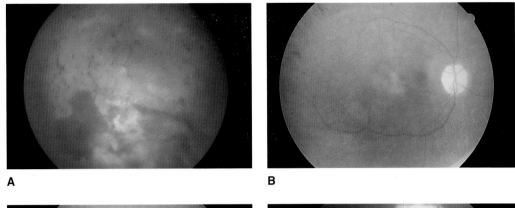

A   B

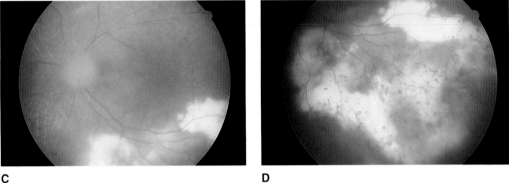

C   D

Intraretinal and subretinal exudate and associated hemorrhage are present in the inferior retina of both the right **(A)** and left **(D)** eyes. The posterior pole of the right eye **(B)** is uninvolved by the exudative process, but subretinal exudate and fluid are entering the posterior pole of the left eye **(C).**

Which of the following statements regarding this patient is *most* correct?

a. The patient's clinical appearance is most characteristic of Coats' retinopathy, which may occur in retinitis pigmentosa.
b. The subretinal exudates most likely are the result of retinal infection with toxoplasmosis.
c. The patient's clinical appearance is most characteristic of familial exudative vitreoretinopathy.
d. The retinal findings most likely result from diabetes mellitus, and a glucose tolerance test should be performed.

Discussion   The clinical picture of telangiectatic retinal vessels and large amounts of subretinal lipid exudate is characteristic of Coats' retinopathy. Classic Coats' retinopathy, however, is typically seen unilaterally in young males. Coats'-type changes have been reported in patients with long-standing retinitis pigmentosa of all inheritance patterns.[7] The condition may be unilateral or bilateral, may occur in patients of either sex, and is often noted in siblings who are also affected by retinitis pigmentosa. The telangiectatic changes are usually located in the inferior quadrants. Visual loss from this condition is variable, depending on whether the macula is affected by edema, exudate, hemorrhage, or subretinal fluid. Treatment of the telangiectatic retinal vessels with either laser photocoagulation or cryotherapy may be considered. In advanced cases, exudative retinal detachment may occur. Other conditions such as diabetes mellitus, familial exudative vitreoretinopathy, or toxoplasmosis may result in intraretinal or subretinal hemorrhage or exudate. The peripheral location of the lesions and lack of prior history of diabetes mellitus would make diabetic retinopathy an unlikely diagnosis in this patient. Familial exudative vitreoretinopathy has not been found to be associated with retinitis pigmentosa; typically, patients with familial exudative vitreoretinopathy present in childhood with an avascular peripheral retina, retinal neovascularization, and temporal dragging of the retina similar to patients with retinopathy of prematurity. Retinitis caused by toxoplasmosis rarely causes exudative retinal changes and typically has old chorioretinal scars present, which are not seen in this patient.

Preferred Response

a. The patient's clinical appearance is most characteristic of Coats' retinopathy, which may occur in retinitis pigmentosa.

A 60-year-old hypertensive woman presents with sudden loss of vision in her right eye. Her visual acuity is counting fingers OD and 20/30 OS. Ophthalmoscopy of the left eye reveals arteriolar narrowing and severe arteriovenous crossing nicks. No drusen are seen OS. The right fundus (part A) and fluorescein angiogram (part B) are shown in the figures.

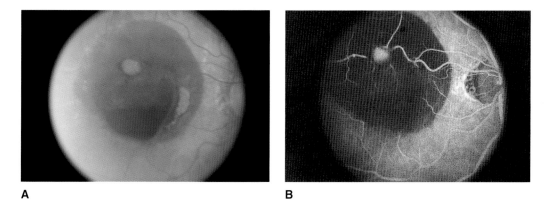

A   **B**

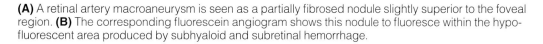

(A) A retinal artery macroaneurysm is seen as a partially fibrosed nodule slightly superior to the foveal region. **(B)** The corresponding fluorescein angiogram shows this nodule to fluoresce within the hypofluorescent area produced by subhyaloid and subretinal hemorrhage.

The *most* likely diagnosis is

a. age-related macular degeneration
b. retinal artery macroaneurysm
c. idiopathic choroidal neovascular membrane
d. choroidal rupture

Discussion

Although age-related macular degeneration is the most likely cause of acute subretinal hemorrhage, it is not the most likely diagnosis for this patient. Age-related macular degeneration is a bilateral condition, and drusen were not seen in the contralateral eye. Furthermore, while choroidal neovascularization from any cause frequently produces subretinal hemorrhage and occasionally vitreous hemorrhage, the combination of subretinal and preretinal hemorrhage is more common in retinal artery macroaneurysms. Systemic hypertension is seen in most patients with retinal artery macroaneurysms;[7] however, systemic hypertension is common among the American population and does not help make the diagnosis. Identification of the macroaneurysm as a fibrous nodule that is hyperfluorescent on fluorescein angiography makes the patient's diagnosis definitive. Idiopathic choroidal neovascularization is unusual in elderly patients. The diagnosis of choroidal rupture requires a visible circumlinear depigmentation or at least some stigmata of ocular trauma.

Preferred Response   b. retinal artery macroaneurysm

A 65-year-old woman presents for evaluation of recent visual loss in her right eye. Her visual acuity is 20/40 OD and 20/20 OS. Biomicroscopy of the macula is shown in the figure.

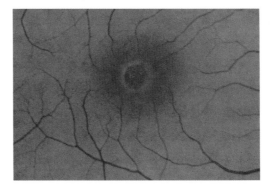

Stage I macular hole.

All of the following are true *except*

a. Amsler grid examination is likely to show metamorphopsia.
b. Posterior vitreous detachment is unlikely to be present in the right eye.
c. There is a 40% to 50% chance that the lesion will resolve spontaneously.
d. The patient has a greater than 50% chance of developing a similar problem in the fellow eye.

Discussion   The condition pictured is an impending, or Stage I, macular hole. Most common in older women, idiopathic senile macular hole typically begins with acute-onset metamorphopsia and central visual blurring or scotoma. In the absence of posterior vitreous detachment, the early macular lesion is characterized by loss of the foveal depression and a yellow foveal ring.[39] As many as 40% to 50% of patients with an impending macular hole will have spontaneous separation of the vitreous from the fovea with resolution of symptoms and no further progression. It is estimated that less than 10% of fellow eyes are at risk for future macular hole development. Although the role of vitrectomy in the management of idiopathic macular hole continues to evolve, many vitreoretinal surgeons favor close observation for impending macular holes. Vitrectomy and fluid–gas exchange are considered for eyes that progress to full-thickness macular holes.

Preferred Response

d. The patient has a greater than 50% chance of developing a similar problem in the fellow eye.

A 70-year-old woman complains of progressive blurring in her right eye. Examination is unremarkable apart from mild vitreous cell and the nodular, shallowly elevated lesion shown in the figures (part A, temporal retina; part B, posterior pole).

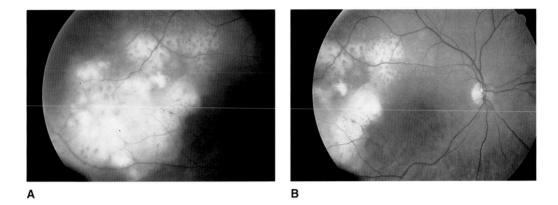

A   **B**

Intraocular large-cell lymphoma seen as sub-RPE infiltration in the temporal retina of the right eye **(A)** that extends into the posterior pole **(B).**

The *most* likely diagnosis is

a. amelanotic melanoma of the choroid
b. tuberculous choroiditis
c. intraocular lymphoma
d. carcinoma metastatic to the choroid

Discussion

Although all of these entities can cause nonpigmented lesions beneath the retina, multiple or confluent yellow tumefactions under the RPE are most characteristic of intraocular large-cell lymphoma (reticulum cell sarcoma). The pigment speckling seen on the surface of the mounds is a clue to their sub-RPE location. Vitreous cells occasionally may be present, masquerading this condition as uveitis. Amelanotic choroidal melanoma is generally a single, dome-shaped, more highly elevated lesion, often with a visible vascular supply. Tuberculous choroidal granulomas are typically multifocal and smaller. Choroidal metastatic lesions have subtler borders, are often multiple, and frequently are associated with overlying subretinal fluid. Bilateral involvement eventually develops in most cases of intraocular lymphoma, and the disease generally confines itself to the eyes and central nervous system. The diagnosis can often be confirmed by diagnostic vitrectomy and lumbar puncture. MRI of the head may be used to detect asymptomatic central nervous system lesions.

Preferred Response

c. intraocular lymphoma

A 10-year-old girl is brought to see you with complaints of decreased vision and headache over the preceding 4 to 6 weeks. Fundus findings are shown in the figures.

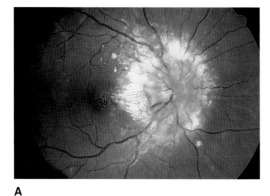

A

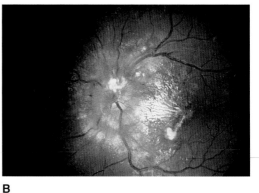

B

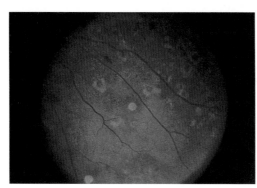

C

Severe bilateral disc edema with exudate extending into the macula in the right **(A)** and left **(B)** eyes. **(C)** Elschnig spots are present in the peripheral fundus of the right eye.

Which of the following tests should be performed *first*?

a. CT scan of the head
b. systemic blood pressure measurement
c. lumbar puncture
d. FTA-ABS test

Discussion   Although all of the above tests have a role in the evaluation of optic disc swelling, measurement of the blood pressure, even in a young patient, is an important part of the workup. This girl, whose blood pressure measured 215/145 mm Hg, demonstrated classic findings of severe (Grade 4) hypertensive retinopathy, including arteriolar narrowing, disc swelling, flame-shaped hemorrhages, cotton-wool patches, hard exudates, and choroidal infarcts (Elschnig spots). Blood pressure determination in this case prompted emergency medical evaluation, leading to the diagnosis of an acute renal disorder. Although CT scan of the head and lumbar puncture are indicated to exclude intracranial mass lesions and other causes of increased intracranial pressure in patients with papilledema, these tests are usually unnecessary after the detection of severe hypertension as the cause of optic disc swelling. Syphilis must also be considered in the differential diagnosis of patients with unexplained disc edema.

Preferred Response   b. systemic blood pressure measurement

An otherwise healthy, emmetropic 45-year-old man reports gradually diminishing vision in his right eye. There is no history of surgery, trauma, or laser treatment. Ocular examination demonstrates dilated episcleral veins, normal intraocular pressure, mild vitreous cells, shallow peripheral ciliochoroidal detachment, nonrhegmatogenous retinal detachment with markedly shifting subretinal fluid, and the pigment alterations shown in the fundus photograph (see the figure, part A) and fluorescein angiogram (see the figure, part B). There are no intraocular masses or signs of significant ocular inflammation.

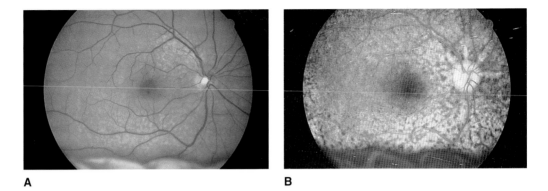

A   **B**

(A) Idiopathic uveal effusion syndrome with an inferior exudative retinal detachment. **(B)** The fluorescein angiogram best demonstrates the irregular RPE pigmentation, which is typical later in this syndrome.

All of the following are true *except*

a. B-scan echography is likely to show diffuse choroidal thickening.
b. The untreated natural history is that of progressive, usually bilateral, visual decline.
c. Scleral buckling is likely to be curative.
d. A surgical procedure to thin the sclera is likely to result in resolution of the retinal detachment.

Discussion   Idiopathic uveal effusion syndrome is characterized by spontaneous ciliochoroidal detachment followed by nonrhegmatogenous retinal detachment in otherwise healthy middle-aged men. The diagnosis is made when the clinical characteristics listed above are present and other known causes of ciliochoroidal effusion have been excluded, including hypotony; nanophthalmos; arteriovenous fistula; uveal, scleral, or orbital inflammation; history of surgery or trauma; and choroidal neoplastic infiltration. B-scan ultrasonography shows diffuse choroidal edema (thickening), which is typically more prominent peripherally. Although the associated exudative subretinal fluid may initially come and go, most untreated patients eventually develop bilateral chronic nonrhegmatogenous retinal detachment with progressive visual decline. Scleral buckling surgery generally worsens the clinical picture. The disorder is hypothesized to result from an abnormality of transscleral protein transport, and a scleral thinning procedure is curative in a large percentage of patients.[40]

Preferred Response   c. Scleral buckling is likely to be curative.

A 23-year-old woman complains of unilateral paracentral scotomas and photopsias. Visual acuity is 20/40 in the left eye, and visual field testing shows enlargement of the physiologic blind spot on the left. Fundus appearance (part A) and fluorescein findings (part B) are shown in the figures. The right eye is normal.

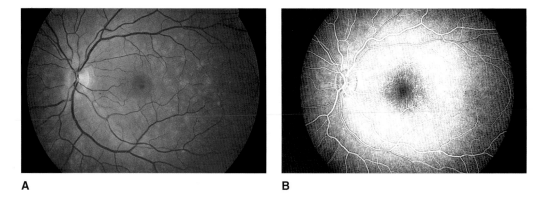

A   **B**

Multiple evanescent white dot syndrome with characteristic gray-white outer retinal/RPE lesions **(A)**, which hyperfluoresce early in the fluorescein angiogram **(B)**.

This clinical presentation is *most* characteristic of

a. idiopathic central serous chorioretinopathy
b. multiple evanescent white dot syndrome
c. acute posterior multifocal placoid pigment epitheliopathy
d. serpiginous choroiditis

Discussion   Multiple evanescent white dot syndrome[41] typically affects one eye of a healthy young woman. The patient may present with photopsias and scotomas. There may also be an enlarged physiologic blind spot in the absence of disc swelling. The fundus characteristically has subtle, small, gray-white lesions at the level of the outer retina/RPE (see the figure, part A), sometimes accompanied by mild disc swelling and/or orange mottling in the fovea. Fluorescein angiography demonstrates early hyperfluorescence of the white lesions in a wreath-like pattern (see the figure, part B), with variable amounts of late staining. Electroretinographic abnormalities suggest outer retinal dysfunction. The white dots disappear within weeks of onset and the visual symptoms gradually resolve over weeks to months. No treatment is necessary. The acute lesions in both acute posterior multifocal placoid pigment epitheliopathy and serpiginous choroiditis are larger, cream colored, placoid, and hypofluorescent in the early phases of the fluorescein angiogram. Idiopathic central serous chorioretinopathy is characterized by serous detachments of the neurosensory retina and/or RPE with fluorescein angiographic evidence of leakage through the RPE.

Preferred Response   b. multiple evanescent white dot syndrome

A 35-year-old man presents with recurrent bilateral iridocyclitis, sometimes including hypopyon. He reports recurrent genital ulcers and reddish bumps on his skin. Examination reveals the oral ulcers (see the figure, part A) and posterior segment findings (see the figure, part B).

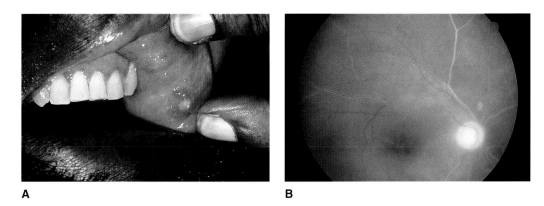

A   **B**

Behçet's disease with oral ulcers **(A)** and occlusive vasculitis **(B).**

All of the following are true *except*

a. This disease is most common in the Middle and Far East.
b. Pricking the skin with a needle may help confirm the diagnosis.
c. Immunosuppressive agents are frequently used for treatment of the associated retinal vasculitis.
d. Untreated patients have an excellent prognosis.

Discussion

Behçet's disease is a multisystem vasculitis, most prevalent in the Middle and Far East. The most common clinical features include recurrent crops of oral ulcers, genital ulcers, ocular disease, and skin disease (especially erythema nodosum). Large-joint polyarthritis and central nervous system involvement may also occur. The most common ocular manifestations include iridocyclitis, retinal vasculitis, and retinal necrosis.[7] The phenomenon of pathergy (formation of a pustule after breaking the skin with a needle) is frequently present. Although the untreated natural history of ocular Behçet's disease is poor, immunosuppressive drug therapy may result in stabilization and long-term remission.

Preferred Response

d. Untreated patients have an excellent prognosis.

References

1. Duker JS, Blumenkranz MS: Diagnosis and management of the acute retinal necrosis (ARN) syndrome. *Surv Ophthalmol* 1991;35:327–343.

2. Blumenkranz MS, Culbertson WW, Clarkson JG, et al: Treatment of the acute retinal necrosis syndrome with intravenous acyclovir. *Ophthalmology* 1986;93:296–300.

3. The Eye Disease Case-Control Study Group: Risk factors for neovascular age-related macular degeneration. *Arch Ophthalmol* 1992;110:1701–1708.

4. Macular Photocoagulation Study Group: Visual outcome after laser photocoagulation for subfoveal choroidal neovascularization secondary to age-related macular degeneration: the influence of initial lesion size and initial visual acuity. *Arch Ophthalmol* 1994;112:480–488.

5. Greenwald MJ: The shaken baby syndrome. *Sem Ophthalmol* 1990; 5:202–215.

6. Elner SG, Elner VM, Arnall M, et al: Ocular and associated systemic findings in suspected child abuse: a necropsy study. *Arch Ophthalmol* 1990;108:1094–1101.

7. Gass JDM: *Stereoscopic Atlas of Macular Diseases: Diagnosis and Treatment.* 3rd ed. St Louis: CV Mosby Co; 1987.

8. Kuppermann BD, Petty JG, Richman DD, et al: Correlation between CD4+ counts and prevalence of cytomegalovirus retinitis and human immunodeficiency virus-related noninfectious retinal vasculopathy in patients with acquired immunodeficiency syndrome. *Am J Ophthalmol* 1993;115:575–582.

9. Jabs DA: Treatment of cytomegalovirus retinitis—1992. *Arch Ophthalmol* 1992;110: 185–187.

10. Sanborn GE, Anand R, Torti RE, et al: Sustained-release ganciclovir therapy for treatment of cytomegalovirus retinitis: use of an intravitreal device. *Arch Ophthalmol* 1992;110:188–195.

11. Diaz-Llopis M, Chipont E, Sanchez S, et al: Intravitreal foscarnet for cytomegalovirus retinitis in a patient with acquired immunodeficiency syndrome. *Am J Ophthalmol* 1992;114:742–747.

12. Brown GC: Retinal arterial obstructive disease. In: Ryan SJ, ed-in-chief: *Retina.* Vol 2. St Louis: CV Mosby Co; 1989.

13. Shields JA, Wright DM, Augsburger JJ, et al: Cryptococcal chorioretinitis. *Am J Ophthalmol* 1980;89:210–218.

14. Diabetic Retinopathy Study Research Group: Four risk factors for severe visual loss in diabetic retinopathy: the third report from the Diabetic Retinopathy Study. *Arch Ophthalmol* 1979;97:654–655.

15. Early Treatment Diabetic Retinopathy Study Research Group: Photocoagulation for diabetic macular edema: Early Treatment Diabetic Retinopathy Study report number 1. *Arch Ophthalmol* 1985:103:1796–1806.

16. Early Treatment Diabetic Retinopathy Study Research Group: Early photocoagulation for diabetic retinopathy: ETDRS report number 9. *Ophthalmology* 1991;98: 766–785.

17. The Diabetes Control and Complications Trial Research Group: The effect of intensive treatment of diabetes on the development and progression of long-term complications in insulin-dependent diabetes mellitus. *N Engl J Med* 1993;329: 977–986.

18. Meisler DM, Mandelbaum S: *Propionibacterium*-associated endophthalmitis after extracapsular cataract extraction: review of reported cases. *Ophthalmology* 1989; 96:54–61.

19. Mandelbaum S, Forster RK: Endophthalmitis associated with filtering blebs. *Int Ophthalmol Clin* 1987;27:107–111.

20. Brown RH, Yang LH, Walker SD, et al: Treatment of bleb infection after glaucoma surgery. *Arch Ophthalmol* 1994;112:57–61.

21. *Diabetic Retinopathy.* Preferred Practice Pattern. San Francisco: American Academy of Ophthalmology; 1993.

22. *Precursors of Rhegmatogenous Retinal Detachment in Adults.* Preferred Practice Pattern. San Francisco: American Academy of Ophthalmology; 1994.

23. Folk JC, Arrindell EL, Klugman MR: The fellow eye of patients with phakic lattice retinal detachment. *Ophthalmology* 1989;96:72–79.

24. Sternberg P: Trauma: principles and techniques of treatment. In: Ryan SJ, ed-in-chief: *Retina.* Vol 3. St. Louis: CV Mosby Co; 1989.

25. Smith RE: Pars planitis. In: Ryan SJ, ed-in-chief: *Retina.* Vol 2. St. Louis: CV Mosby Co; 1989.

26. Mieler WF, Aaberg TM: Further observations on cryotherapy of the vitreous base in the management of peripheral uveitis. *Dev Ophthalmol* 1992;23:190–195.

27. Tornambe PE, Hilton GF, Brinton DA, et al: Pneumatic retinopexy: a two-year follow-up study of the multicenter clinical trial comparing pneumatic retinopexy with scleral buckling. *Ophthalmology* 1991;98:1115–1123.

28. Brod RD, Lightman DA, Packer AJ, et al: Correlation between vitreous pigment granules and retinal breaks in eyes with acute posterior vitreous detachment. *Ophthalmology* 1991;98:1366–1369.

29. Novak MA, Welch RB: Complications of acute symptomatic posterior vitreous detachment. *Am J Ophthalmol* 1984;97:308–314.

30. Yoshizumi MO, Kreiger AE, Sharp DM: Risk factors associated with the development of massive periretinal proliferation. In: Ryan SJ, Dawson AK, Little HL, eds: *Retinal Diseases.* Orlando, FL: Grune & Stratton; 1984.

31. American Academy of Pediatrics, American College of Obstetricians and Gynecologists: Clinical considerations in the use of oxygen. In: *Guidelines for Perinatal Care.* 2nd ed. Elk Grove Village, IL: The Academy; Washington, DC: The College; 1988; 244–248.

32. The Cryotherapy for Retinopathy of Prematurity Cooperative Group: Incidence and early course of retinopathy of prematurity. *Ophthalmology* 1991;98:1628–1640.

33. Byer NE: Long-term natural history study of senile retinoschisis with implications for management. *Ophthalmology* 1986;93:1127–1137.

34. Gass JDM: Vitiliginous chorioretinitis. *Arch Ophthalmol* 1981;99:1778–1787.

35. Gass JDM: Hemorrhage into the vitreous, a presenting manifestation of malignant melanoma of the choroid. *Arch Ophthalmol* 1963;69:778–779.

36. Vine AK, Schatz H: Adult-onset foveomacular pigment epithelial dystrophy. *Am J Ophthalmol* 1980;89:680–691.

37. Gass JDM, Blodi BA: Idiopathic juxtafoveolar retinal telangiectasis: update of classification and follow-up study. *Ophthalmology* 1993;100:1536–1546.

38. Barr CC, Glaser JS, Blankenship G: Acute disc swelling in juvenile diabetes: clinical profile and natural history of 12 cases. *Arch Ophthalmol* 1980;98:2185–2192.

39. Gass JDM: Idiopathic senile macular hole: its early stages and pathogenesis. *Arch Ophthalmol* 1988;106:629–639.

40. Johnson MW, Gass JDM: Surgical management of the idiopathic uveal effusion syndrome. *Ophthalmology* 1990;97:778–785.

41. Jampol LM, Sieving PA, Pugh D, et al: Multiple evanescent white dot syndrome. I. Clinical findings. *Arch Ophthalmol* 1984;102:671–674.

Additional Resources From the AAO

Academy Statements

Detection and Control of Diabetic Retinopathy. Public Health Note. 1992.

Eye Care of Patients with Diabetes Mellitus. Policy Statement. 1991.

Laser Surgery. Policy Statement. 1993.

Ophthalmic Management of AIDS & HIV-Infected Patients. Public Health Note. 1993.

Progression of Diabetic Retinopathy. Clinical Handout. 1993.

The Repair of Rhegmatogenous Retinal Detachments. Ophthalmic Procedures Assessment. 1990. (Item No. 112012)

Use of Laser Surgery in Ophthalmology. Information Statement. 1993.

Basic and Clinical Science Course

Retina and Vitreous. Section 12. Updated annually.

Focal Points

Bressler NM: *Laser Management of Choroidal Neovascularization.* Vol XI, Module 5. 1993. (Item No. 029011)

Bressler SB: *Age-Related Macular Degeneration.* Vol XIII, Module 2. 1995. (Item No. FP95)

Brown GC: *Retinal Arterial Obstruction.* Vol XII, Module 1. 1994. (Item No. 029012)

Byer NE: *Lattice Degeneration of the Retina.* Vol VII, Module 5. 1989. (Item No. 029007)

Culbertson WW: *Viral Retinitis.* Vol VI, Module 12. 1988. (Item No. 029006)

Finkelstein D, Clarkson JG, The Branch Vein Occlusion Study Group: *Branch and Central Vein Occlusions.* Vol V, Module 12. 1987. (Item No. 029005)

Flynn HW Jr, Blankenship GW: *Proliferative Diabetic Retinopathy.* Vol III, Module 12. 1985. (Item No. 029003)

Folk JC, Pulido JS, Wolf MD: *White Dot Chorioretinal Inflammatory Syndromes.* Vol VIII, Module 11. 1990. (Item No. 029008)

Ginsburg LH, Aiello LM: *Diabetic Retinopathy: Classification, Progression, and Management.* Vol XI, Module 7. 1993. (Item No. 029011)

Holland GN: *AIDS: Ophthalmic Considerations.* Vol II, Module 9. 1984. (Item No. 029002)

Holland GN: *An Update on AIDS-Related Cytomegalovirus Retinitis.* Vol IX, Module 5. 1991. (Item No. 029009)

Hooper PL: *Pars Planitis.* Vol XI, Module 11. 1993. (Item No. 029011)

Isenberg SJ: *How to Examine the Eye of the Neonate.* Vol VII, Module 1. 1989. (Item No. 029007)

Jacobiec FA, Levinson AW: *Choroidal Melanoma: Etiology and Diagnosis.* Vol III, Module 5. 1985. (Out of print)

Jacobiec FA, Levinson AW: *Choroidal Melanoma: Prognosis and Treatment.* Vol III, Module 6. 1985. (Out of print)

Little HL: *Nonproliferative Diabetic Retinopathy.* Vol III, Module 11. 1985. (Item No. 029003)

Mandelbaum S, Forster RK: *Infectious Endophthalmitis.* Vol I, Module 9. 1983. (Item No. 029001)

Palmer EA: *Retinopathy of Prematurity.* Vol II, Module 12. 1984. (Item No. 029002)

Monographs and Manuals Berkow JW, Orth DH, Kelley JS: *Fluorescein Angiography: Technique and Interpretation*. Ophthalmology Monograph 5. 1991. (Item No. 0210012)

Fishman GA, Sokol S: *Electrophysiologic Testing in Disorders of the Retina, Optic Nerve, and Visual Pathway*. Ophthalmology Monograph 2. 1990. (Item No. 0210020)

Hilton GF, McLean EB, Chuang EL: *Retinal Detachment*. Ophthalmology Monograph 1. 1989. (Item No. 0210069)

Michels RG: *Vitreous Surgery*. 1982. (Item No. 0210132)

Preferred Practice Patterns *Age-Related Macular Degeneration*. 1994. (Item No. 110021)

Diabetic Retinopathy. 1993. (Item No. 110020)

Precursors of Rhegmatogenous Retinal Detachment in Adults. 1994. (Item No. 110022)

Slide-Script Kincaid MC: *Diabetic Retinopathy*. Eye Care Skills for the Primary Care Physician Series. 1992. (Item No. 0240379)

Videotapes Chen CJ: *Management of Suprachoroidal Hemorrhage With Perfluorophenanthrene*. Annual Meeting Series. 1994. (Item No. 0252033)

DRSR Group, ETDRSR Group: *Management of Diabetic Retinopathy for the Primary Care Physician*. Clinical Skills Series. 1990. (Item No. 0250893)

DRSR Group, ETDRSR Group, DRVSR Group: *Evaluation and Treatment of Diabetic Retinopathy*. Clinical Skills Series. 1990. (Item No. 0250903)

ETDRSR Group: *Photocoagulation for Diabetic Macular Edema*. Clinical Skills Series. 1987. (Item No. 0250623)

Kelly MP: *Basic Techniques of Fluorescein Angiography*. Clinical Skills Series. 1994. (Item No. 0250973)

Palmer EA: *Clinical Management of Retinopathy of Prematurity*. Clinical Short Subjects Series. 1988. (Item No. 0251063)

OPTICS, REFRACTION, CONTACT LENS, AND VISUAL REHABILITATION

An intraocular lens (IOL) placed in the capsular bag following phacoemulsification and continuous-tear capsulorrhexis has moved axially toward the cornea over the first 6 weeks after surgery as a result of contraction of the capsule. The refractive change that would be expected from the anterior axial movement of an IOL is

a. hyperopic shift
b. no effect
c. myopic shift
d. not determinable

Discussion

The anterior movement of any plus corrective lens (spectacle lens, contact lens, crystalline lens, or IOL) increases the effective power of the lens.[1] The shift in refraction is therefore always in a myopic direction with anterior displacement. For a 20.0 D intraocular lens in the posterior chamber, the myopic shift is approximately 1.9 D of myopia for every millimeter of anterior displacement. For a 20.0 D anterior chamber lens, the shift is approximately 1.2 D of myopia for every millimeter of anterior displacement. An axial posterior displacement would have exactly the opposite effect, causing a hyperopic shift. Some of the variability of IOL calculations is due to our inability to predict the exact final axial position of the IOL prior to surgery.

Preferred Response

c. myopic shift

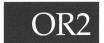

Five years ago, a patient underwent bilateral 16-incision radial keratotomy with a 3 mm optical zone. This patient has now developed 4 mm posterior subcapsular cataracts in each eye. His vision is limited to 20/50 visual acuity OU due to the cataracts, and IOL implantation is planned. The *least* accurate method for determining the corneal K readings to be used for IOL calculation in this patient is

a. manual keratometry
b. automated keratometry
c. calculation of change in refraction with and without a hard contact lens
d. calculation of K readings from preoperative radial keratometry K readings and the change in refraction

Discussion

Manual keratometry is the least accurate of all methods for determining corneal power.[2] The manual keratometer measures two points approximately 3.2 mm apart to determine the corneal power in a given meridian. The nearer the optical zone of the keratorefractive procedure is to the 3.0 mm diameter, the more inaccurate the manual keratometer. Automated keratometers use a slightly smaller sample diameter of approximately 2.6 mm, which is why automated instruments perform slightly better. The change in refraction with and without a contact lens can be very accurate, but it is limited by the patient's visual acuity as a result of the cataract.[3] Although calculating K readings from the corneal power prior to the keratorefractive procedure and the change in refraction is very accurate, the values are not always available to the cataract surgeon. Some corneal topographic instruments do provide accurate corneal power measurements of irregular corneas, but these systems are not always available.

The patient's course following the cataract surgery is often similar to the acute postoperative period following radial keratotomy, with an immediate hyperopic overcorrection that decreases over a few days or weeks. Knowledge of these changes helps to prepare the surgeon and patient for the visual changes during the immediate postoperative period.

Preferred Response

a. manual keratometry

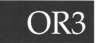

Which of the following statements about antireflection coatings on eyeglasses is true?

a. They are applied by a dipping process.
b. They decrease reflections by producing a matte surface.
c. They work by destructive interference of reflected light.
d. They are always clear and colorless.

Discussion

Tints can be applied by a dipping process, but antireflection coatings can not. Antireflection coatings are thin-film crystalline substances applied by vacuum evaporation/deposition techniques. The surface created is entirely smooth and specular, not matte; a matte surface would interfere with vision. Reflection is decreased by destructive interference of light reflected from the front and back surfaces of the coating. Destructive interference is only maximal at a peak wavelength for a given coating, and wavelengths at the ends of the visible spectrum are often partly reflected, giving a slight purple color to these coatings.

Preferred Response

c. They work by destructive interference of reflected light.

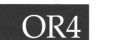

All of the following are indications for planned replacement of soft contact lenses *except*

a. mucus formation and secretions
b. 3 and 9 o'clock staining
c. giant papillary conjunctivitis
d. limbal epithelial hypertrophy

Discussion

By definition, planned replacement of soft contact lenses refers to daily-wear lenses that are worn for a limited time (1 day, 2 weeks, 4 months) before they are discarded and replaced with identical lenses. Soft-lens spoilage or dirty lenses can contribute to decreased vision, discomfort, and tissue problems. In addition to routine replacement of soft contact lenses, there are other conditions that require earlier replacement of a lens. Subclinical adhesions caused by an aged, tight lens may result in localized peripheral epithelial hypertrophy (see the figure) with resulting loss of epithelial adhesion. Protein coatings and mucus formation and secretions set the stage for the tarsal conjunctival response known as giant papillary conjunctivitis. Staining at 3 and 9 o'clock is a complication most frequently associated with rigid lens wear.

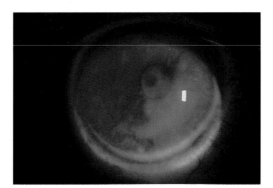

Limbal epithelial hypertrophy secondary to aged soft contact lens.

Preferred Response

b. 3 and 9 o'clock staining

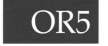

Closed-circuit television systems provide great assistance for many individuals with low vision. Which of the following statements is true?

a. Like many magnification systems, closed-circuit television requires the user to be at a specific distance for proper usage.
b. Closed-circuit television systems have the ability to present black letters on a white background or white letters on a black background. This reverse polarity is useful for patients with photophobia, who prefer to read black letters on a white background.
c. Patients who can no longer benefit from standard magnification systems also cannot be helped with closed-circuit television systems.
d. Many people who successfully use closed-circuit television systems also use other optical aids for specific tasks.

Discussion

A closed-circuit television (CCTV) reading system consists of a television camera that relays a magnified image to a television monitor screen. The patient therefore can adjust magnification for a relatively comfortable (and variable) reading distance. Patients find that using CCTV is less tiring than other aids because of the more comfortable distance from the screen. Advantages include the greater range of magnification, the use of binocularity in patients who benefit from using both eyes, and the ability to do useful work more easily than with regular spectacle or other magnifiers. There are disadvantages as well, including slow reading speed, the weight of the CCTV units, and the expense of these units in comparison with other magnifying devices. Reverse polarity is an important feature of CCTV; patients who experience photophobia prefer white letters on a black background, since the illumination can be intense and a white background causes a glare effect. Many patients, particularly young patients who have considerable difficulty with standard magnification systems, are able to work full or part time using the CCTV system. Many people successfully use a combination of regular low-vision optical aids and the CCTV system.[4,5]

Preferred Response

d. Many people who successfully use closed-circuit television systems also use other optical aids for specific tasks.

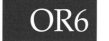

Monocular diplopia, in which the patient sees a ghost image adjacent to the primary image, can arise from any of the following *except*

a. immature cataract
b. age-related maculopathy
c. early keratoconus
d. uncorrected refractive error

Discussion

Monocular diplopia most commonly arises from optical irregularities in the crystalline lens such as those that develop with early cataracts. Retinal lesions such as epiretinal membranes sometimes cause monocular diplopia, but age-related maculopathy at most causes distortion, not the ghost-image vision disorder of monocular diplopia. Corneal irregularity such as in keratoconus is another common cause of monocular diplopia. Uncorrected refractive error also can cause monocular diplopia, apparently resulting from diffractive effects or from an accentuation of the mild optical irregularities that are present in practically every eye.[6,7]

Preferred Response

b. age-related maculopathy

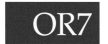

Nine months after successful cryotherapy to a peripheral retinal tear, a patient develops slightly decreased vision in the treated eye and what appears to be 1 prism diopter of vertical diplopia that disappears when either eye is closed. A 1 prism diopter vertical prism, taped to the glasses, immediately relieves the diplopia, but it recurs 10 seconds later. Several trials with additional prisms are similarly unsuccessful, with the diplopia recurring in minutes to hours.

What is the *most* likely cause of the diplopia?

a. a decompensating vertical phoria
b. the top of the bifocal segment covering part of the pupil
c. an epiretinal membrane with vertical foveal dragging and central diplopia
d. monocular diplopia from an early cataract

Discussion   It is very rare to have true strabismus with only 1.0 prism diopter of symptomatic vertical diplopia. Vertical fusional amplitudes are usually sufficient to compensate for such small vertical deviations. Monocular diplopia could be caused by the top of the bifocal segment covering part of the pupil, but the diplopia would persist when the other eye is closed, rather than disappear as in this patient. Monocular diplopia from an early cataract would likewise persist when the other eye is closed, and neither type of monocular diplopia would be relieved, even momentarily, with a prism taped to the glasses. The symptoms and findings in this patient are typical of mild vertical foveal dragging from an epiretinal membrane, chorioretinal scar, or laser treatment scar. A small degree of true binocular diplopia occurs in these patients in central vision only, with normal peripheral fusion maintaining ocular alignment in the rest of the visual field. Relief of the diplopia with low-power prisms is typically only temporary. Often there is no treatment possible for this condition, other than partial or complete occlusion.[8]

Preferred Response   c. an epiretinal membrane with vertical foveal dragging and central diplopia

OR8

Which of the following intraocular lens designs would be *most* affected by a 15° lens tilt?

a. convexoplano (convex anterior)
b. planoconvex (convex posterior)
c. biconvex
d. meniscus

Discussion   The intraocular lens design that minimizes spherical aberration and is least sensitive to lens tilt and decentration is the biconvex design.[9] The IOL design most sensitive to lens tilt and decentration is the meniscus design. A meniscus IOL can exhibit 2.00 to 3.00 D of induced astigmatism, shifting the refraction in a myopic direction from the original target refraction. This design may also limit visual acuity to less than 20/20 when tilted more than 15°. The easiest clinical method for detecting refractive astigmatism induced by IOL tilt is to compare the corneal astigmatism (determined by keratometry) and the refractive astigmatism (determined by refraction). If there is significant disparity in the magnitude and axis of astigmatism of these two measurements, the induced astigmatism from the tilted or decentered IOL must be significant. In the most severe cases, in which the visual acuity is limited by the poor optics, replacing the IOL is the only effective treatment.

Preferred Response   d. meniscus

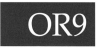

A 21-year-old male college student ruptured his penetrating keratoplasty incision 3 months ago in his right eye. Although this eye is beginning to stabilize after surgical repair, visual recovery is still incomplete. He reports several episodes of corneal abrasion on his left keratoconic eye.

You might attempt contact lens fitting for the left eye by using

a. disposable soft lens for comfort even though the vision would not be optimal
b. a reusable soft lens for comfort
c. a soft basement lens (reusable or disposable) with a rigid lens on top ("piggyback" system)
d. limited wearing time of a traditional gas-permeable lens

Discussion

Soft contact lenses alone, although comfortable, cannot provide adequate vision for the keratoconic eye. A traditional gas-permeable lens will not allow apical vaulting, whereas a keratoconus-style lens (Soper lens) might achieve this status. However, the patient has a low level of tolerance due to recurrent abrasions. A basement soft lens, either disposable or reusable, may provide the comfort level this patient requires. A rigid lens can then be designed to ride over the soft lens to provide for the rest of the optical needs (see the figure). This dual lens system ("piggyback") requires highly oxygen-transmissible materials.

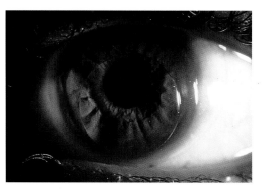

"Piggyback" system: soft basement disposable lens for daily wear with rigid gas-permeable lens on top.

Preferred Response

c. a soft basement lens (reusable or disposable) with a rigid lens on top ("piggyback" system)

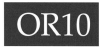

What trial reading add would be a good initial approximation in a base prescription for a patient who has a distance visual acuity in the range of 20/200?

a. +2.00 D lens
b. +5.00 D lens
c. +10.00 D lens
d. +20.00 D lens

Discussion   Low vision with subnormal visual acuity (or significantly abnormal visual fields) presents problems in vision that cannot be corrected by conventional spectacle lenses or contact lenses. Usually, a visual acuity of 20/70 or worse is considered low vision. In the initial attempt to find the correct lens for reading, one takes the reciprocal of the Snellen distance visual acuity (Kestenbaum's rule). Thus, with a distance visual acuity of 20/200, Kestenbaum's rule yields 200/20, so one would start a patient with a trial +10.00 D reading add, knowing that this amount of correction most likely underestimates the usual dioptric requirement for near work.[4,5,10]

Preferred Response   c. +10.00 D lens

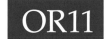

After cataract surgery with IOL implantation, a patient obtains a new plastic spectacle lens and complains of double vision through the reading segment. Which of the following is the *best* therapeutic approach?

a. Prescribe a slab-off prism based on calculations involving the powers of the pre- and postoperative spectacle lenses.
b. Prescribe a slab-off prism based on measurement of the vertical misalignment in down gaze.
c. Prescribe a reverse-slab prism based on calculations involving the powers of the pre- and postoperative spectacle lenses.
d. Prescribe a reverse-slab prism based on measurement of the vertical misalignment in down gaze.

Discussion   A change in the power of the vertical meridian from the preoperative spectacle lens to the postoperative spectacle lens can induce enough vertical prism in down gaze to cause symptomatic diplopia. A slab-off prism or reverse-slab prism can be prescribed to realign the eyes in down gaze. The amount of prism prescribed should be based on measurement of the deviation through the new spectacle lenses in down gaze, rather than on calculations involving the spectacle lens powers, for there is no guarantee that the patient's ocular alignment behind the glasses is the same in down gaze as in primary position. In fact, patients often adapt partially or fully ("orthophorization") to peripherally induced prism in anisometropic spectacle corrections, and the ophthalmologist cannot know the extent of this adaptation without measuring the residual deviation. Reverse-slab prisms are most commonly used with modern plastic spectacle lenses. For these the slab-off prism effect is ground off the mold, thus *adding* base-down prism effect to the lower portion of the molded plastic spectacle lens. The reverse-slab prism is generally put on the more plus, or less minus, spectacle lens rather than the other way around as for slab-off prisms.[11]

Preferred Response   d. Prescribe a reverse-slab prism based on measurement of the vertical misalignment in down gaze.

OR12

An aphakic patient with a refraction of +12.00 +3.00 × 180 at a vertex distance of 14 mm is considering a secondary implant. If the secondary implant surgery has no effect on the corneal astigmatism and the postoperative target is emmetropia, the expected postoperative refraction would be

a. plano
b. −1.50 +3.00 × 180
c. −1.50 +3.00 × 90
d. −2.25 +4.50 × 180

Discussion

The vertex distance of a refraction affects not only the magnitude of the sphere, but also the magnitude of the astigmatism.[1] It should be noted that this patient's aphakic refraction is actually +12.00 × 90 and +15.00 × 180 at a vertex distance of 14 mm. If this refraction is adjusted for the vertex distance to the plane of the cornea, the refraction would be +14.42 × 90 and +18.99 × 180, yielding an astigmatism of +4.57 × 180. In this aphakic patient, the final refraction should have a spheroequivalent of zero, and the astigmatism is approximately +4.50 × 180. The resultant refraction would be −2.25 +4.50 × 180. This effect is just the opposite for high myopia, in which the astigmatism at the corneal plane is *less* than the astigmatism at the spectacle plane.

Preferred Response

d. −2.25 +4.50 × 180

OR13

Which of the following statements about fixed-focus stand magnifiers is true?

a. To reduce peripheral aberrations, the lens is set closer to the page than its focal length. Therefore, a moderate reading add or accommodative effort is required to bring the image into focus.
b. When a patient is using a stand magnifier and a reading add, the combined power of the lens system is that of a simple lens system and can be determined by adding the powers of the add and the magnifier.
c. The field of a stand magnifier is not dependent on the viewing distance.
d. Stand magnifiers are less useful than hand magnifiers for patients who are tremulous.

Discussion

Stand magnifiers are commonly used in the rehabilitation of low-vision patients and have the advantages of a rigid lens mounting and a predictable focus. A fixed-focus stand magnifier lens has been set by the manufacturer closer to the page than its focal distance to reduce peripheral aberrations. The rays emerging from the stand magnifier are no longer parallel but divergent, requiring accommodative effort or a moderate reading add to bring the image into focus. The resultant virtual image is intended to be viewed from a normal distance (40 cm) with a +2.50 D add, although a stronger bifocal will also be effective at closer distances.

The magnification gained from using a stand magnifier and a reading add is always less than the sum of the two lenses because of the separation of the lenses. The field of the stand magnifier becomes greater when patients use a stronger reading add that allows them to get closer to the stand magnifier and thereby to gain a wider field. People with tremors or poor coordination may be uncomfortable holding an unsupported hand magnifier and may find it much easier to read with a fixed-focus stand magnifier.[5,10]

Preferred Response

a. To reduce peripheral aberrations, the lens is set closer to the page than its focal length. Therefore, a moderate reading add or accommodative effort is required to bring the image into focus.

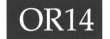

Which of the following statements about round-top bifocal segments is true?

a. They cause significant image jump on plus lenses but not on minus lenses.
b. They increase image displacement on plus lenses.
c. They are generally preferred over flat-top segments for use on minus lenses.
d. They are generally preferred for use on plus lenses.

Discussion

Round-top bifocal segments have their optical centers relatively far down on the lens, at the center of the round curve. This produces a base-down prism effect, especially at the top of the segment, where a significant image jump is produced whether the segment is placed on a plus lens or a minus lens. Adding the base-down, round-top segment to the base-down lower portion of a minus lens increases image displacement, whereas adding such a segment to the base-up lower portion of a plus lens decreases image displacement. For this reason, round-top segments are generally preferred for use on plus lenses, even though there is image jump. For most people, the image jump is less bothersome than image displacement.

Preferred Response

d. They are generally preferred for use on plus lenses.

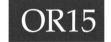

A 25-year-old patient presents with a refraction of −6.00 D in the right eye with 20/20 visual acuity and −9.00 D in the left eye with 20/200 visual acuity. The visual acuity has decreased in the left eye over the last year because of a traumatic cataract, and the refraction in the right eye has been stable for many years. The patient cannot tolerate contact lenses.

What should the target refraction be for the left eye?

a. plano
b. −0.50 D
c. −1.00 D
d. −4.50 D

Discussion

A patient with a refraction of −6.00 D in the right eye will not be able to tolerate a refraction more than 3.00 D different in the vertical meridian of that eye. Because there is some tolerance in the precision of the IOL calculation and final refraction in the left eye, most experts recommend targeting the refraction for 1.00 D or 2.00 D nearer emmetropia when there is a monocular cataract.[12] The primary reason for this limitation is the induced prism difference that is created in the vertical meridian by anisometropia, not the aniseikonia. It is possible to target for emmetropia or mild myopia if the patient can tolerate a contact lens or monovision. The ability to tolerate a contact lens or monovision must be determined preoperatively to avoid problems postoperatively. In this contact lens–intolerant patient, the only choice is to target for −4.00 D to −5.00 D of myopia.

Preferred Response

d. −4.50 D

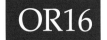

Which of the following statements about chromatic aberration of prisms, lenses, or the eye is true?

a. It represents a well-known exception to Snell's law, with different angles of refraction occurring with the same angle of incidence.
b. It causes the blue rays to come into focus anterior to the red rays in the eye (closer to the crystalline lens).
c. It is minimized in spectacle lenses by using high-index glass or plastic.
d. It is the basis of the duochrome (red-green) test commonly used for binocular balancing.

Discussion

Blue rays are refracted more strongly than red rays by prisms and lenses, because the refractive index is different for different wavelengths of light. Snell's law is inviolate. The eye has a large amount of chromatic aberration (1.50 D to 3.00 D, depending on the spectral range measured), with the blue rays coming into focus anterior to the red rays. High-index glass or plastic lenses usually have high values of dispersion (the change of refractive index with wavelength) and thus have more chromatic aberration than ordinary glass or plastic spectacle lenses. With high-index lenses, colored fringes are often seen on bright objects when they are viewed through the periphery of the lenses. The duochrome (red-green) test exploits the chromatic aberration of the eye for refinement of the spherical component of refraction under monocular conditions; it is inappropriate to use for binocular balancing.

Preferred Response

b. It causes the blue rays to come into focus anterior to the red rays in the eye (closer to the crystalline lens).

All of the following are good indications for rigid bifocal contact lenses *except*

a. successful monovision (one contact lens at reading refraction and one contact lens at distance refraction)
b. previous successful contact lens wear
c. normal external examination
d. failure of monovision

Discussion

While presbyopic contact lens corrections are a compromise as compared with spectacles, the increased availability of better lens designs improves the chances for successful fitting. Alternating and simultaneous designs (see the figure) in various rigid materials are now available. Alternating designs rely on translation of the lens to move the appropriate lens segment in front of the pupil. In primary gaze, the top of the near segment sits at or below the pupil so that it does not interfere with distance viewing. When near vision is needed, the eye is lowered and the lower eyelid holds the lens, pushing it up slightly so that near vision is available.

Careful attention to refractive error, occupational demands, and realistic expectations coupled with fitting experience may help to identify such situations as a hyperopic patient who accepts an aspheric design when progressive add power might be better tolerated because of a latent hyperopia. Myopic patients often prefer binocularity and may not accept a monovision approach; they would be better satisfied with a true bifocal design. Those patients who are already happy with monovision are less likely to become candidates for bifocal lenses.

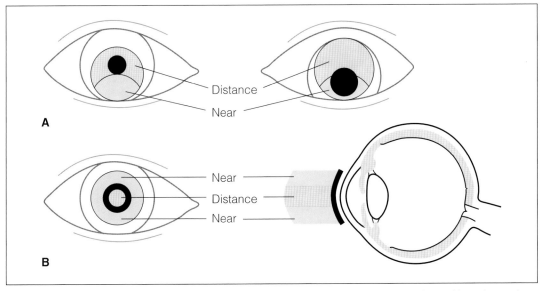

Rigid bifocal contact lens designs. **(A)** For alternating vision, the distance segment is positioned over the pupil (left); as the patient looks down toward the reading position, the lower lid pushes up the contact lens so that the near segment covers the pupil for reading (right). **(B)** For simultaneous vision, the distance (or near) optical portion of the lens is made smaller than the pupil so that light rays from distance and near pass through the pupil simultaneously. The lens wearer chooses either the central portion of the lens for distance vision or the peripheral portion for near vision.

Preferred Response

a. successful monovision (one contact lens at reading refraction and one contact lens at distance refraction)

OR18

For a physician not currently performing low-vision examinations, what is required to initiate low-vision services in a private office?

a. a well-stocked low-vision cabinet, costing several thousand dollars, containing most of the magnification devices
b. a technician trained in low-vision services
c. a preassembled low-vision kit, costing several hundred dollars, available through retail outlets
d. closed-circuit television aids

Discussion

Low-vision services begin with the prescribing of bifocals above a +3.00 D add. All ophthalmologists have the essential skills to provide basic and uncomplicated low-vision services. New and established ophthalmologists, even if they do not wish to provide low-vision services on a regular basis, are able to help many of their low-vision patients by using a pre-assembled, inexpensive low-vision kit that contains basic magnifiers, illuminated devices, and high-plus spectacles. This kit enables them to treat many of their low-vision patients in the office, while sending some patients with more serious problems to a low-vision referral center.[5,10]

Preferred Response

c. a preassembled low-vision kit, costing several hundred dollars, available through retail outlets

OR19

A patient complains of a starburst pattern and haze around lights at night with her pseudophakic eye. Her vision is correctable to 20/50. The pupil dilates to 8 mm, revealing an opacified posterior capsule. A 2 mm Nd:YAG laser posterior capsulotomy is subsequently performed and the patient's visual acuity returns to 20/20. Although her symptoms improve, she still complains of haze and starburst with oncoming headlights at night.

The *most* likely cause is

a. IOL optically damaged with the Nd:YAG laser
b. capsular opening too small for scotopic pupil
c. vitreous floaters in visual axis
d. positioning holes in IOL optic within the capsular opening

Discussion

A starburst image can only be produced by some alteration in the optical system of the eye that results in a Bagolini lens effect, such as proliferating lens fibers on the posterior capsule.[13,14] The streaks will be oriented transverse to the axis of the proliferating fibers. In this patient, the most likely cause of the persistent starburst image at night is a capsular opening too small for the scotopic pupil. Optically, the opening in the posterior capsule should be as large as the scotopic pupil to avoid any remaining light scatter. Mechanically, however, this size opening may not be safe to create because the opening should never extend beyond the perimeter of the IOL to avoid allowing vitreous into the anterior chamber and/or weakening of the support for the IOL. The typical limit is therefore approximately 4 to 5 mm. Pitting an intraocular lens with the Nd:YAG laser causes wide-angle, diffuse glare that makes lights appear to have a diffuse halo. Vitreous floaters will cause shadows of varying intensity, depending on the proximity of the floater to the retina, ie, the closer to the retina, the darker the floater. The patient will also notice movement of the floater and fading away over time. When positioning holes in an IOL are within the capsular opening, the patient sees additional images of a point for every positioning hole.[15] For example, if four holes are exposed, the patient will see four additional pinpoint images around a light. Because of the problems with positioning holes, the posterior capsule should never be opened in a manner that would expose a positioning hole. Gradual opacification of the capsule behind these positioning holes sometimes causes these unwanted images to disappear with time after cataract surgery.

Preferred Response   b. capsular opening too small for scotopic pupil

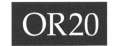

Moving a plus spectacle lens forward (away from the cornea) when viewing a distant object

a. decreases the size of the retinal image
b. cannot be compensated for by an increase in accommodation
c. decreases the effective plus power of the lens
d. will blur objects viewed at intermediate distances

Discussion   Moving a plus spectacle lens forward moves its secondary focal point forward as well, increasing the effective plus power of the lens when viewing a distant object. Because accommodation can only add plus power, increased accommodation cannot compensate for this increase in the effective plus power of the spectacle lens. The increased effective plus power will bring intermediate-distance objects into better focus. The retinal image of the distant object will become blurred but will also increase in size because of the increased Galilean-telescope effect when the plus lens is moved forward.

Preferred Response   b. cannot be compensated for by an increase in accommodation

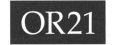

A 42-year-old male with a history of severe diabetic retinopathy has had secondary glaucoma and enucleation of his left eye. He presents in your office with an extended-wear aphakic soft lens in place that has not been removed for many months because of lack of family support. The patient's refraction is +11.75 D sphere to correct visual acuity to 20/40. His keratometric readings are spherical, and the mire images are free of distortion. His current soft contact lens corrects his visual acuity to 20/60.

The *best* approach to provide a safer fitting regimen as well as to improve vision would be

a. aphakic spectacles
b. disposable soft contact lens
c. gas-permeable contact lens
d. extended-wear soft contact lens of corrected power

Discussion

The risk/benefit rationale for fitting a diabetic patient with contact lenses must be carefully weighed. Aphakic spectacles might be an option, but limiting the field of vision for this monocular patient would not be satisfactory. Disposable soft contact lenses are not currently available in this high-plus power range, and extended-wear soft lenses would continue to leave the patient at risk for developing ulcerative keratitis. With careful attention to handling technique, the patient could be taught to insert, remove, and care for a tinted daily-wear gas-permeable lens. Better oxygenation, improved corneal health, and reduced risk of infection make the gas-permeable contact lens the best choice for overall visual rehabilitation.

Preferred Response

c. gas-permeable contact lens

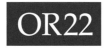

A 26-year-old emmetrope with ocular albinism, foveal hypoplasia, and moderate low vision has visual acuities of 20/200 in each eye separately but 20/140 visual acuity binocularly. His preferred reading distance is 8 cm, but he complains of significant eye fatigue and headaches. For near reading performance, the preferred low-vision aid is

a. a +12.00 D aspheric spectacle
b. a +10.00 D prismatic half-eye spectacle
c. a high-add bifocal (+5.00 D) on a plano carrier
d. a hand-held 4× magnifier

Discussion

A brisk reading speed at 8 to 10 cm is common with foveal hypoplasia. Since this patient is binocular, a low-vision aid that incorporates the improved bifoveal performance is preferred. A hand-held magnifier is helpful for spotting isolated images but is limited for sustained reading by the restricted visual field and the movement artifact. A +12.00 D aspheric spectacle, although correctly powered for 8 cm (assuming no accommodative amplitude), must be used monocularly because of lost accommodative convergence and thus offers only 20/200 best-corrected visual acuity in this patient. A high-add bifocal still requires 7.00 D of accommodation and again diminishes the convergence amplitude necessary for bifoveal reading. The off-the-shelf +10.00 D prismatic half-eye spectacle with 12 prism diopters base-in provides sufficient optical convergence while permitting bifoveal viewing in the 10 cm and closer range.[4,5,16]

Preferred Response

b. a +10.00 D prismatic half-eye spectacle

OR23

An uncorrected bilateral 2.00 D hyperope with an accommodative amplitude of 3.00 D

a. will probably have asthenopic symptoms, even for distance vision
b. will see comfortably at 40 cm with single-vision reading glasses of +1.50 D
c. has a far point 50 cm in front of the eyes
d. has a near point 20 cm in front of the eyes

Discussion

A 2.00 D hyperopic eye has a virtual far point 50 cm behind the eye. Of the 3.00 D accommodative amplitude, 2.00 D will be used in neutralizing the hyperopia to focus clearly at infinity. Only 1.00 D of accommodative power remains to try to focus on near objects, but this brings the near point to only 1 m in front of the eyes. With +1.50 D single-vision reading glasses, the patient will be able to see clearly at 40 cm but only when exerting maximal accommodation. A well-accepted rule of thumb is that only half of the accommodative amplitude can be sustained comfortably for near tasks. This amount of accommodation will leave this patient still "focused" 0.50 D beyond infinity. The patient will most likely be asthenopic even for distance viewing, and single-vision reading glasses of +3.00 D will be necessary for comfortable reading at 40 cm (+0.50 D to overcome the residual hyperopia and +2.50 D to focus from infinity to 40 cm).

Preferred Response

a. will probably have asthenopic symptoms, even for distance vision

OR24

A 20.0 D biconvex IOL is tilted 20° about the vertical axis (90°). This situation would result in which of the following spectacle prescriptions if the patient were emmetropic with no lens tilt?

a. $-0.75 -2.00 \times 90$
b. $-0.75 +2.00 \times 90$
c. $+0.75 -2.00 \times 90$
d. $+0.75 +2.00 \times 90$

Discussion

Any lens tilted about an axis will increase the power of the lens and induce an astigmatism about that axis with the same sign as the lens.[1] An intraocular lens tilted about the vertical axis would therefore increase in its effective plus power and induce a plus astigmatism at an axis of 90°. For a 20.0 D biconvex IOL, the induced astigmatism is approximately 0.50 D for a 10° tilt, 2.00 D for a 20° tilt, and 5.00 D for a 30° tilt. The increase in the spherical magnitude is approximately one-third of these amounts for the respective lens tilt.[12] The intraocular lens would therefore induce a reading of +0.75 +2.00 × 90 in this patient. The corrective lens in the spectacle must have the opposite sign to neutralize the induced sphere and cylinder. The final spectacle prescription would thus be −0.75 −2.00 × 90 or −2.75 +2.00 × 180.

Preferred Response

a. $-0.75 -2.00 \times 90$

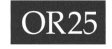

A 68-year-old woman presents with age-related macular degeneration, atrophic foveae with 20/200 visual acuity, +3.50 D of hyperopia, and moderate cataract with heavy vacuoles and mild posterior subcapsular opacities. Regarding the low-vision aspects of cataract surgery in this individual, which of the following is *least* accurate?

a. Worsening of cataract symptoms and functional impairment with increased illumination is common and helps to justify cataract surgery.
b. Leaving the patient aphakic and thus wearing aphakic spectacles will give 25% image magnification and enhance low-vision performance.
c. Selecting IOL power for a –2.50 D target postoperative refraction is functionally preferred over emmetropia.
d. With nuclear sclerosis, the addition of mild posterior subcapsular cataract changes or vacuoles can significantly and disproportionately increase the cataract's effect on functional vision.

Discussion

Cataract surgery can often help low-vision patients who are troubled by lenticular glare and reduced contrast sensitivity along the edge of the macular scotoma. Mild increases in needed illumination can constrict a pupil and can aggravate intraocular light scatter. At the same time, subtle worsening of the cataract can amplify the cataract symptoms. In addition, 20/200 visual acuity with hyperopia complicates low-vision adaptation because spectacle-induced aberrations from higher plus lenses—which are required to neutralize the hyperopia and then to focus the image very close—are often poorly tolerated. Choosing a myopic postoperative refraction is more favorable, offers casual near-point focus, facilitates higher plus adds, and does not interfere with peripheral visual acuity or with mobility. Although aphakic spectacles classically provide 25% image enlargement, the near acuity with aphakic bifocal adds or additional high-plus lenses significantly handicaps low-vision adaptation and prevents a glasses-free option for less demanding close activities such as hygiene, grooming, and routine mobility.[4,10]

Preferred Response

b. Leaving the patient aphakic and thus wearing aphakic spectacles will give 25% image magnification and enhance low-vision performance.

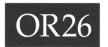

A 31-year-old patient with soft contact lenses in place has an initial corrected visual acuity of 20/400 OU. She wears glasses over her lenses for the rest of her needed correction to provide a best-corrected visual acuity of 20/50 OD and 20/80 OS. She had worn gas-permeable contact lenses 2 years ago but, because of protein buildup, was converted to soft contact lenses. She was advised that her astigmatism would make glasses necessary to refine her vision. Her refraction OD is –16.75 +2.00 × 105 to achieve 20/20 +2; refraction OS is –17.25 +2.00 × 75 to achieve 20/20. Keratometry reveals readings of OD 48.12 D × 93°/46.12 D × 3°, OS 50.00 D × 74°/48.00 D × 164°. Biomicroscopy confirms no corneal thinning. Computerized corneal analysis displays a pattern of with-the-rule astigmatism. The remainder of her ophthalmologic exam is unremarkable.

This patient can *best* be helped visually by

a. keratoconic-design gas-permeable contact lenses
b. reverse-aspheric gas-permeable contact lenses
c. hyperflange gas-permeable contact lenses aided by spectacles
d. hyperflange gas-permeable contact lenses

Discussion

Although some soft contact lens manufacturers do provide spherical power up to about –20.00 D, this patient's findings suggest the need for a custom toric soft lens. However, delivery time would be several weeks. The keratometric readings reveal steep corneas but all data suggest no evidence of keratoconus. The reverse-aspheric design is used in an attempt to provide an optimal lens-cornea relationship for the refractive surgical results after radial keratotomy. The more powerful lens requirements of aphakia or extreme high myopia require special edge flanges. The edge of the contact lens is ground to the opposite of the lens power. A myopic carrier is added to an aphakic lens (myoflange) and a hyperopic carrier is added to a myopic lens (hyperflange). High-myopic gas-permeable contact lenses could be designed with the full correction in the lenses without the need for spectacles for full distance correction.

Preferred Response

d. hyperflange gas-permeable contact lenses

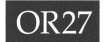

An elderly patient with age-related macular degeneration, parkinsonism, and 20/200 visual acuity in her better eye wishes to keep and wear her current +3.00 D add bifocals and resists holding material closer than 25 cm. The low-vision aid *most* likely to be accepted for near work (such as reading bills or writing) is

a. +4.00 D prismatic half-eye spectacles
b. 4× open-stand magnifier
c. 6× hand-held aspheric magnifier
d. 2.8× loupe hung on the current spectacles over the better eye

Discussion

Since this patient desires to use her current spectacles, prismatic half-eye spectacles are excluded. Parkinsonism results in tremulous upper extremities, neck and head motion, and impaired oculomotor tracking. A hand-held magnifier is thus problematic, as is a telescopic device mounted on her spectacles, because these devices would produce exaggerated movement artifact with each tremor. A self-supporting stand magnifier (see the figure on page 306) is excellent in a monocular situation, offering stability and adequate image size for 20/200 visual acuity and permitting discrete near tasks such as those mentioned. The open side allows handwriting under magnification.[4,5,10]

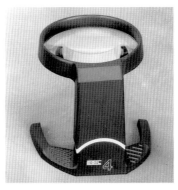

Stand magnifier with stable viewing configuration and side opening for external illumination and under-lens writing.

Preferred Response   b. 4× open-stand magnifier

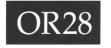

Which of the following is true about an eye that has a spherical cornea but has 1.00 D of with-the-rule simple myopic astigmatism after cataract and IOL surgery?

a. The intraocular lens is undoubtedly tilted about its vertical axis.
b. The astigmatism can be decreased by loosening one or more sutures in the horizontal meridian if the wound has been closed in that manner.
c. The astigmatism can be corrected with a minus cylinder with its axis placed vertically.
d. The patient may not desire any correction of the astigmatism.

Discussion   With a spherical cornea, with-the-rule astigmatism can only arise because the IOL is tilted forward or backward about its horizontal axis, thus inducing increased plus power in the vertical meridian. This astigmatism could be decreased by loosening sutures in the vertical meridian, if such sutures have been placed. If a minus cylinder is used for correction, its axis will have to be placed horizontally. This amount of simple myopic astigmatism is close to the optimal amount for the best compromise between distance and near vision with pseudophakia,[17] and the patient may not wish any additional correction at all.

Preferred Response   d. The patient may not desire any correction of the astigmatism.

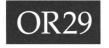

A 43-year-old man underwent bilateral radial keratotomy in 1982. He suffered significant overcorrection of the left eye, creating unacceptable anisometropia, which was corrected by soft contact lenses in both eyes. Neovascularization of two of the superior radial incisions—at the 11 and 1 o'clock positions—occurred in the left eye. Subsequently, large-diameter, rigid gas-permeable lenses were fitted but eventually they were discontinued because of concerns about further superior neovascularization. After discontinuation of these lenses, a circumferential-incision suturing procedure was performed in the left eye in an effort to reduce the patient's residual left hyperopia. This procedure was not successful, and several suture knots are still buried in the stroma. The patient's current refraction OD is +2.25 −0.25 × 151 to achieve 20/20, and OS is +8.50 −0.50 × 156 to achieve 20/25. He is an emerging presbyope and is using reading glasses. This patient is a private pilot and needs to maintain binocular vision.

Which of the following nonsurgical options could be used to achieve binocularity?

a. spectacles with less plus correction for the left eye
b. disposable soft contact lenses aided by glasses for residual correction
c. a single soft contact lens for the left eye and reading glasses
d. gas-permeable contact lenses with reverse-curve design aided by reading glasses

Discussion

Because of the degree of anisometropia, spectacles alone will not provide maximum vision for this patient. Soft contact lenses, whether reusable or disposable, are less acceptable due to the superior neovascularization of the left cornea. Gas-permeable contact lenses with reverse peripheral curves allow for steeper-than-normal secondary curves (usually 2.00 D) that aid in stability of fit and also allow for a wide power range to maximize full visual potential. These lenses can be fabricated in a material of high oxygen permeability and designed to ride more inferiorly to minimize further superior corneal insult (see the figures). Reading glasses could be used for near vision requirements.

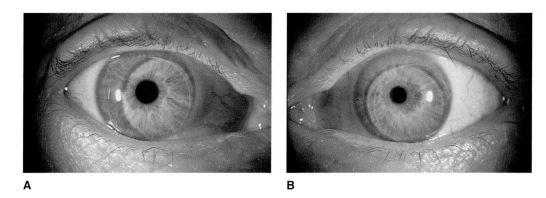

A   **B**

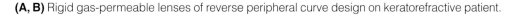

(A, B) Rigid gas-permeable lenses of reverse peripheral curve design on keratorefractive patient.

Preferred Response

d. gas-permeable contact lenses with reverse-curve design aided by reading glasses

OR30

Regarding general low-vision rehabilitation, which of the following is *least* effective?

a. repositioning and enlarging the available visual field using selective prisms
b. increasing angular magnification by moving the object closer to the lens
c. enhancing target contrast by manipulating background color and object saturation
d. augmenting the illumination source with greater wattage and broader-spectrum output

Discussion

The essential means for low-vision enhancement are magnification (optical aids or electronic devices), improved contrast (by selecting background versus object colors or by electronically manipulating text), and greater illumination (more light yields more retinal detail). Repositioning and enlarging the available visual field with prisms or using reverse telescopic devices to expand the field (causing image size to decrease) both have significant drawbacks with few benefits and have very limited acceptance by patients.[5,10,16]

Preferred Response

a. repositioning and enlarging the available visual field using selective prisms

OR31

Surgical loupes are designed for a given working distance. This working distance may be

a. increased by omitting habitual myopic correction in the surgeon's glasses
b. increased by adding a plus lens to the front of the loupe
c. increased by adding a plus lens to the rear of the loupe
d. effectively increased by choosing a lower-power loupe with the same nominal working distance

Discussion

A surgical loupe may be thought of as a Galilean telescope with a reading add on the front, with the focal length of the reading add being equal to the nominal working distance of the loupe. Adding a plus lens anywhere in the system (or omitting the myopic correction in the surgeon's glasses) will *decrease* the working distance. If one thinks of light traveling backward from a point on the retina, the place where light comes to focus through the loupe establishes the working distance. Adding plus power will pull this point of focus against the light, thus decreasing the working distance. Lower-power telescopes have a greater depth of field than higher-power telescopes, so choosing a lower-power loupe will allow the surgeon to sit slightly farther from the patient and still keep the operative field in focus.

Preferred Response

d. effectively increased by choosing a lower-power loupe with the same nominal working distance

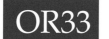

The fabricated add on a −15.00 D pair of spectacles is +2.00. The 45-year-old patient complains that near vision is still blurry. The glasses are measured on a lensmeter with the posterior surface against the lensmeter, and the add is measured to be +1.50 D. Why is the measured add weaker than the prescription?

a. The optician made the add power incorrectly.
b. The effective add is always less than the fabricated add in high-minus glasses.
c. The effective add is always less than the fabricated add in high-plus glasses.
d. Image minification by high-minus lenses causes the effective add and the fabricated add to be different.

Discussion

The correct method for measuring bifocal spectacles is to measure the distance correction using the posterior vertex, but the add should be measured by (1) turning the glasses around and measuring the front vertex power, (2) finding the power at the center of the add, and then (3) subtracting to find the difference. In prescriptions of less than ±4.00 D, the effect is negligible. Between 4.00 D and 8.00 D, there is approximately 0.25 D difference between the fabricated add and the effective add. For lenses between 8.00 D and 12.00 D, the disparity is approximately 0.50 D. For plus lenses the effective add is always greater than the fabricated add, and for minus lenses it is just the opposite.[1] In this patient with high myopia, the effective add is less than the fabricated add. For this reason, in aphakic spectacles the average add is approximately +2.50 D whereas in pseudophakic spectacles, in which the patient is near plano, the add averages +3.00 D. The clinician must keep this difference in mind when writing a prescription to make sure the patient gets the correct effective add. Also, since patients vary in their working distance for various tasks, each patient should be checked for the proper near add at the specific working distance.

Preferred Response

b. The effective add is always less than the fabricated add in high-minus glasses.

OR33

Neutralization of the retinoscopic reflex with the streak retinoscope and trial lenses

a. places the far point of the combination of the patient's eye and the trial lenses at infinity
b. locates the far point of the patient
c. is not affected by the patient's accommodation
d. places the circle of least confusion on the retina

Discussion

Neutralization of the retinoscopic reflex with the streak retinoscope and trial lenses locates the far point of the patient's eye by moving the far point of the eye/lenses combination to the peephole of the retinoscope. Later, mathematical compensation for the working distance will place the far point of the eye/lenses combination at the far wall or at infinity. The patient's accommodation interferes diopter-per-diopter with the retinoscopic finding, but the examiner's refractive error does not interfere at all provided that the examiner can clearly see the patient's pupil. The concept of the circle of least confusion is neither useful nor used when performing or analyzing retinoscopy. Rather, the conoid of Sturm is collapsed by bringing each focal line to the retina in turn.

Preferred Response

b. locates the far point of the patient

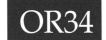

When a patient cannot read the 20/400 line on a standard eye chart at the standard distance, what should the ophthalmologist do?

  a. Measure the visual acuity by having the patient count fingers at the maximum distance possible.
  b. Obtain a numeric visual acuity score by testing with a chart at a closer distance.
  c. Record the visual acuity as "less than 20/400."
  d. Record the visual acuity as "hand movements only."

Discussion

Accurate visual acuity assessment is of great value in predicting functional implications of vision loss and in predicting the magnification devices that may allow a person to read and do other detail discrimination tasks. Counting fingers notation is inherently inaccurate, as it actually covers a wide range of measurable visual acuity scores. Visual acuity can be repeatedly and accurately measured to as low as 20/1000 by moving a letter chart closer to the patient.[4,5,10]

Preferred Response

b. Obtain a numeric visual acuity score by testing with a chart at a closer distance.

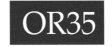

Because of the large optical corrections required for extremely high-myopic patients, glasses have poor cosmetic appearance and limited function (see the figure). Yet the manufacturing limitations of contact lenses also make them challenging for realizing the full visual potential.

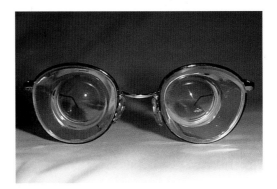

High-myopic spectacles are cosmetically unacceptable to many patients.

An example of best design and usage would be

a. spherical soft contact lenses aided by glasses
b. tinted soft contact lenses aided by glasses
c. tinted gas-permeable contact lenses with special edge design
d. hybrid contact lenses with rigid center and soft skirt

Discussion

Mass-produced soft contact lenses are limited for spherical correction beyond –20.00 D. Custom soft lenses can be obtained beyond this power, as well as for any cylinder power needed up to 16.00 D, but they become increasingly difficult both to manufacture and obtain. Replacement lenses for these designs often require a wait of at least 2 weeks. The hybrid contact lens design—a rigid center with a soft skirt—is not currently available in extremely high powers (over –20.00 D). However, gas-permeable designs are obtainable (see the figures below). Careful attention to proper contact lens design by using lenticulation and plus carriers in combination with tinted polymers of varying oxygen permeability can provide a safe and effective fit, achieving best vision with minimal delays for replacement in case of loss or damage. Most laboratories will provide overnight delivery within 1 to 2 days of request, once American National Standards Institute (ANSI) fabrication standards are met.

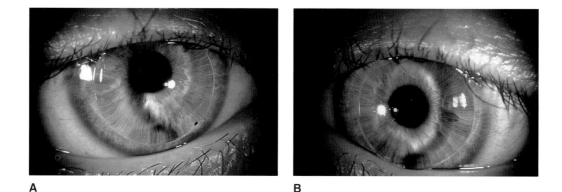

A　　　　　　　　　　　　　　**B**

(A, B) Gas-permeable contact lenses with special edge design can be worn successfully by many patients with extremely high myopia.

Preferred Response

c. tinted gas-permeable contact lenses with special edge design

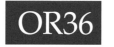

A patient who wears rigid gas-permeable contact lenses has developed bilateral posterior subcapsular cataracts that have decreased the visual acuity to 20/60 OU. Keratometry readings and axial lengths are measured for IOL calculations. The K readings are spherical at 45.00 D for each eye with no irregularity; the axial lengths are 23.5 mm. The contact lenses were fitted elsewhere so pre–contact lens K readings are unavailable.

For this patient, it would be appropriate to

a. use the present spherical K readings and recommended IOL powers
b. discontinue the contact lenses for 24 hours and repeat K readings
c. discontinue the contact lenses for 1 week, repeat K readings, and use the average of the two measurements
d. discontinue the contact lenses and repeat K readings weekly until stable (two consecutive measurements the same)

Discussion

Rigid contact lenses can significantly alter the corneal power and consequently the K readings for several weeks. Most studies have shown that corneal power stabilizes by 3 weeks, but in some patients who have been wearing these lenses for many years the corneal power may not stabilize for even longer. The only way to be certain that the cornea is no longer changing is to establish that the K readings are the same in consecutive measurements. In most cases, the rigid contact lens temporarily increases the power of the cornea, so that if these K readings are used the patient will shift in a hyperopic direction as the cornea stabilizes, causing a hyperopic error in the actual postoperative refraction. Because hyperopic errors following cataract surgery are poorly tolerated, serious problems can result if an accurate K reading is not identified preoperatively.[12]

Preferred Response

d. discontinue the contact lenses and repeat K readings weekly until stable (two consecutive measurements the same)

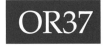

A 75-year-old man has a stable but profound reduction in vision, having previously developed subfoveal choroidal neovascular membranes in both eyes. His best-corrected visual acuity is 20/480 in each eye. A central visual field defect with a diameter of approximately 7° is noted in both eyes. The peripheral visual field is intact.

All of the following statements are true *except*

a. The patient may be able to read continuous text by using a video magnifier (closed-circuit television).
b. The patient's ability to use residual vision may be improved by training in eccentric viewing techniques.
c. A +10.00 D add would be the minimum add necessary to resolve 20/40 near vision (newsprint size, Jaeger 3, or 1M in metric system).
d. The patient may experience difficulty with negotiating street crossings and have other mobility concerns.

Discussion

Individuals with profound visual impairment may still be able to read continuous text with a video magnifier (closed-circuit television), which allows a high level of magnification with good luminescence and contrast enhancement. After a central scotoma develops in an elderly patient, skills in using an eccentric location for fixation can be improved by training and practice; considerable plasticity still exists in the geriatric visual system. Kestenbaum's rule states that the reciprocal of the visual acuity gives the theoretical minimum add, ie, 480/20 or +24.00 D. Therefore, a patient with 20/480 visual acuity would require a minimum of a +24.00 D add to resolve typical newsprint (20/40, J3, 1M). A patient with a full peripheral field may still have significant mobility problems. A decrease in central visual acuity or visual field will often decrease a person's confidence with routine mobility tasks and orientation in new environments.[10]

Preferred Response

c. A +10.00 D add would be the minimum add necessary to resolve 20/40 near vision (newsprint size, Jaeger 3, or 1M in metric system).

OR38

A patient who wants to be fitted with contact lenses has a spectacle refraction of −8.00 +3.00 × 90 bilaterally and K readings of 45.00 D × 90°/42.50 D × 180° bilaterally. Which type of lens would be *most* appropriate?

a. a bitoric, rigid gas-permeable contact lens
b. a soft, nontoric, disposable contact lens
c. a spherical, rigid gas-permeable contact lens
d. a toric soft contact lens without prism ballast

Discussion

The astigmatism in the spectacle refraction (3.00 D) arises primarily from the cornea (2.50 D). Since astigmatism accompanying high-minus corrections measures less at the cornea than in the spectacle plane (the reverse is true for astigmatism accompanying aphakia), a spherical, rigid gas-permeable contact lens will neutralize the corneal astigmatism completely and a bitoric design is not required. A spherical soft contact lens will mold itself to the cornea and will not correct the corneal astigmatism. Adding a toric front surface to the soft contact lens will work but not without prism ballast to keep the lens from rotating.

Preferred Response

c. a spherical, rigid gas-permeable contact lens

OR39

An 8-year-old phakic boy has a quiet eye following repair of traumatic corneal laceration. His fellow eye is emmetropic. An aspheric gas-permeable contact lens has been suggested to correct the moderate amount of irregular astigmatism of the injured eye.

Which of the following would be a reasonable choice for providing best visual acuity with adequate protection for both eyes?

a. spectacles only; too young for contact lens
b. soft toric contact lens with ultraviolet protection
c. gas-permeable contact lens during school hours only
d. ultraviolet-absorbing gas-permeable contact lens worn with sports goggles for outside activities

Discussion

As long as the injured eye is otherwise healthy and the ocular surface is stable, age is not a factor in lens selection. While soft contact lens manufacturers are now incorporating ultraviolet protection into spherical lenses, soft toric ultraviolet-absorbing lenses are not yet available. Ultraviolet protection is available in rigid contact lens designs but part-time wear is impractical and unnecessary. Researchers have documented that sunlight causes damage to every part of the eye that absorbs it. Photokeratoconjunctivitis, pinguecula and pterygium, nodular band keratopathy, cataract, solar retinopathy, and macular degeneration are some of the known sunlight-related diseases. Visual corrections, whether spectacles or contact lenses, should therefore contain ultraviolet absorbers when available. Ambient light from around the sides and top of glasses or sunglasses will still reach the eyes. The dark lenses of sunglasses cause the pupils to dilate, allowing even more light to enter the eye. In this patient, as well as in any non-injury patient, an ultraviolet-absorbing rigid contact lens can be designed to be worn with sports goggles during athletic events. The polycarbonate lenses in the sports goggles not only provide protection from physical contact but also have additional built-in protection from ultraviolet radiation.

Preferred Response   d. ultraviolet-absorbing gas-permeable contact lens worn with sports goggles for outside activities

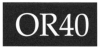

A 75-year-old man with atrophic age-related macular degeneration has a visual acuity of 20/70 in both eyes. As a retired newspaper editor, he expresses great frustration with his inability to read the newspaper; he can see the characters on a page but has difficulty making the letters into words and words into sentences. After completing a line of text, he has difficulty finding the next line at the left margin; he frequently finds he is rereading the same line or has missed a line of text. His reading rate is too slow to make reading enjoyable. He has tried using magnifiers but they have not helped much.

The *most* likely cause of his reading difficulty is

a. early dementia
b. ring scotoma surrounding fixation
c. insufficient magnification
d. a poor attitude

Discussion   Patients who have greater difficulty reading than might be expected from their visual acuity alone may have a ring scotoma surrounding central fixation. Stronger magnification often enlarges letters onto the scotomatous retina, worsening the functional symptoms. Recent studies have shown that 17% of all patients with low vision have their fixation located within a central island of vision with a diameter of less than 5° and surrounded by an absolute or relative scotoma. Individual motivation or cognitive skills will affect visual performance and reading stamina, but these issues should not be considered too early in the evaluation.[10]

Preferred Response   b. ring scotoma surrounding fixation

OR41

Which low-vision enhancement technique would be expected to offer the *greatest* benefit for the patient in Question OR40?

a. enhancing magnification by using loupes for near tasks
b. adjusting image contrast with a closed-circuit television that uses reverse-polarity letter projection and computer-sharpened image enhancements
c. increasing illumination with a broad-spectrum fluorescent light
d. arranging for Library of Congress books on tape for auditory access to printed material

Discussion

As discussed previously, magnification of reading material is problematic when letters are enlarged onto scotomatous retinal areas surrounding central fixation. Contrast enhancement through closed-circuit television image refinement and reverse-character polarity yields improved visual processing without inducing glare or magnification problems. Increased illumination, frequently valuable to the low-vision patient, offers modest gains in functional reading performance; often the patient is already using maximum-wattage lightbulbs in work areas. Some low-vision patients prefer broad-spectrum fluorescent light sources while others prefer incandescent. The Library of Congress produces books on tape but does not have equivalent resources for contemporary news.[5,10]

Preferred Response

b. adjusting image contrast with a closed-circuit television that uses reverse-polarity letter projection and computer-sharpened image enhancements

OR42

A patient with age-related macular degeneration has developed nuclear sclerotic cataracts. The best-corrected visual acuity in each eye is counting fingers at 1 foot, but with the potential acuity meter the retinal acuity is 20/200. Current spectacles and best refraction are nearly plano. The *best* target for the postoperative refraction would be

a. target +8.00 D so that the patient can get magnification from the high-plus glasses
b. target plano to give the best-uncorrected visual acuity
c. target −3.00 D to provide near vision with no significant effect on distance acuity
d. use negative IOL to create a Galilean telescope with high-plus glasses

Discussion

Targeting the refraction for +8.00 D would be similar to leaving the patient aphakic. The slight amount of magnification (+16%) is not even enough to increase the visual acuity by one line (each line on the Snellen acuity chart represents +25%). Furthermore, the problems with ring scotoma, jack-in-the-box phenomenon, and pincushion distortion are very annoying and far outweigh the effects of the magnification. Using a negative IOL simply exaggerates this condition and does not work well either. Because the patient's retina is only capable of 20/200 acuity, the distance acuity will not be affected by up to 3.00 D of myopia. In addition, this correction will allow the patient to hold things very close with normal reading glasses (+4.00 D). For working distances at arm's length, the eye is already in best focus with no correction. Targeting for plano does not give the patient an optical advantage at intermediate and near distances.[18]

Preferred Response

c. target −3.00 D to provide near vision with no significant effect on distance acuity

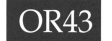

After cataract and IOL surgery, an eye has a refraction of −1.00 +1.50 × 90 and K readings of 43.00 D/43.00 D. The astigmatism may be caused by

a. decentration of the IOL
b. an eccentric pupil
c. a tilted IOL
d. a tilted retina

Discussion

A decentered intraocular lens causes only prismatic displacement, not astigmatism. When an eccentric pupil restricts the light to an eccentric portion of the IOL, no astigmatism is caused because the light rays follow a portion of the same paths to the image as they would if the pupil were wide open and centered. Tilting the retina cannot cause astigmatism but rather causes a type of "curvature of field." Tilting a spherical lens such as an IOL causes the well-known aberration of astigmatism of oblique incidence, enough to cause the amount of astigmatism measured here.

Preferred Response

c. a tilted IOL

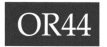

A 6-week-old patient with monocular aphakia has a correction of +18.00 D at a vertex distance of 12 mm. Even though keratometry is not available for this spherical eye, you want to proceed with contact lens fitting for visual rehabilitation.

Which of the following lens powers *best* meets the optical power requirements?

a. +26.00 D
b. +23.00 D
c. +18.00 D
d. +19.00 D

Discussion

Aphakia is an absolute indication for contact lens fitting in the pediatric population. Ideally, keratometry should be obtained presurgically or later during evaluation under anesthesia, but contact lens fitting can be attempted without this information. The use of a portable slit lamp, a Burton lamp (hand-held ultraviolet-lamp magnifier), diagnostic lenses, and patience can often yield excellent results. Pediatric silicone and hydrogel lenses work especially well under these conditions. The contact lens–cornea relationship can be observed with a high-molecular-weight fluorescein that does not stain soft contact lenses (Fluorosoft) on the initial fitting as well as on the refitting that will be necessary as the eye changes in curvature with age. A vertex distance of 12 mm with a power requirement of +18.00 D yields +23.00 D at the corneal plane. However, to allow for the loss of accommodation in this eye, an additional +3.00 D is required for a total need of +26.00 D. At a later age, glasses can be incorporated for bifocal correction and the power adjusted to infinity.

Preferred Response   a. +26.00 D

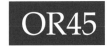

An 82-year-old woman who is undergoing cataract and IOL surgery in her right eye has a preoperative refraction of +3.00 D sphere = 20/60 OD and +3.50 D sphere = 20/25 OS. Postoperatively, the refraction OD is −2.50 +1.00 × 80, yielding a visual acuity of 20/20. On receiving the new corrective lens, she may experience difficulty from any of the following problems *except*

a. diplopia on side gaze
b. diplopia on down gaze
c. monocular diplopia
d. unequal image sizes

Discussion   A 5.00 D shift in spherical equivalent in the spectacle refraction after cataract and IOL surgery is enough to cause significant symptoms from the induced prism in side gaze as well as in down gaze, resulting in "anisotropia" with double vision as the patient looks away from the center of the glasses in various directions. A 5.00 D shift in the spectacle-corrected refraction will cause a change in magnification of about 10%, easily enough to cause symptoms from aniseikonia (different image sizes in the two eyes), which can interfere with fusion. There is no particular reason why monocular diplopia should arise when the new corrective lens is obtained.

Preferred Response   c. monocular diplopia

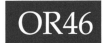

A patient with severe bilateral cataracts has been emmetropic in both eyes most of his life. He undergoes uneventful cataract surgery with implantation of a +20.0 D biconvex IOL in his first eye. The final correction in the first eye is 20/20 with a −0.50 D refraction. Surgery is performed on the second eye 2 months later with implantation of the same power and style of IOL. On the first day postoperatively the patient shows a visual acuity of counting fingers at 3 feet with no correction but refracts to 20/40 with a −12.00 D sphere.

The *most* likely explanation for this large refractive surprise is

a. mismeasured axial length
b. mismeasured K reading
c. lens optic is implanted upside down
d. mislabeled IOL

Discussion Large refractive surprises of 10.00 D or more are almost always the result of a mislabeled IOL. The only exception is with highly myopic patients who have large staphylomas and in whom the length of the visual axis is much different than the length of the optical axis. Such errors can be as much as 2 mm or 3 mm off, resulting in 6.00 D to 9.00 D of refractive error. In this case, with a good result in the first eye, it is unlikely that the patient could have this much anisometropia or that the K readings or axial length reading could have been mismeasured in one eye by this amount, particularly with a lifelong history of emmetropia. An intraocular lens that is reversed (implanted upside down) could not cause this amount of myopia. For a +20.0 D biconvex lens, reversal rarely causes more than 3.00 D or 4.00 D of difference. The problem cases are those with a 3.00 D or 4.00 D surprise, in which the causes may be a cumulative result of small errors all leading in the same direction. There is a method for measuring lens power while the IOL is in the eye,[19] but it is difficult to perform clinically. The best method is to be prepared to measure the IOL in a water bath at the time of its removal to confirm the mislabeled power and then to exchange the IOL with another lens of appropriate power.

Preferred Response d. mislabeled IOL

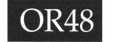

Fluctuating visual function after radial keratotomy is seen because of any of the following *except*

a. fluctuating macular edema
b. a decentered optical zone
c. a small optical zone
d. fluctuating refractive error

Discussion As the pupil dilates in the presence of a decentered or small optical zone, areas of surgical scarring or irregular astigmatism will often be uncovered, causing fluctuation in visual function. The actual refractive error of the eye can also fluctuate with changes in corneal hydration during the day. Fluctuating macular edema as a cause of altered visual function is not linked to radial keratotomy.

Preferred Response a. fluctuating macular edema

OR48

A first-time wearer of gas-permeable contact lenses complains of blurred vision at the 2-week follow-up visit. Further discussion reveals that visual acuity levels seem to fall as the day progresses and that the lenses are difficult to remove. The patient reports that her eyes are slightly red at the end of the day but that this injection is gone by morning. Slit-lamp observation reveals faint 3 and 9 o'clock staining but is otherwise unremarkable. The lenses appear to meet normal criteria for a satisfactory fit.

Which of the following would be a reasonable procedure?

a. Do not alter the fit, as this is a novice wearer and the absence of significant findings suggests waiting for further follow-up.
b. Switch the patient to soft contact lenses to satisfy comfort and vision issues.
c. Contact lens adhesion may be occurring late in the day; parameter changes should be made.
d. Enlarge the diameter of the lens by 0.4 mm to enhance the stability of vision.

Discussion

Novice gas-permeable contact lens wearers are frequently symptomatic, and logic might suggest waiting for further follow-up, except for the information that vision decreases toward the end of the day and, most notably, that the lenses are difficult to remove. Lens adhesion is not an uncommon finding with gas-permeable contact lenses. Blurred vision occurs with accumulation of debris and stagnation of tears. Either flattening the base curve to align the contact lens more closely with the cornea or reducing the overall diameter of the lens will encourage lens movement. Also, thin contact lenses placed over a highly astigmatic cornea may create suction because of lens flexure over the toric surface. This phenomenon could be eliminated by increasing the thickness at the center of the lens or by using an aspheric design. Refitting the patient in a soft contact lens would reduce symptoms but may not be necessary if appropriate parameters are changed.

Preferred Response

c. Contact lens adhesion may be occurring late in the day; parameter changes should be made.

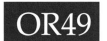

Which of the following is true when macular disease results in loss of foveal function and subsequently produces a dense central scotoma?

a. A preferred retinal locus for fixation will naturally and reliably occur in a paracentral location.
b. Letter recognition is not possible.
c. Color perception is lost.
d. Diplopia is likely to be experienced during training in the use of magnifiers.

Discussion

A preferred retinal locus, an extrafoveal location providing preferential fixation, develops after foveal function is lost. Reading and letter recognition are generally possible using the preferred retinal locus if sufficient magnification and illumination are provided and the locus has adequate functioning juxtapositional retinal tissue. Diplopia is generally not encountered by an individual developing a preferred retinal locus at an eccentric location, unless the preferred retinal loci are at noncorresponding locations in each eye and the patient has binocular vision. Color perception by retinal cone receptors, although most numerous in the central 15° around the fovea, remains intact even with large central scotomas.[10]

Preferred Response
a. A preferred retinal locus for fixation will naturally and reliably occur in a paracentral location.

OR50

Before cataract surgery with IOL placement in the left eye, a patient's glasses measure +1.00 +0.50 × 30 = 20/25 OD and plano +2.50 × 120 = 20/50 OS. Postoperatively, the spectacle refraction of the left eye is +1.00 sphere = 20/20+.

With the new lens in place, the patient is likely to complain of

a. monocular diplopia in the spectacle-corrected left eye
b. decreased visual field in the left eye
c. distortion of vision in the left eye under monocular conditions
d. orientation problems

Discussion
A patient adapted to wearing a moderate oblique cylinder in the glasses will experience spatial distortion when the cylinder is removed upon surgical correction of the astigmatism, the same as a patient will experience spatial distortion when an oblique cylinder is first added to an eye never corrected before.[20] Such distortion is not noticed under monocular conditions unless the astigmatism is very high. Binocularly, however, the spatial distortion often leads to complaints of disorientation, until the patient adapts over time. There is no particular reason why removal of cylinder in the glasses will cause monocular diplopia or a decrease in the visual field.

Preferred Response
d. orientation problems

References

1. Rubin ML: *Optics for Clinicians.* 2nd ed. Gainesville, FL: Triad Scientific Publishers; 1974.

2. Koch DD, Liu JF, Hyde LL, et al: Refractive complications of cataract surgery after radial keratotomy. *Am J Ophthalmol* 1989;108:676–682.

3. Holladay JT: Consultations in refractive surgery. *Refract Corn Surg* 1989;5:203.

4. Faye EE, ed: *Clinical Low Vision.* 2nd ed. Boston: Little, Brown & Co; 1984.

5. *Rehabilitation: The Management of Adult Patients with Low Vision.* Preferred Practice Pattern. San Francisco: American Academy of Ophthalmology; 1994.

6. Guyton DL: Diagnosis and treatment of monocular diplopia. *Focal Points.* Vol II, Module 2. San Francisco: American Academy of Ophthalmology; 1984.

7. Coffeen P, Guyton DL: Monocular diplopia accompanying ordinary refractive errors. *Am J Ophthalmol* 1988;105:451–459.

8. Bixenman WW, Joffe L: Binocular diplopia associated with retinal wrinkling. *J Pediatr Ophthalmol Strab* 1984;21:215–219.

9. Holladay JT, Bishop JE, Prager TC, et al: The ideal intraocular lens. *CLAO J* 1983;9:15–19.

10. Colenbrander A, Fletcher D, eds: *Low Vision and Vision Rehabilitation. Ophthalmology Clinics of North America.* Vol 7, No 2. Philadelphia: W.B. Saunders Co; 1994.

11. Hiatt RL: Diagnostic and therapeutic applications of prisms. *Focal Points.* Vol IV, Module 5. San Francisco: American Academy of Ophthalmology; 1986.

12. Holladay JT, Rubin ML: Avoiding refractive problems in cataract surgery. *Surv Ophthalmol* 1988;32:357–360.

13. Holladay JT, Bishop JE, Lewis JW: Diagnosis and treatment of mysterious light streaks seen by patients following extracapsular cataract extraction. *Am Intraocul Implant Soc J* 1985;11:21–23.

14. Holladay JT, Bishop JE, Lewis JW: The optimal size of a posterior capsulotomy. *Am Intraocul Implant Soc J* 1985;11:18–20.

15. Rosner M, Sharir M, Blumenthal M: Optical aberrations from a well-centered intraocular lens implant. *Am J Ophthalmol* 1986;101:117–118.

16. Gurland JE, Wheeler MB, Wilson ME, et al: Children with low vision: Evaluation and treatment in the 1990s. In: Burde RM, Slamovits TL, eds: *Advances in Clinical Ophthalmology.* Volume 1. St. Louis: Mosby-Year Book; 1994.

17. Sawush MR, Guyton DL: Optimal astigmatism to enhance depth of focus after cataract surgery. *Ophthalmology* 1991;98:1025–1029.

18. Milder B, Rubin ML: *The Fine Art of Prescribing Glasses Without Making a Spectacle of Yourself.* Gainesville, FL: Triad Scientific Publishers; 1978.

19. Holladay JT, Long SA, Lewis JW, et al: Determining intraocular lens power within the eye. *Am Intraocul Implant Soc J* 1985;11:353–363.

20. Guyton DL: Prescribing cylinders postoperatively. In: Ernest JT, ed: *Year Book of Ophthalmology—1985.* Chicago: Year Book Medical Publishers; 1985:63–66.

Additional Resources From the AAO

Academy Statements   *Contact Lens Advisory: Keratitis and Extended-Wear (Overnight) Contact Lens Use.* Clinical Alert. 1989.

Extended Wear of Contact Lenses. Policy Statement. 1992.

Basic and Clinical Science Course   *Optics, Refraction, and Contact Lenses.* Section 3. Updated annually.

Focal Points

Faye EE: *Management of the Partially Sighted Patient.* Vol V, Module 6. 1987. (Out of print)

Gurland JE: *Progressive Addition Spectacle Lenses.* Vol VII, Module 9. 1989. (Item No. 029007)

Guyton DL: *Diagnosis and Treatment of Monocular Diplopia.* Vol II, Module 2. 1984. (Item No. 029002)

Hiatt RL: *Diagnostic and Therapeutic Applications of Prisms.* Vol IV, Module 5. 1986. (Item No. 029004)

Javitt JC, Taylor HR: *Absorptive Lenses: The Need for Ocular Protection.* Vol IX, Module 3. 1991. (Item No. 029009)

Lembach RG: *Aphakic and Myopic Extended-Wear Contact Lenses.* Vol II, Module 6. 1984. (Item No. 029002)

Meltzer DW, Stein HA: *Current Management of Presbyopia.* Vol VI, Module 2. 1988. (Item No. 029006)

Michaels DD: *Accommodation: Clinical Aspects.* Vol V, Module 10. 1987. (Out of print)

Milder B: *Recent Advances in Spectacle Corrections.* Vol I, Module 4. 1983. (Item No. 029001)

Rowsey JJ, Hays JC: *Corneal Astigmatism: Topographic and Surgical Insights.* Vol V, Module 4. 1987. (Out of print)

Stein RM, Stein HA: *Corneal Complications of Contact Lenses.* Vol XI, Module 2. 1993. (Item No. 029011)

Waring GO III: *Radial Keratotomy for Myopia.* Vol X, Module 5. 1992. (Item No. 029010)

Wilkins J, Fraunfelder FT: *Transient Changes in Refractive Error.* Vol VIII, Module 6. 1990. (Out of print)

Monograph

Stamper RL, Sugar A, Ripkin DJ: *Intraocular Lenses: Basics and Clinical Applications.* Ophthalmology Monograph 7. 1993. (Item No. 0210152)

Preferred Practice Patterns

Low to Moderate Refractive Errors. 1991. (Item No. 110013)

Rehabilitation: The Management of Adult Patients with Low Vision. 1994. (Item No. 110023)

Videotapes

Cobo ML: *Intraocular Lens Removal: Indications and Technique.* Clinical Short Subjects Series. 1988. (Item No. 0251043)

Freeman MI, Rakow PL, Campbell RC: *Basic Principles of Contact Lens Fitting.* Clinical Skills Series. 1993. (Item No. 0250953)

Gelender H, Mandelbaum SH: *Postoperative Astigmatism: Prevention and Management.* Clinical Short Subjects Series. 1987. (Item No. 0251083)

Guyton DL: *Aphakic Spectacles in Perspective.* Classic Series. 1980. (Item No. 0250303)

Guyton DL: *Subjective Refraction: Cross-Cylinder Technique.* Clinical Skills Series. 1987. (Item No. 0250653)

Low Vision Patients. Classic Series. 1974. (Item No. 0250033)